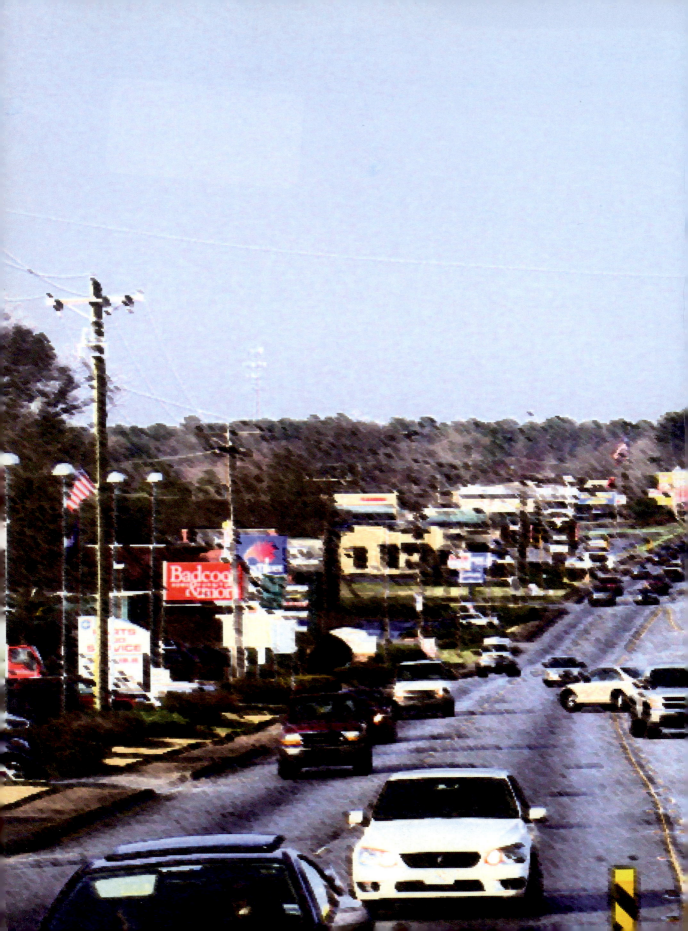

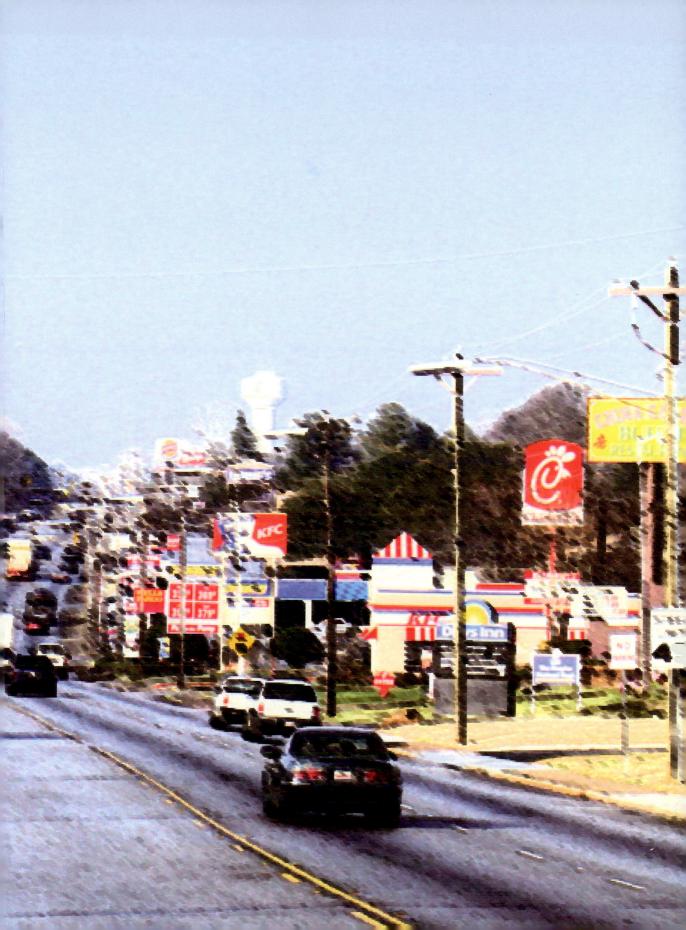

# SPRAWLING CITIES AND OUR ENDANGERED PUBLIC HEALTH

Sprawl is an unsustainable pattern of growth that threatens to undermine the health of communities globally. It has been a dominant mid-to-late 20th century growth pattern in developed countries and in the 21st century has shown widespread signs of proliferation in India, China, and other growing countries. The *World Health Organization* cites sprawl for its serious adverse public health consequences for humans and ecological habitats. The many adverse impacts of sprawl on the health of individuals, communities, and biological ecosystems are well documented. Architects have been rightly criticised for failing to grasp the aesthetic and functional challenge to create buildings and places that mitigate sprawl while simultaneously promoting healthier, active lifestyles in neighbourhoods and communities.

*Sprawling Cities and Our Endangered Public Health* examines the past and present role of architecture in relation to the public health consequences of unmitigated sprawl and the ways in which it threatens our future. Topics examined include the role of 20th century theories of architecture and urbanism and their public health ramifications, examples of current unsustainable practices, design considerations for the creation of health-promoting architecture and landscape urbanism, a critique of recent case studies of sustainable alternatives to unchecked sprawl, and prognostications for the future.

Architects, public health professionals, landscape architects, town planners, and a broad range of policy specialists will be able to apply the methods and tools presented here to counter unmitigated sprawl and to create architecture that promotes active, healthier lifestyles. Stephen Verderber is an internationally respected evidence-based researcher/practitioner/educator in the emerging, interdisciplinary field of architecture, health, and society. This, his latest book on the interactions between our buildings, our cities and our health, is an invaluable reference source for everyone concerned with sustainable architecture and landscape urbanism.

**Stephen Verderber,** Arch. D., NCARB, is Professor at the School of Architecture and Adjunct Professor, Department of Public Health Sciences, Clemson University, USA. He is a Registered Architect in the United States.

# SPRAWLING CITIES AND OUR ENDANGERED PUBLIC HEALTH

*Stephen Verderber*

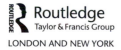
Routledge
Taylor & Francis Group

LONDON AND NEW YORK

First published 2012
by Routledge
2 Park Square, Milton Park, Abingdon, Oxon OX14 4RN

Simultaneously published in the USA and Canada
by Routledge
711 Third Avenue, New York, NY 10017

*Routledge is an imprint of the Taylor & Francis Group, an informa business*

*British Library Cataloguing in Publication Data*
A catalogue record for this book is available from the British Library

*Library of Congress Cataloging in Publication Data*
  Verderber, Stephen.
  Sprawling cities and our endangered public health/Stephen Verderber.
    p. cm.
  Includes bibliographical references and index.
  1. Public health.   2. Architecture—Health aspects.   3. Cities and
  towns—Health aspects—Growth.   I. Title.
  RA566.6.V47 2012
  362.1—dc23
                                                            2011045615

ISBN: 978–0–415–66532–2 (hbk)
ISBN: 978–0–415–66533–9 (pbk)
ISBN: 978–0–203–11921–1 (ebk)

Typeset in Bembo
by RefineCatch Limited, Bungay, Suffolk

Printed and bound in India by Replika Press Pvt. Ltd.

For Elyssa Leigh Verderber and Alexander Verderber

# CONTENTS

# ILLUSTRATIONS

Cover image: ONL (Oosterhuis_Lénárd)/'751 Project'_Hyperbody Research Group, TU Delft, in collaboration with South-East University of Nanjing, 2006

# PREFACE AND ACKNOWLEDGEMENTS

I was raised in a suburb of Chicago. My family's home was 2 miles inland from Lake Michigan and 12 miles north of downtown. My parents' home was a now-classic 1950s suburban ranch with a broad front lawn and backyard. The Edens Expressway linked our suburb to the city center. Commuting was then and remains a way of life in this bedroom suburb, Skokie. The area was settled by mostly German immigrants where, at one time, Native American trading routes crossed. Miles and miles of street were paved, and sanitary systems built, in the 1920s just prior to the 1929 Great Stock Market Crash and the subsequent Great Depression of the 1930s. The budding suburb's private developers and the local government went bust in the Depression. Not much happened until the end of World War II, then basically everything happened all at once. Until then, a few houses and neighborhoods were built here and there, most within walking distance of the old town center and its commuter rail line (North Shore Line) whose passenger stations ran up along Skokie through the Chicago's North Shore suburbs then up to Milwaukee.

America's suburbs were once the land of opportunity. The booming post-war years were filled with hope and optimism for a better life. The post-WWII decades were about expansion in every way: larger lifestyles, larger paychecks, larger career aspirations, larger families, larger automobiles, and larger quantities of mass consumer products. The successive waves of migration outward from the city center to new suburbs ever further out had a negative impact on many inner ring suburbs. This mass out-migration was seen as necessary in the quest to attain the American Dream. The boom began in 1946, with the return of thousands of veterans who were starting families and needed more space than an apartment in the city could provide. By 1970, nearly every vacant lot in Skokie was built-out. There was nowhere for upwardly mobile families to go except to move ever further out into suburbia's more upscale destinations—to one of an ever-expanding array of suburbs that by then stretched outward, radiating like tentacles for miles far into once-open prairie and farmland, up to 50 miles from Chicago. By then, inner ring suburbs such as Skokie were considered passé although the place never fell on hard times because of its excellent location within the suburban matrix.

When I was nineteen, I remember driving with my father, ranting on how for a teenager living in a suburb was like existing in some strange purgatorial state—suburbgatory. I remember repeating to him, "The suburbs will die! They will die! They cannot survive!" It was the middle of the Arab Oil Embargo. Spiking oil prices were causing long lines at the filling station and everyone was grumbling. What they were really complaining about were the first signs of the end of the Age of Suburban Innocence. My father kept saying, in a rising voice, that this is what he and all his family and friends had wanted for their children. It is what they worked so hard for. They did it for us, he was saying. They wanted a better, safer life. I was already disillusioned with all its monotony, always having to drive everywhere it seemed.

That day, and thereafter we debated the merits of faceless subdivisions, generic strip malls, and suburbia's stultifying monoculture. For two years I worked at a large architectural firm in downtown Chicago (Skidmore, Owings & Merrill), commuting by train-subway. I only recall having to drive to work on a handful of days during those two years. After this I lived for three years in Ann Arbor, Michigan, while in graduate school. I had experienced a welcome reprieve from suburbia during these years. I moved to Houston after graduate school. What a shock! What I had experienced growing up in Chicago was nothing compared with the eye-opening, car-centric, Wild West sprawl of Texas's largest city. I was caught totally unprepared for its panoramic vistas of unzoned, ad hoc, pastiche landscapes with everything pushed up against everything else everywhere. In retrospect, I think it looked like a Photoshop-created collage. A few months after my arrival, I recall telling my Father how I actually would begin to feel nauseous while driving through Houston's endless and visually chaotic commercial strip-scapes. Houston to me was one immense *sprawl machine* that seemed to revel in devouring everything in its path. It became so depressing that I had to leave after four years. New Orleans was the antithesis of Houston. My attraction to New Orleans was based largely on its compactness, its unshakable self-identity, and its celebrated indigenous culture. Its older neighborhoods were walkable. New Orleans's comparatively land-locked suburbs featured their fair share of sprawl, but nowhere near to the extent of either Houston or Chicago, each with their endlessly flat expanses of open farmland there for the taking. It would be twenty-one years until the next move.

In 2007, my wife and I and our two children (then 16 and 19) relocated to the Upstate of South Carolina. It would be disingenuous to say that Hurricane Katrina had played no role in this. The 2005 catastrophe left New Orleans utterly transformed, and since 2005 I have worked there *pro bono* in the arena of historic landmark preservation, and I wrote a book about the place (*Delirious New Orleans: Manifesto for an Extraordinary American City*, 2009). In the Upstate, we dove once again into a growing sprawl machine. Here too the once-rural landscape was being devoured at an alarming rate. The sprawl was not as intensive as Houston's, although everything pointed in that direction. The Great Recession mercifully brought the Upstate's sprawl machine down to low gear but it remains very hard for local developers to accept the reality that sprawl may not be a good thing for everybody all the time. Local and regional grassroots groups now call for smart growth policies. One such organization, Shared Upstate Growth Vision, predicts the Upstate will continue to be one of America's fastest growing corridors throughout this century.

Greenville County is in the heart of the Upstate. Its population grew by 19 percent, to 451,225, in the first decade of the 21st century and is expected to top 542,000 by 2030. In the past twenty years the Upstate's population grew by more than 300,000, to 1,362,000 in the 2010 U.S. Census. One third of South Carolina's population now lives within this ten-county region. By 2030 the region is expected to have 1.6 million residents. The Upstate's sprawl will soon consume the entire length of Interstate 85, which crisscrosses the region connecting Charlotte to Atlanta and beyond. Various smart growth groups' reports focus on the region's history of stubborn resistance to planned growth and how residents see any land use planning as a governmental infringement on private land ownership rights. However, there is a growing consensus that sporadic planning in a piecemeal manner will only further exacerbate disjointed land uses and the needless consumption of open space and non-renewable natural resources. If the Upstate is to survive, it must hold onto and enhance its considerable natural charms and recreational amenities. The award-winning advocacy group Upstate Forever strives to preserve the natural beauty of the Upstate. It remains a pitched battle over individual rights versus the public good. It will remain difficult and contentious because sprawl dies hard.

For South Carolina, and for sprawling landscapes everywhere, it is not too late.

The subject of this book has become of national importance in the United States and increasingly in many other parts of the world. The future viability of suburbia is under unprecedented scrutiny. The Museum of Modern Art's timely 2011 initiative, Foreclosed: Rehousing the American Dream, targeted the deep challenges facing suburbia and the consequences of unmitigated hyper-suburbanization. Its underlying premise was to examine the American Dream of home ownership in the suburbs and how the national foreclosure crisis and the Great Recession have broken it. It was launched by a panel discussion in May of 2011 when five interdisciplinary teams were created, each charged with addressing a different American suburban sprawl setting and making proposals for its reinvention. The composition of the teams themselves reflected a long-overdue need to blur the unsustainable disciplinary boundaries that for too long have separated the fields of architecture, urban design, and landscape architecture from one another. This initiative and others like it provide hope that our gridlocked, entrenched universities will follow suit and move beyond tedious intra-disciplinary ivory tower rivalries.

In 2007, I joined the faculty of the School of Architecture and Public Health Sciences (adjunct status) at Clemson University. Prior to this I had been a professor of Architecture at Tulane University, where I was an adjunct professor in its School of Public Health and Tropical Medicine. The project that evolved into this book began in a graduate level design studio at Clemson in January 2010 in the Graduate Program in Architecture + Health. I am indebted to the support provided by Jose Caban, Kate Schwennsen, and the Richard McMahan Fund for Excellence in the School of Architecture. I took everyone in the studio down to New Orleans to document the case study (Chapter 5), and to immerse them in that city's uniqueness. The students in the studio were Katie Yohman, Derrick Simpson, Heather Bachman, Eva Behringer, Patrick Willke, Lindsay Wagner, and Colleen Herr. We walked through many neighborhoods including Uptown, the CBD, Central City, the Vieux Carre', the Upper and Lower Ninth Wards, and Mid-City. My research assistant, Annette Himelick, worked diligently on this project for fifteen months. Clay Phillips provided additional research support, and Ryan Ramsey provided a prototype of the book's cover. I am also indebted to my editors at Routledge, including Alex Hollingsworth, Georgina Johnson, and Louise Fox. Caroline Malinder, consulting editor to Routledge, had a key role in this book's genesis.

I am fortunate to have held an interdisciplinary academic appointment between architecture and public health continuously for twenty-five years. I remain surprised that it was the first and only one of its kind. This is a first attempt to examine the public health consequences of sprawl through the specific lens of architecture rather than through the lens of its closely allied disciplines, urban design and landscape architecture. A number of recent books and published research articles in planning and design have examined the urban design and planning ramifications, including *Retrofitting Suburbia: Urban Design Solutions for Redesigning Suburbs*, by Ellen Dunham-Jones and June Williamson, and Paul Lukez's provocative *Suburban Transformations* (2007). However, these books have tended to overshoot the sort of boots-on-the-ground attitude or call-to-arms sensibility that is so urgently needed at this time, while Dolores Hayden's pithy *A Field Guide to Sprawl* (2004) hits closer to the mark in this regard. Another insightful book is *Seven Rules for Sustainable Communities: Design Strategies for the Post-Carbon World* (2010), by Patrick M. Condon and Robert Yaro. In the field of public health, the recent books *Making Places Healthy: Designing and Building for Health, Well-Being, and Sustainability*

(2011), edited by Andrew L. Dannenberg, Howard Frumkin, and Richard J. Jackson, and the earlier book *Urban Sprawl and Public Health: Designing, Planning, and Building for Healthy Communities* (2004) by Frumkin, Jackson, and Lawrence Frank, each admirably make the case from the public health perspective. The work being done in this field at the U.S. Centers for Disease Control and Prevention, in Atlanta, has also been a source of inspiration, as well as the work of Congress for the New Urbanism (CDC). The CDC indeed deserves credit for kick-starting the present discourse in 1993 that Jane Jacobs launched with her classic *The Death and Life of Great American Cities* (1961) and in recent books on its global ramifications such as Elizabeth Farrelly's insightful *Blubberland: The Dangers of Happiness* (2008). I am sick and tired of the status quo. What is needed, is a book that examines the various and at times convoluted discourses and their associated literatures, including that of the nascent discipline of landscape urbanism.

This book has six parts. Chapter 1 provides an overview of the current public health crisis, its parameters, and the threats it poses by examining the phenomena of *sprawl machines*. Chapter 2 consists of a brief history of the role of architecture in sprawl and the specific role of architecture in creating unhealthy sprawl communities. Chapter 3 is an essay on the threat of global sprawl machines that are currently consuming vast amounts of open farmland and related non-renewable natural resources in developing parts of the globe. Chapter 4 consists of a compendium of seventy-five planning and design considerations intended to help guide the amelioration of sprawl machines, and their transformation—transfusion—into livable and walkable *ecohumanist* communities. Chapter 5 focuses on the aforementioned case study for a suburban section of post-Hurricane Katrina New Orleans; its narrative is accompanied by intervention referred to here as *sprawl transfusion*. Chapter 6 is largely a cautionary tale of the consequences of unchecked sprawl, and the actions that will be needed to counter its negative impacts on public health and on our planet's ecological health.

In most places, sadly, sprawl itself remains an unmitigated phenomenon. Meanwhile, the world's population grows at an accelerated rate and more people cannot simply consume more and more open land and nonrenewable resources. The United Nations recently raised its "low" population projection estimates for 2050 by 177 million more than it projected a mere two years ago. The world's population is now projected by the UN to reach 9.2 billion people by 2050, up from nearly 6.8 billion today. The insatiable global thirst for speculative land development, its conspicuous consumption, and discarded landscapes cannot have a happy ending unless something dramatic is done. Any community that values and promotes the health of its citizens cannot sit by idly on the sidelines, either. This book—along with other recent, related books, reports, conferences, and exhibits on this subject—represents an attempt to raise awareness. This is a cautionary tale of how we can promote intelligent growth and prosperity and avoid a coming calamity if preemptive action is not taken. It is no coincidence that efforts are now underway in many cities to bestow historic landmark status on the best examples of commercial vernacular architecture, suburban architecture, and suburban community design. This should occur, as it is a subject deserving in-depth treatment. The dysfunctionality of unchecked sprawl will harm us all sooner or later. Genuinely healthy communities possess regenerative qualities and an undeniable spirit, grit, determination, and soul that is clearly and proudly expressed in its physical character. Unhealthy communities, by contrast, do not express these qualities, because they physically appear as and indeed are fatigued, spent, listless. As my mother often said, "Health is wealth." Without opportunities to engage in healthy, physically active lifestyles, we will all be that much poorer.

*Stephen Verderber*
*Greenville, South Carolina, October 2011*

# 1

# INTRODUCTION: AN EPIDEMIC ON OUR DOORSTEP

Sprawl is unsustainable. It threatens to undermine the health and well being of communities globally. It was the predominant 20th century growth pattern in developed countries and now, in the 21st century it proliferates in the developing world. The World Health Organization (WHO) cites sprawl as a source of serious adverse public health consequences for humans and for natural ecological habitats. Its adverse consequences for individuals, communities, and biological ecosystems have been well documented, particularly since 2000, and have drawn increasing attention in global mainstream and cyberspace mass media.[1] A number of non-communicable diseases (NCDs), specifically obesity, heart disease, stroke, diabetes, asthma, hypertension, depression, chronic kidney disease, osteoporosis, and cancer, are the most prevalent unhealthful outcomes empirically associated with sprawl, to date. An NCD is defined as a medical condition or disease of a non-infectious nature, and are generally diseases of long duration and of generally slow progression. The WHO reports NCDs as by far the leading cause of annual mortality rates, representing over 60 percent of all deaths globally. Out of the 35 million people who died worldwide from NCDs in 2005, half were under the age of seventy and half were women. Risk factors such as lifestyle and the built environment are increasingly being linked with NCDs.[2]

The world is becoming a heavier place, especially the most affluent Western nations. Chronic NCDs were once a problem limited to high-income countries and were known as "diseases of affluence." Among developed nations, Americans are the heaviest, and the Japanese the slimmest. But global obesity rates have doubled in the past three decades even as blood pressure and cholesterol levels in these parts of the world have dropped. Every year, at least 5 million die globally around the world due to tobacco use and more than 2.8 million die from being overweight. By 2030, global deaths due to chronic NCDs are expected to increase to 52 million per year while deaths caused by infectious diseases, maternal and perinatal conditions, and nutritional deficiencies are expected to decline by 7 million per year during the same period. In response, in 2009 the WHO established the Global Non-Communicable Disease Network (NCDnet) to better coordinate the worldwide battle against this emerging public health challenge.[3] In 1980, about 5 percent of men and 8 percent of women worldwide were obese. By 2008, the rates were nearly 10 percent for men and 14 percent for women. This translates into 205 million men and 297 million women. Another 1.5 billion adults were overweight, according to recent studies using body mass index (BMI), cholesterol levels, and blood pressure as key metrics.[4]

Epidemiologists warn that the increasing numbers of obese could lead to a global "tsunami" of cardiovascular disease, and diabetes. By 2011, obesity alone was linked to more than 3 million deaths annually.[5] Especially since 2010, international attention has been solidly trained on combating this epidemic, e.g. the Pan American Conference on Obesity, held in Aruba, the XI International Conference on Obesity, held in Stockholm, the European Association Conference for the Study of Obesity, held in Munich, the UN Standing Committee on Childhood and Adolescent Nutrition and Obesity Conference, held in Abu Dhabi, a WHO Summit on global NCDs, held in Oslo, Norway, and a UN/WHO first-time High level Meeting on Non-communicable Disease Prevention and Control, held in New York City.

In the U.K., the number of people with NCDs, including diabetes, soared by 150,000 in a single year (2009). One in twenty adults in the U.K. is now afflicted and almost one in ten adults, or 5.5 million people, are obese, with nearly one quarter of all adults now classified as clinically obese, and 24 percent of children aged two through fifteen in the U.K. are now classified as such.[6] About 90 percent of diabetics—2.5 million people in the U.K.—suffer from the Type 2 condition. Ten percent of the total National Health Service (NHS) budget is now consumed by treatment for NCDs and this figure is expected to significantly rise in the coming decade unless preventive measures are put in place.[7] A London-based not-for-profit organization, C3 Collaborating for Health, focuses on health promotion initiatives in the U.K. It functions as a clearinghouse for the review of public policy and on increasing public awareness. This organization posted a 2011 Lords report on the national need for more extensive health-promoting policies and new public health incentives for people to take better care of themselves in this regard in the face of the U.K.'s current epidemic.[8]

The U.S. population alone is predicted to reach nearly 600 million by 2100, about double its current population. Its society is aging rapidly—and its future healthcare costs will be staggering; the deleterious consequences of unmitigated sprawl will be a major contributory factor, unless something is done. What is it like to live in a post-WWII suburban sprawl landscape that fosters sedentary lifestyles, and as a consequence, poor health? Too many of us already know what it's like. Everyday life is nearly entirely automobile dependent. Families typically live in subdivisions with neither sidewalks nor destination points within a walkable distance. In these places, persons of all ages develop feelings of isolation and alienation. As for the automobile, since 1982, the U.S. population has increased by 20 percent but the time Americans spend in traffic has increased by an astonishing 236 percent. The average U.S. driver now spends 443 hours each year behind the wheel—the equivalent of fifty-five nine-hour days or eleven workweeks per year. By 2010, the average U.S. household owned 2.8 cars, and approximately half of all Americans lived in suburbia. Meanwhile, between 1986 and 1998, obesity among children in the U.S. doubled; 14 million (24 percent) between the age of two and seventeen became obese. Children in the U.S. who reside in neighborhoods with disproportionately fewer recreational facilities and lacking in amenities such as sidewalks tend to be more overweight than children who live in neighborhoods with more recreational facilities and related amenities.[9]

The planet's roadways are becoming clogged with fuel-consuming vehicles. By 1997, smog pollution was responsible for more than 6 million asthma attacks in the U.S., 159,000 visits to emergency departments for treatment, and 53,000 hospitalizations; this number has grown significantly since.[10] As for the health costs of sprawl, the nation's obesity bills are ramping up. Annual obesity-related healthcare expenditures are expected to rise by nearly $265 billion a year between 2011 and 2018, while annual Medicare expenditures are expected to increase by about $360 billion during this same period. The U.S. Centers for Disease Control and Prevention (CDC) recently attributed $147 billion a year in U.S. medical costs to obesity alone—over 9 percent of all U.S. healthcare spending. And obese Americans are living longer due to factors such as cholesterol-reducing medicines, but many of these added years are lived in poor health; annual medical bills are nearly 42 percent higher than those of the non-obese.[11] The cohort of clinically obese rose from 24 percent of adults in 1960 to 47 percent in 1980 to 64 percent by 2000. Obese persons are nearly forty times more likely to develop diabetes compared to the non-obese, and this includes overweight children.[12]

Researchers have measured the effects of sprawl in relation to age, socio-economic status, travel behaviors, air quality, density, urban infrastructure, water quality, behavioral typologies, and morphological attributes of transport catchment areas as a means to predict ridership probabilities.[13] Special constituencies with disabilities, including the poor, the medically underserved, the extreme aged, and children and adolescents, are particularly susceptible to the deleterious public health consequences of sprawl.[14] The health of our children and adolescents is in peril due to sedentary lifestyles and poor nutrition. Of course, sprawl alone cannot account for the obesity epidemic and yet it is a fact that children in developed countries are spending less time outdoors engaged in healthful behaviors such as walking, running, cycling and swimming, than before. This unhealthful trend is in part attributable to the lure of technology, i.e. computers and video games. Traditional play outdoors is in steep decline. The consequences of outdoor play avoidance can be profound—it itself is a growing crisis. As outdoor play declines, fitness levels decline, waistlines expand, and a host of other health problems can follow. For centuries, outdoor play was an essential ingredient in aiding children in their physical and emotional development, and in their acquisition of essential Vitamin D from sunlight exposure.[15]

Physicians know they are on the front line in the fight against global obesity, but they also know they alone cannot reverse this epidemic and its associated highly sedentary lifestyles. Education and consistent reinforcement are necessary on the part of parents, schools, and by the support provided by the neighborhoods and buildings where they live.[16] In a recent study of 290 primary care physicians, 89 percent of respondents believed it was their responsibility to help their patients lose weight, although 72 percent claimed they were not properly trained to provide weight loss education; only 45 percent indicated they regularly discussed weight with their patients. In another recent study of 1,002 adults in the U.S., only one-third of those who were obese (defined as weighing roughly 30 or more pounds over their normal healthy weight level) indicated their healthcare professional had informed them they were overweight.[17] The healthcare system itself is too often the culprit. Highly hospital-centric healthcare systems over-rely on hospital-dispensed care. They have historically tended to undervalue sickness prevention in public education and awareness. In such a system a patient may not take "ownership" of his/her health condition until it is far too late—by then accruing, by default, very costly hospital-based emergency care that could have otherwise been avoided at far less expense.[18]

## Battling the Status Quo

A century ago, the nascent fields of planning and public health converged over the need to mitigate the unhealthful effects of slums and tenements constructed literally at the doorsteps of dirty, noisy factories. Workplaces spewed billowing clouds of highly toxic substances into their surrounding neighborhoods.[19] As is discussed in later chapters, this resulted in the establishment of zoning laws now viewed as archaic and in need of a total overhaul. After decades of the status quo, with relatively little serious discourse between these disciplines, they have recently re-converged.[20] During this "lost period," decades of inattention and ineffectiveness, combined with careless actions on the part of developers, politicians, and others resulted in the construction of vast stretches of suburbia that seemingly had no beginning, no middle, nor end, not unlike a very poorly fitted shag carpet stretched beyond its reasonable limits across the landscape. One tool developed by public health specialists working in consort with urban planners has been the Health Impact Assessment (HIA) developed by the CDC in the U.S. It parallels the environmental impact statement of the U.S. Environmental Protection Agency (EPA).[21] HIAs generally focus on aggregate community-wide data, however, not on the micro-behaviors and mobility patterns of individuals at the scale of the architectural or immediate neighborhood environment. While efforts to quantify the behaviors of suburbanites may smack of social re-engineering, efforts are underway on the part of some physicians anyway, in consort with urban planners, to develop metrics that can assess and correlate caloric intake, caloric expenditures, and physical movement patterns in suburbia during a person's typical 24-hour living cycle.[22]

At one time in America, sprawl was considered virtuous, even visionary. It symbolized a new universe of lifestyle and job opportunities, unfettered expansion, and an abundance of anything and everything we could possibly desire. Case in point: the population of the State of Nevada grew by 35 percent between 2000 and 2010, making it the fastest growing state in the U.S. By any measure, this would have ordinarily been cause for great celebration. Instead, it deteriorated into yet another reminder of how bad things had become. Since the start of the Great Recession in early 2008, people have been moving out due to having lost their job, or foreclosure in a housing market with the highest foreclosure rate in the nation. Unemployment rose sharply, to nearly 15 percent, also the highest in the nation. Meanwhile, thousands of homes, strip centers, and related vestiges of sprawl sit empty on the hot, treeless, desert floor and subdivisions with names like Vantage Lofts on Horizon Ridge Road (the latter completely abandoned in mid-construction).[23] This occurs while the rate of suburban poverty has risen across the U.S. as its suburbs become more and more racially diverse.[24]

Sprawl apologists such as Wendell Cox claim that things are not so bad in suburbia just as they are.[25] Nonetheless, the politics of sprawl have become more polarized than ever and are now enmeshed in such thorny, highly contentious issues as global climate change and geopolitical events in once seemingly far-off places such as China and India.[26] Other sprawl apologists go further and assert that the so-called anti-suburban zealots are merely an expression of an elitist, left-wing conspiracy to undermine Western economies. However, everyone seems to agree that, for example, the sheer number of dead shopping malls and roadside strip centers, i.e. vacant or abandoned, which has drawn the attention of many cultural observers whether conservative, liberal and in-between, should be of equal concern to anti-sprawlites and pro-sprawlites alike.[27] Against this backdrop, still others single out and condemn the practices of bureaucratic, highly centralized states and dysfunctional healthcare systems that preside over increasingly fragmented, isolated suburban landscapes. They argue against failed policies towards sprawl in a call for completely new, grassroots-initiated realignments centered around suburban economies and lifestyle priorities. However, it is precisely this type of planning process that is being proposed in the U.K. at this time, and many fear its consequences will include too much local control by unscrupulous developers, resulting in the rise of unprecedented, rampant private development across the U.K., devouring once-scenic landscapes.[28]

## Sprawl Machines: What Are They?

The way a human experiences a sprawling metropolis is not unlike the inseparable relationship between a fish and the water in which it swims—both are immersive experiences insofar as one exists within the other. In the U.S., suburbia is widely seen as a libertarian right, personifying a "live and let live" culture and attitude. The right to use one's land as one wishes has always been seen as an unassailable freedom. This "leave us alone" suburban ethos has been taken to the extreme, whereby private landowners and for-profit developers deeply resent being told how to use to any extent the land they own. The term *sprawl* itself denotes a thing, object, or set of objects that are spread out randomly. In an animal or human, it denotes a rather random spreading out of sprawled limbs, irregularly or awkwardly, an act having occurred in a sprawling manner not unlike a child's building blocks turned upside down, falling out from their storage box and sprawling across the carpet. In stark contrast, a *machine* is a highly precise, mechanized apparatus consisting of interrelated parts with separate yet interdependent, highly coordinated functions. It is a device or entity that dispenses a type of product or service such as an automobile, dishwasher, or a semi-automatic machine gun. The word machine is frequently applied metaphorically to a complex agency or operating system, such as a *political machine* that carries out predetermined operative functions, or a political agenda executed by a government or for that matter any entity otherwise seeking to attain and/or maintain control. It therefore, by extension, is applicable to any entity that controls regional or local land use, such as a cartel of powerful private developers who, in turn, may either intentionally or inadvertently exert undue influence over their architects and those they view as having been elected to serve *them* first and foremost.

A *sprawl machine* is the outcome of irregular, minimally coordinated yet interdependent and systemic development patterns that occur across time and space. It is a curious and highly ironic amalgam of both randomness and intensely mechanized precision. Organizationally, it functions as a self-perpetuating entity which feeds upon itself in order to exist, thrive, and in/organically expand in the loosest sense, with its progenitors and benefactors often functioning (as actors) autonomously from one other and yet often interdependently, in consort, even lock-step, i.e. the Wal-Mart cannot be built without *some* coordination with the Hampton Inn next door, with the new mega-gas station/casino/truck stop across the street, the McDonald's next door to it, and soon, an assortment of fast (fat) food outlets, the new roads built leading to it with public taxpayer dollars, and so on yet they together share a very clearly defined common goal. Its commercial components are single-mindedly affixed on the maximization of profit. In its broadest definition, the term *sprawl machine* extends the work of Harvey Molotch's 1976 essay "The city as a growth machine." In it, Molotch called attention to the manner in which local power elites construct a system with land reconstituted as a market commodity providing power and wealth to a select few, referring to planned, minimally coordinated sprawl as "growth machines."[29]

Sprawl machines are paradoxical. They at once synthesize and express both order and corrosive disorder, and as the architect Robert Venturi pointed out nearly fifty years ago, in 1966, profound complexities and contradictions.[30] Sprawl machines evolve organically over time and space not unlike the erasable plant species known as *kudzu*. Both lack a genuine physical center or any particular sense of place. With the possible exception of a small subset of large, vaguely iconic, post-WWII shopping malls and their attendant collections of generic strip malls, the "centers" or cores of sprawl machines typically lack uniquely definable characteristics which set them apart from anywhere else. Sprawl machines tend to be homogenous, placeless, whether in the suburbs of Paris, Tokyo, Beijing, San Francisco, Atlanta, Houston, or Chicago. People increasingly eat the same foods everywhere, buy the same clothes, and drive the same cars. Yet on the other hand, people are always searching to find that which is deeply personal and authentic. This human fascination with authenticity/inauthenticity drives the global tourism industry and has an equally profound influence on public health. Once place-uniqueness and authenticity becomes corroded, eradicated, or replicated everywhere else, be it through the promotion of inauthentic, non-vernacular-based architecture, poor nutritional food quality, or encroaching sedentarianism, it is difficult if not impossible to reverse. How many sprawl machines can be described as unique, authentic, or, for that matter, places that genuinely promote human health?

Sprawl machines destroy natural ecological systems and habitats, dismiss local historic architecture, and often run roughshod over local grassroots attempts to solicit genuine public input in the local planning process. The result is a visually chaotic patchwork quilt of uncoordinated, non-walkable, anti-pedestrian spatial aggregations. Its non-profit cogs, such as the public library branch or the primary care outpatient health clinic next door to it, are just as auto-dependent, and exist for these same sedentary constituencies. Progress is a double-edged sword. What came first, the chicken or the egg? Does the new hospital built on formerly open pasture way out on the edge of town attract sprawl, or vice versa? Most sprawl is internally synchronized only minimally to the extent it is subject to regulation through zoning laws. Many currently dead and dying regional malls and strip centers could not have been constructed without the massive zoning variances and rezoning favors granted to their developers.[31]

Sprawl is nearly entirely autocentric. Its vehicular arteries function as tentacles, reaching outward from an existing older urban core or from a crossroads or geographic feature, becoming an expansive stretched canvas, continuously or discontinuously via leapfrogging across open landscapes—as a benign *horizontalism*.[32] The post-WWII Las Vegas strip evolved, for example, as an extension of Fremont Street in the historic main street/rail station nexus of what once was a remote railroad town in the American West. Westheimer Street, in Houston, was extended multiple times as Houston sprawled rapidly west of the CBD from the 1960s through the 1980s. Sprawl also can infill between two independent urban cores with the connecting artery soon becoming lined with endless strip development such as the infill sprawl between Dallas and Fort Worth, Chicago and Milwaukee, Charlotte and Atlanta to name but a few examples in the U.S.

Regional shopping malls and megamalls (see Chapter 2) may function as the core engine of sprawl. They often form their centers, spawning myriad attached and freestanding fast food outlets, strip malls, and gas stations, along seemingly endless aggregations of mind-numbing roadside strips. In the 2000s, yet another wave of generic mini-sprawl machines—low-cost hotel chains, gas stations, and seas of fast food outlets, invaded the last of the Interstate highway interchanges that had somehow up to then remained sprawl-free in the American South and elsewhere in the U.S. Because two core attributes of a sprawl machine are its striking placelessness and its surreal inauthenticity, it lives and dies in relation to the relative happiness of the mass consumer who provides the lubricant that keeps it operational. And this has become a dicey proposition in an economy where consumer spending now accounts for more than two-thirds of all economic activity.[33]

### Sprawl Machines and the Public's Health: How Are They Interrelated?

The mechanical inner workings of sprawl machines and their deep relationship to public health is intensely complex and contradictory. The earliest suburban malls were initially touted as walking-friendly although in no way did they promote any degree of genuinely community-based or inter-connected culture of pedestrianism.[34] Albeit, no two sprawl machines are precisely alike and their inner workings and influences on public health is a relationship tempered by many local determinants. With this said, an attempt is made at this point to capture some essential underlying constructs that define the tenets and parameters of this relationship and its interdependencies, as they manifest through the prism of everyday life. These constructs are portrayed within an interactive space (Figure 1.1) and each is defined by the endpoints of two principal crossing bipolar axes—the first of these axes, Axis 1/3, denotes the essential importance of there being in place a viable, supportive, health-promoting urban civic context and, on its opposing endpoint, the

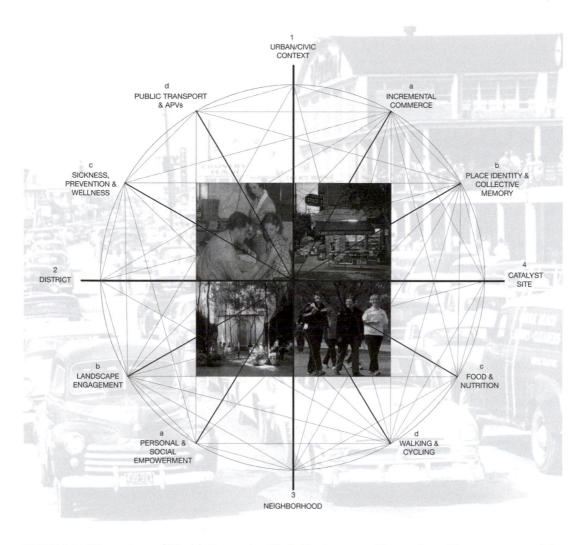

**FIGURE 1.1** Dimensions of Health Promotion/Built Environment Transactions. Photo courtesy of the United States Library of Congress

importance of those attributes which collectively define a health promoting, safe, culturally and economically viable neighborhood. A horizontal axis, Axis 2/4, defines the horizontal parameters of this diagram, and denotes the importance of the district as the site context, or unit of inquiry and analysis, for subsequent interventions aimed at increasing the health status of a community. On its opposing endpoint, the importance is denoted of carefully weighing and maximizing the amenity of any catalyst site. Together, these cross-axes can provide a conceptual foundation to classify and to examine health-promoting interventions in the built environment at any scale of inquiry, be it at the interventional scale of a given room, building, neighborhood, city, and so on.

A further distinction is worth noting with regards to this conceptual model. Public health specialists, particularly epidemiologists, have historically tended to use pathogenic perspectives, i.e. disease-based conceptualizations of the built environment, to examine the neighborhood and, by extension, the region, rather than to focus on the therapeutic or health-promoting role of the architectural environment per se. Such pathogenic models are in need of recalibration to include *salutogenic*, as opposed to strictly pathogenetic factors, and that include in their scope architecture as a contributory factor in the improvement of a community's overall healthfulness. The term salutogenic was put forth in the 1990s to capture the need to focus far more on the health-promoting dimensions of healthcare versus the typical disease-response-treatment model of care that continues to dominate Western medicine.[35] An emergent field, *salutogenesis*, encompasses this broader, emerging area of discourse.[36] With this said, the vertical and the horizontal axes of the salutogenic model yield four quadrants. Within each quadrant are two bi-polar constructs that traverse the horizontal/vertical cross-axes. These constructs are similar in structure to the aforementioned two principal axes, and are similarly interconnected. This operative framework therefore is an attempt to link architecture with the aforementioned broader perspectives of health promotion in the built environment. While sprawl's effects on human health has garnered increasing attention in the medical and public health disciplines as of late, effective solutions will require the combined energies, skill sets, and influence of health professionals, planners, and architects, speaking as one, acting in tandem. Four principal dimensions of this conceptualization are described below in direct relation to their *architectural ecologies*, and are reprised in later chapters:

### A. Incremental Commerce as a Function of a Community's Degree of Genuine Personal and Social Empowerment, and Its Architecture

In the post-WWI decades, sprawl machines prospered at the expense of the more than 25,000 Main Street commercial districts which fell into decline across America alone during this period. Many traditional, pedestrian-centric towns and cities that were built in the late 19th and early to mid-20th centuries in particular fell on hard times as sprawl advocates set their sights on superseding the traditional town core itself in a grand-scale experiment to reinvent and supplant the traditional commercial core in its own generic, faceless image, i.e. big box stores, outlet centers, and strip malls. My home town/suburb was one of these places, once a rural community near to but wholly autonomous from Chicago. Its present origins date from the late 19th century, where two Native American dirt-path trading trails crossed, and later, as unpaved farm-to-market roads. This town, Niles Center, Illinois, was later renamed "Skokie" in honor of its original Native American settlers. Originally, Niles Center was separated from the nearby city by forests, mills, and dairy farms. Niles Center grew steadily through to the late 1950s and early 1960s but would succumb to being just another bedroom community within Chicago's interconnected sprawl machines. The construction of the Old Orchard Shopping Center, 3 miles to the north of the traditional town center, was the major blow. Designed by Victor Gruen & Associates, it was a prototype post-WWII open-air American suburban mall, with its acres of free parking. Its opening in 1956 had an eviscerating effect on the old town as it simply could not compete. In response, it began devouring itself, tearing down one after another of its most historic buildings in order to clear land—all in the name of free parking. It was this I experienced, firsthand, as a child and later adolescent: the push–pull dialectics of an expanding sprawl machine. One by one, the small shops that figured so prominently in my childhood closed, including the local mom and pop toyshop and my dad's favorite pub. The old town's rebirth would not begin in earnest for thirty more years and still continues to this day.

## B.  Place Identity and Collective Memory as a Function of Citizens' Engagement with the Natural Landscape

The physical properties of sprawl machines tend to deny the important civic function of sustaining a community's collective memory with respect to nature and landscape. They deny the importance of history, sentiment, and emotional attachment to particular landscape experiences. These form a person's worldview from the earliest age and shape one's lifelong habits, outlook, and perceptions as a contributing member of society. They also deny the importance of nature and landscape in relation to buildings in the construction of collective memory. In general, the apparatus of a sprawl machine does not easily make concessions to nor establish set-asides of open space for parks, wetland preserves, water elements, gardens and the like. Until very recently, amenities such as these were not perceived as profit-generating and hence not to be valued when the goal was to jam as many big box outlet stores as economically feasible onto a single parcel of land. Too often, landscape and nature set-asides do not do well as "highest and best" recommended land uses in market forecasters' prognostications and in the reports commissioned by the developers who hired them. Why create a park? "Why not build more homes there instead?" "Why preserve that frontage along the main artery versus putting in a speculative strip center?" The block my family lived on when I was young was comprised of mostly open prairie. Our spec ranch house was completed in 1954. The open prairie was just referred to as "the prairie", perhaps in reference to the Midwestern open prairies that once carpeted the region. It was a last remaining vestige, a holdout parcel. Soon, speculative houses were built crowded together on the block to squeeze out every square foot of sellable land. The prairie was gone. We were then forced out to a formal public park nearby, with its basketball and tennis courts, baseball field, formal play equipment and large shady trees. But it wasn't the same. By far, we preferred the raggedness of that vanished natural ecology.[37]

## C.  Community's Wellness as a Function of Its Nutritional Health, and Its Architecture

The automobile-dependent supermarket is a suburban architectural creation. Conventional wisdom has it that these places in the U.S. with their often-strange names, such as Winn-Dixie, Publix, Harris Teeter, and Piggly Wiggly, were major component parts of sprawl machines. At the same time they sold foods of generally poor nutritional quality. These businesses were (are) housed in monolithic big boxes one level in height on large greenfield sites without consideration for meaningful connections with walking, cycling, or public transport. The traditional suburban grocery store of the 1950s–1990s period is now in many places anachronistic: supermarket big boxes with their paved parking lots filled with now-vacant free parking. They required everyone to drive to them. But history has a funny way of repeating itself. Wal-Mart is currently attempting to become the major center for suburban food distribution. It is an unfortunate public health consequence that too many suburbs suffer from too few options for people to purchase healthy food locally. This food is of poor nutritional quality although it has been amply demonstrated that proper food and diet have a major positive impact on a community's public health outcomes. Nutritional health education seems to be an equally scarce commodity and especially in medically underserved suburbs, urban neighborhoods, and small towns. Where ample options exist nearby in terms of a coordinated mix of primary care clinics, wellness centers, hospitals, together with key public health-based amenities such as parks, and fresh food markets, improved nutritional health can be fostered. The design of fresh food market and agricultural distribution facilities is interweavable with local food production and distribution systems. Architecture can have a significant role in this, just as it did with the invention of the suburban supermarket. The local fresh food market, as a building type, warrants reappraisal, along with mixed use, trans-programmatic typologies with housing and small shops and community gardens, with close connections to walking, cycling, and pubic transport as a means to ameliorate the occurrence of non-communicable diseases associated with unmitigated sprawl.

## D. Walking and Cycling Behaviors as a Function of the Efficacy of Public Transport, Alternative Personal Vehicles (APVs), and Architecture

Suburbanites depend on the private automobile for nearly every facet of everyday life. In 2008, nearly 57 percent of the petroleum consumed in the U.S. was imported oil. And in that year the U.S. consumed nearly 23 percent of all the oil drilled and refined in the entire world. Private autos accounted in that year in the U.S. for 34 percent of all fossil fuel oil used for transportation.[38] Destination points are often not easily reachable by walking or cycling. Wherever travel distances, inclement weather, or one's personal limitations due to accident or disability render it impossible to walk or bike, the provision of supportive and user-responsive public transport systems can fill this demand gap. Electric personal vehicles, e-bikes, and other in-development products are viable alternatives. However, the issue of range anxiety with respect to alternative APVs will be a limiting factor in their acceptance until a dependable network of electro-charging stations is built within and between towns and regions. These new products and new consumer travel behaviors alone are not predicted to have any significant ameliorating effect on sprawl or its associated unhealthful public health outcomes. In other words, owning an APV alone will probably not necessarily reduce the current excessive rate of NCDs such as obesity, chronic heart disease, diabetes, or hypertension rates—since people may still be in their cars driving just as much and as far as before. Once again, architecture can perhaps contribute much in this regard, with buildings that facilitate home-based electrocharging functions so that APVs can be cleverly integrated with aesthetic concerns. As for the scale of a given building or complex, it is not beyond reason to design internal and external circulation systems to promote more walking within and between buildings, and to correspondingly rely less on mechanical lifts and escalators.

## Summary

A public health crisis is on our doorstep. Individual citizens and communities can and will become motivated to act to ameliorate the unhealthful consequences of unmitigated sprawl. The stakes are high because our endangered human health and well-being, and the endangered ecological health of our planet calls for new, integrative, *eco-humanist* paradigms. This book is premised on the belief that massive change in the everyday built environment is possible in this regard but it will be extremely difficult for most people to grasp its importance in their daily lives. In Chapter 2, the history of this subject is briefly reviewed. The coming transformations will be particularly difficult for the apologists of sprawl machines. The framework presented in this chapter on person/environment transactions with respect to public health and the functions of architecture is reprised in later chapters. An older suburban community that currently suffers from a poor level of public health, acute care health services, and a deteriorating urban infrastructure is examined from the standpoint of designing and implementing a *suburban transfusion* of its community and architectural infrastructure. The need for such measures at this time underscores the core theme of this book because too often, globally, it is the poor whose public health remains most marginalized as they become increasingly engulfed in unmitigated sprawl and its unhealthful consequences. In Chapter 3, rapidly proliferating sprawl machines in the Middle East, India, Southeast Asia, and in China are discussed in detail. They exist in Australia, in South Africa, in Egypt, Russia, Brazil, in Argentina and in many other parts of the world. *Sprawling Cities and Our Endangered Public Health* seeks to examine the past, present, and future of architecture, planning, and landscape architecture in relation to the public health consequences of sprawl and how it threatens our future. It examines 20th-century theories of architecture and urbanism in direct relation to current unsustainable practices, design considerations in creating a health-promoting language of *ecological architecture* and requisite landscape urbanism.

## Notes

1 Ewing, R., Schmid, T., Killingsworth, R., Zlot, A., and Raudenhush, S. (2003) 'Relationship between urban sprawl and physical activity, obesity, and morbidity,' *American Journal of Health Promotion*, 18(1): 47–57.

2 World Health Organization (2011) *Chronic Diseases*. Online. Available at www.who.int/topics/chronic_diseases/en/html (accessed 20 July 2011).

3 World Health Organization (2005) *Preventing Chronic Diseases: A Vital Investment*. Geneva. Also see World Health Organization (2002) *The World Health Report 2002—Reducing Risks, Promoting Healthy Life*. Geneva. Online. Available at www.who.int/whr/2002/en/html (accessed 19 July 2011), and World Health Organization (2009) 'New network to combat non-communicable diseases.' Geneva, 8 July.

4 Body mass index is a measurement based on weight and height. People with a BMI of 18–24 are considered to have a healthy weight. Those with a BMI of 25 or above are overweight and those with a BMI over 30 are classified by epidemiologists as obese.

5 Finucane, Mariel M., Stevens, Gretchen A., Cowan, Melanie J., Danaei, Goodarz, Lin, John K., Paciorek, Christopher J., Singh, Gitanjali, Gutierrez, Hialy R., Lu, Yuan, Bahalim, Adil N., Farzadfar, Farshad, Riley, Leanne M., and Ezzati, Majid (2011) 'National, regional, and global trends in body-mass index since 1980: Systematic analysis of health examination surveys and epidemiological studies with 960 country-years and 9.1 million participants," *The Lancet*, 377 (9765): 557–567.

6 Bates, Claire (2011) 'Fat Britain: Tackling the obesity epidemic,' *The Daily Mail*, 21 July. Online. Available at www.dailymail.co.uk/health/article-301419/Fat-Britian-Tackling_Obesity.html (accessed 22 July 2011).

7 Carter, Helen (2010) 'Diabetes and obesity rates soar to shocking levels,' *The Guardian*, 25 October. Online. Available at www.guardian.co.uk/society/2010/oct/25/uk.html (accessed 20 July 2011).

8 Summary article 'A nudge or a shove?' on *Behaviour Change, Report of the Lords Select Committee*, London, 19 July 2011. C3 Collaborating for Health. Online. Available at www.c3health.org/alerts/alerts-diet/a-nudge-or-shove/html (accessed 21 July 2011).

9 Gordon-Larsen, Penny, Nelson, Melissa C., Page, Phil, and Popkin, Barry M. (2006) 'Inequality in the built environment underlies key health disparities in physical activity and obesity,' *Pediatrics*, 117(2): 417–424.

10 Andersen, Glen (2002) 'The built environment: Is there a connection between sprawl and public health?' *Public Health News. State Health Notes*, 6 May, pp. 3–6.

11 Stipp, David (2011) 'Obesity—not aging—balloons health care costs,' *Miller-McCune*, 7 June. Online. Available at www.miller-mccune.com/health/obesity-aging-cause-ballooning-health-care-costs-31879/.html (accessed 15 June 2011).

12 Frumkin, Howard, Frank, Lawrence, and Jackson, Richard (2004) *Urban Sprawl and Public Health: Designing, Planning, and Building for Healthy Communities*. Washington, D.C.: Island Press.

13 Ibid., pp. 12–42.

14 Ibid., pp. 186–199.

15 Dunlap, Eleanor and Teachey, Michael (2010) 'Now go outside and play,' *The Greenville News*, 11 April, p. 10A.

16 American Academy of Pediatrics, Committee on Environmental Health (2009) 'The built environment: Designing communities to promote physical activity in children,' *Pediatrics*, 123(6): 1591–1598. Also see Ogden, C., Carroll, M.D., and Flegal, K. (2008) 'High body mass index for age among U.S. children and adolescents: 2003–2006,' *JAMA*, 299(20): 2401–2405.

17 Hellmich, Nanci (2010) 'Doctors need tools to help patients slim down,' *The Greenville News*, 18 March, p. 2C.

18  Wells, Nancy M., Evans, Gary W., and Yang, Yizhao (2010) 'Environments and health: Planning decisions as public health decisions,' *Journal of Architectural and Planning Research*, 27(2): 124–142.

19  Frumkin et al., *Urban Sprawl and Public Health*, pp. 26–64.

20  Duany, Andres and Speck, Jeff (2010) 'Plan to reduce sprawl will boost health, environment,' *The New York Times*, 16 October. Online. Available at www.washingtonpost.com/wp-dyn/content/article/2010/10/15ar2010101505197.html (accessed 18 October 2010).

21  Lerner, Jonathan (2010) 'How urban planning can improve public health,' *Miller-McCune*, 28 April. Online. Available at www.miller-mccune.com/health/how-urban-planning-can-improve-public-health-11408/html (accessed 5 May 2010).

22  Hoyt, Clark (2009) 'The health care sprawl,' *The New York Times*, 11 October. Online. Available at www.nytimes.com/2009/10/11/opinion/11pubed.html (accessed 12 November 2009).

23  Nagourney, Adam (2010) 'Behind census figures showing boom in Nevada, a story of bust,' *The New York Times*, 22 December. Online. Available at www.nytims.com.html (accessed 10 January 2011).

24  Yen, Hope (2010) 'In new "white flight," affluent return to cities,' *The Greenville News*, 9 May, p. 12A. One result of this is that megachain store outlets and big box 'Power Malls' are now invading urban neighborhoods.

25  Cox, Wendell (2006) *War on the Dream: How Anti-Sprawl Policy Threatens the Quality of Life*. New York: iUniverse.

26  Goodyear, Sarah (2010) 'Is there a war between cities and suburbs? Does there have to be one?' *Grist*, 20 October. Online. Available at www.grist.org/article/2010-20/html (accessed 12 November 2010).

27  The deadmall.com web site contains lists of hundreds of closed malls across the United States. It also posts recollections provided by people who frequented these shuttered malls. Many are touching, filled emotional testimonies that attest to the enduring power of these once-vibrant places in their lives.

28  Doward, Jamie (2011) 'Apathy over planning law changes could put countryside in danger,' *The Guardian*, 10 September. Online. Available at www.guardian.co.uk/politics/2011/sep/10/html (accessed 14 September 2011). Also see Blond, Philip (2009) 'Rise of the red Tories,' *Prospect*, 28 February. Online. Available at www.prospectmagazine.co.uk/2009/02/riseoftheredtories/html (accessed 15 July 2011), and Brooks, David (2010) 'The broken society,' *The New York Times*, 18 March. Online. Available at www.nytimes.com/2010/03/19/opinion/19brooks.html (accessed 15 July 2011).

29  Molotch, Harvey (1976) 'The city as growth machine: Toward a political economy of place,' *American Journal of Sociology*, 82(9): 309–332. Also see Hayden, Dolores (2004) *A Field Guide to Sprawl*. New York: W.W. Norton & Company.

30  Venturi, Robert (1966) *Complexity and Contradiction in Architecture*. New York: Museum of Modern Art. Also see Lindsay, Greg (2010) 'How much longer can shopping malls survive?' *FastCompany.com*, 23 February. Online. Available at www.fastcompany.com.html (accessed 12 March 2011).

31  Anon. (2009) 'Urban planning experts skewer Englewood CityCenter project,' *Face the State*, 1 June. Online. Available at www.facethestate.com/articles/16482-urban-planning-experts-skewer-englewod-citycenter.html (accessed 14 August 2010).

32  Berger, Alan (2006) *Drosscape: Wasting Land in Urban America*. New York: Princeton Architectural Press.

33  Non-growth economies will very likely become a permanent fixture of our everyday life in the most developed countries with the most aged populations. This is becoming evident within sprawl landscapes and is inextricably linked to steeply rising oil prices, exhausted fresh water sources, and the slow death-by-suffocation and overfishing of the oceans.

34  The systematic study of pedestrian flow and typologies—pedestrianism—is emerging as a field to provide metrics in the efficacy of public space rights of ways, destination points, how they are regulated, user attributes and preferences, encoded, rendered legible, and navigable.

35  Antonovsky, Aaron (1996) 'The salutogenic model as a theory to guide health promotion,' *Health Promotion International*, 11(1): 11–18.

36  Suominen, Sakari and Lindstrom, Bengt (2008) 'Salutogenesis,' *Scandinavian Journal of Public Health*, 36(4): 337–339.

37  The early 20th-century organic architecture of Frank Lloyd Wright through to the best work of Emilio Ambaz, Antoine Predock, Glenn Murdock, and Frank Gehry provides baseline precedents from which to extend holistic, carbon neutral approaches into new frontiers.

38  Brooks, Jeanne (2010) 'Oil spill calls for taking long view,' *The Greenville News*, 18 June, p. B1.

# 2

# SPRAWL, ARCHITECTURE, AND HEALTH: A BRIEF HISTORY

The cities will be part of the country; I shall live 30 miles from my office in one direction, under a pine tree; my secretary will live 30 miles away from it too, in the other direction, under another pine tree. We shall both have our own car. We shall use up tires, wear out road surfaces and gears, and consume oil and gasoline. All of which will necessitate a great deal of work. . .enough for all.

*Le Corbusier (1935)[1]*

The situation today in many sprawl machine communities is a story of unfinished subdivisions, deserted neighborhoods, a sea of foreclosures, and shattered dreams. Timothy Egan refers to California's current dystrophic condition as *Slumburbia*:

Drive along foreclosure alley, through new planned communities that look like tile-roofed versions of a 21st century ghost town, and you see what happens when people gamble with houses instead of casino chips. Dirty flags advertise rock bottom discounts on empty starter mansions. Foreclosure signs are tagged with gang graffiti. Empty lots are untended, cratered with mud puddles. . .nobody is home in the cities of the future. In a decade, they saw real property defy reality in real time in these instant-neighborhoods that sprouted in what had been some of the world's most productive farmland, the population nearly doubled in ten years, and home prices tripled. After inhaling all this real estate helium, some developers and their apologists in urban planning circles hailed the boom as the new America. . .every citizen a home-owner! Half-acre lots for all! No credit, no problem! Others saw it as the residential embodiment of the Edward Abbey line that "growth for the sake of growth is the ideology of the cancer cell." Now median homes prices have fallen from $500,000 to $150,000—among the most precipitous drops in the nation—and still the houses sit empty. . .in nearby strip malls tenants seem to last no longer than the life cycle of a gold fish, and the bottom feeders have moved in.[2]

Is this what happens when money, investor–driven greed, and markets alone guide how we live? How can a community possibly be healthy when one in eight houses is in foreclosure, when unemployment is 16 percent? In 2010, a record 2.8 million U.S. homes were in foreclosure and more than 5 million homeowners (one in ten mortgages) owed more than their houses were worth. Many homeowners simply walk away leaving their "investment" to fall into ruin.[3] In an influential article "The next slum" in *The Atlantic* in 2008, Christopher B. Leinberger predicted the catastrophic collapse of a new home market that has turned McMansion subdivisions into 21st-century post-industrial tenement districts.[4] In the case of California, the state's dysfunctional tax system compelled cash-starved towns to expand into farmland, as a means to generate desperately needed new tax revenue. Developers, who had been given *carte blanche*, rejoiced, while zombie banks mindlessly propelled an unregulated loan-fest.

Sprawl apologists claim these ghost suburbs will eventually fill up as the U.S. population soars by an expected 100 million by 2050. This despite the unhealthful ramifications associated with their excessive carbon footprints and auto-dependency. To find out how things got so out of whack, the origins of sprawl machines need to be traced back to their late 19th-century roots. In the U.S., the origins of current debates over the future of cities and their surrounding sprawl machines lie in the transformative years following World War II, when millions of middle-class families fled cities for cheap, spacious new houses on the outskirts of town.

The following discussion is structured according to five time periods, or epochs, in an attempt to chronologize key architectural developments from the late 19th century to the present. These periods are: 1. Pre-Automobile Suburbanization, 2. Roadside Commercial Vernacular Typologies, 3. Post-War Sprawl Machines, 4. The Rise of the Megamall, and 5. Ecological Architecture and Urbanism. This chronology is not to be construed as definitive or all-inclusive, as space allows for no more than a brief outline of a subset of major developments. This author is well aware of the pitfalls of timelines, including their perhaps sounding didactic or too simplistic.[5] Regardless, the focus here is on the work of architects, the relationship between architecture and its allied fields, urban design and landscape architecture, and by extension the relationship between architecture and its allied disciplines to community-based public health. As Dolores Hayden has adroitly pointed out, most histories of suburbia in America have been singularly preoccupied with tracing improvements in transportation technologies, as these are seen as the fundamental progenitors of suburban expansion and form.[6] This is true but only to a certain extent. This historical overview is, by and large, recounted from an American perspective although it remains a subject of international interest and debate.[7] All societies, of course, have their own parallel histories of growth, architecture, and health. It is acknowledged from the outset that U.S. free market attitudes toward land use deregulation have historically differed greatly from top-down land use controls practiced in the U.K. and in many other parts of the world. Land use planning remains far more centrally controlled in these places.[8] These five periods, or *waves*, address continuities and discontinuities across time and space and across sprawl-based building types and trends. This conceptualization will, it is hoped, aid in seeking to make sense of the complex, contradictory, and, at times, paradoxical interrelationship between sprawl, architecture, and public health.

## 1. Pre-Automobile Suburbanization (1880–1900)

The ancient agoras and medieval piazzas of European and Middle Eastern cities are antecedents of the contemporary strip mall. The Industrial Revolution of the 19th century produced the department store, among other commercial typologies, at a time when central cities were becoming overcrowded, unhealthy places. Rural spas were built near cities to accommodate the upper classes who could afford to escape the deadly epidemics that ravaged urban communities at this time. Public officials and private philanthropists sought to improve public health and safety by providing an alternative to the dense central city's unhealthful conditions, thereby giving birth to the modern suburb. Ironically, the earliest suburbs of the Industrial Age themselves were often considered undesirable places to live. As recently as the 1880s, many working-class and lower middle-class families resided at the urban periphery where the land was cheapest and least desirable. The outskirts of 19th-century cities frequently were where noxious industries such as slaughterhouses and glue factories, charity institutions such as asylums, orphanages, and poorhouses, contagious disease hospitals, prisons, as well as sites for temporal land uses, i.e. circuses, and in the American South, lynchings, were located. Squatters lived on this marginal land in substandard dwellings. Later, the development of upscale suburban precincts was made possible only through the successful marketing of the virtues of restriction and exclusion, implemented through developers' deed restrictions, banks' red lining practices, and related discriminatory practices. In 1898, Ebenezer Howard published *To-Morrow: A Peaceful Path to Real Reform*, his treatise on the Garden City, whose mission was to outline the precepts of a safe, healthier haven far from industry and its associated urban public health evils.[9] The field of epidemiology was rapidly developing at this time in urban medical centers in Europe and in North America.

In a 1903 report, the New York Tenement House Commission focused on the "greatest evil of the day," the lack of natural light and fresh air. It concluded tuberculosis had reached an epidemic level in these overcrowded settings.[10] Inner city immigrant families lived in overcrowded tenements lacking in proper hygiene amenities, and many would later move out to streetcar suburbs as soon as they could afford to do so. This would soon have a major impact on the ethnic mix of the newly built suburbs prior to 1920.[11] Proponents of zoning went further, claiming it inadequate to simply designate various segregated districts by land use, i.e. residential, commercial, industrial. Residential districts were to be sub-zoned further, i.e. single-family, and multifamily. It was argued that tenements constituted a quantitatively different type of dwelling versus single-family dwellings in terms of their structure as well as the social class they housed. Leaders in the real estate industry zealously supported the views of public health experts because they knew that segregated land use zoning could stabilize metro housing markets and make it possible to simultaneously market to multiple niche markets in different neighborhoods. Los Angeles, in establishing the first U.S. segregated land use zoning statute in 1908, assuaged the fears of upper-class homebuyers that their investment would not be eroded by the construction of multifamily housing in the immediate neighborhood.[12] Frederick Law Olmsted's Central Park in New York City set the standard for a generation of new urban parks that served as respites from their harsh surroundings. Electric streetcar lines and inter-urban railway lines also contributed to the growth of segregated income-level neighborhoods in suburbia in the late 19th and early 20th centuries. Entrepreneurs subdivided lots and constructed houses and commercial structures on every acre of buildable land along these routes, connected to bedroom suburbs, for niche market homebuyers (this is discussed in greater depth in Chapter 5). This spawned the fist wave of transit-oriented development in the U.S. (TOD-1).

## 2. Roadside Commercial Vernacular Typologies (1900–1945)

By the early years of the 20th century, picturesque upscale suburban bedroom suburbs such as Oak Park, Illinois, were firmly established, where the social elite thrived. By World War I, many urban streetcar lines began to wane in profitability because the lines suffered from a combination of build-out, overextension, poor management, and aging equipment. The proliferation of automobiles, low-cost fuel, and new waves of subdivisions made auto travel more feasible than long streetcar commutes to and from downtown. After 1910, developers encouraged people with autos to move to even more distant areas far beyond the reaches of many public transport lines. Market Square, the first

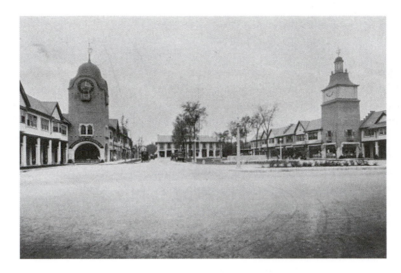

**FIGURE 2.1** Market Square, Lake Forest, Illinois, 1916. Photo courtesy of the United States Library of Congress

"planned" shopping mall in the U.S., opened in 1916 in Lake Forest, Illinois. This U-shaped mall fused Tyrolean and Italian Renaissance motifs (Figure 2.1). Chicago architect Arthur Aldis persuaded wealthy residents of Lake Forest, and investors such as Cyrus H. McCormick, Jr., to form the Lake Forest Improvement Trust, to build an integrated, mixed-use shopping complex of twenty-eight stores, twelve office units, thirty apartments, gym, clubhouse, and gardens. The auto was central to its planning as most local residents owned autos at an early date. The earliest suburban malls for the elite classes sought to express neoclassical architectural styles and periods, the dialectic between nature and urbanity, and were influenced by Garden City precepts.[13] Market Square's origins, however, dated back to 1908 to Baltimore's Roland Park.[14]

The largest percentage growth in auto ownership in U.S. history occurred in the 1920s, the decade in which Detroit manufacturers began to lobby intensely for federal highway construction funds. By 1930, virtually every American city had rings of suburbs and commercial arteries and downtown was where the family's breadwinner worked.[15] Meanwhile, developers and their architects were building strip malls such as Houston's upscale River Oaks, and new commercial vernacular building types emerged to accommodate a new class of auto commuters. In the U.S., the Urban Land Institute was founded in 1936, when many American cities were experiencing suburbanization as well as inner city decay, with limited public sector planning and no guidance available to the private sector. Soon thereafter, the U.S. auto companies, led by General Motors, began to strategize to buy out and shut down the privately owned and municipally owned urban streetcar lines. The streets leading to and within the new residential suburban enclaves began to be lined with gas stations, dry cleaners, shopping strips, motels, diners, drive-in theaters, supermarkets, banks, and myriad other commercial businesses with bold forms, imagery, colors, and neon signs all competing to capture the eye of the passing motorist, no differently than today. Architects jumped at these commissions, in the heart of the Great Depression. Roadside strip development stretched far into the once-rural countryside, soon to be filled in with subdivisions. The gas station was the earliest commercial vernacular roadside building type, having evolved from livery stables. While the gas station serviced a new wave of motorists, powered by cheap oil, prosperous grocery chains built supermarkets in strip centers surrounded by seas of pavement, and soon put their smaller competitors out of business.[16] In 1940, only 15 percent of the U.S. population resided in the suburbs. Seventy years later, more than 50 percent of the population was considered suburban.

*Landscape* magazine's editor, the enigmatic landscape theorist J.B. Jackson, published many seminal essays in the 1950s, giving new voice to the critical re-appraisal of this new wave of unselfconscious roadside architecture rapidly expanding along America's highways: Jackson celebrated this movement as a breath of fresh air, an antidote to the severe minimalism of the International Style. He referred to this type of building as an *other-directed architecture*.[17] The best architectural examples were cleverly composed and expressed evocative, often whimsical and highly iconic, memorable imagery (Figure 2.2). California personified the growth and evolution of this type of pre-World War II commercial vernacular architecture. The streets of Los Angeles in the period between the two world wars were once dotted with these diners, gas stations, supermarkets, and a wide assortment of inimitable commercial establishments, i.e. a piano store shaped as a piano, a camera store configured as a camera, a giant donut sitting atop the Donut Hole drive-in.[18] Seaside resorts such as Myrtle Beach, South Carolina, also flourished at this time as new within-driving-distance meccas for throngs of middle-class tourists who now could afford to own a car (Figure 2.3). This rising tourist class gave rise to ever more numerous diners and roadside attractions across the U.S. (Figures 2.4–2.6) including in and near to amusement arcades along the Atlantic Ocean (Figure 2.7). Little did the architect know at the time that he (very few women were architects at the time) was contributing to a coming national obesity and non-communicable disease epidemic.

Meanwhile, Le Corbusier's views on urbanism, within the strict confines of the International Style, would profoundly (if often inadvertently) influence suburbanization in industrialized Western countries. An advocacy arm of the movement, CIAM (Congress Internationaux d'Architecture Moderne), had been founded in Switzerland in 1928. It was an avant-garde association of architects who sought to advance both modernism and internationalism in architecture. CIAM was strongly influenced by the Bauhaus academy, in Dessau, Germany, widely considered a cradle of modernism and the International Style. The Bauhaus opened in 1919 and was shut down by Hitler in 1933. Meanwhile, CIAM saw itself as an elite group seeking to revolutionize architecture to better serve the interests of society. Its membership numbered in the hundreds, and included Le Corbusier, Walter

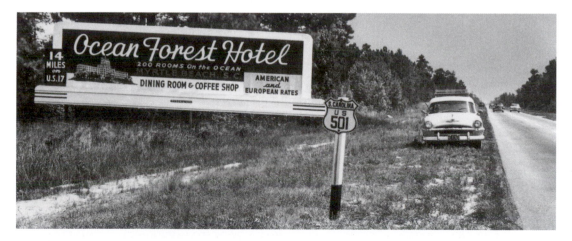

**FIGURE 2.2** Old South Carolina Highway 501, 1950s. Photo courtesy of the Jack Thompson Photographic Trust

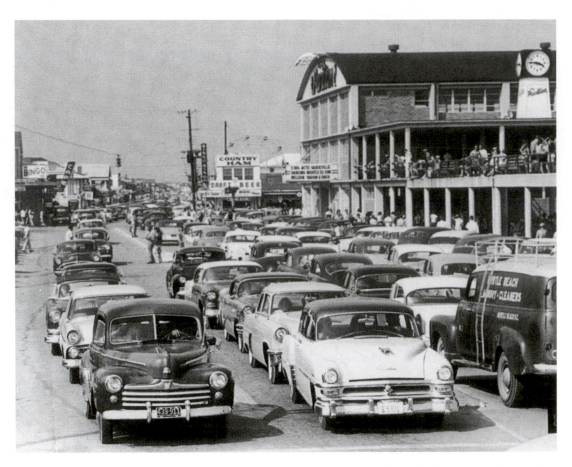

**FIGURE 2.3** Myrtle Beach, South Carolina, 1950s. Photo courtesy of the Jack Thompson Photographic Trust

Gropius, and Richard Neutra; the theories promoted at the Bauhaus, and the "Functional City" (1931–1939). CIAM sought to radically influence public policy and after World War II led to the creation of Team 10, which sought to somewhat temper CIAM's singular advocacy on behalf of the International Style, and did so in a more socially engaged manner. CIAM itself dissolved in 1959.[19] Le Corbusier's initial vision of the modern city-as-machine inspired the clearance of dense inner city slum neighborhoods in countless industrial cores. Concurrently, the collective civic memory of the inhabitants who had lived, worked, and worshiped in these lost neighborhoods was trampled. Place, and tradition, was devalued in the process. In retrospect, this period was a-historical, anti-pedestrian, auto-dependent, ungrounded in health-promoting precepts, all deficiencies to later incite the ire of the great 20th-century urbanists Lewis Mumford, and Jane Jacobs, who stridently called for reinvigorated, vibrant urban neighborhoods and street life.

## 3. Post-War Sprawl Machines (1946–1975)

With populations between 50,000 and 80,000, the largest post-World War II suburbs looked and felt like overblown subdivisions. In Levittown, New York, begun in 1946, model homes on generic streets housed homogenous sedentary populations whose lifestyles were reflected in national TV sitcoms. The 1956 Interstate Highway Act led to the construction by 1980 of 42,500 miles of a "National System of Interstate and Defense Highways" across the country at an estimated cost of $27 billion. In fact, there was no real concern for defense because the highway engineers never actually consulted with the military. In the mid-1950s, a new term, *Googie Architecture*, was coined to capture the wave of "space age ultramodern" roadside commercial vernacular.[20] By 1970, more and more Americans lived in the suburbs than in either central cities or rural areas. Architects contributed much to roadside vernacular architecture and the coming fast food epidemic, i.e. the prototype McDonald's drive-in in 1955 in Des Plaines, Illinois, but they never got a handle on sprawl itself. Nor did architects acknowledge the profoundly adverse public health outcomes that the food served from these buildings spawned. The landmark 1972 book, *Learning from Las Vegas*, documented the messy, unorthodox, "vital" strip iconography and aesthetic language of the Las Vegas strip, without any mention of any of this.[21]

The mid-1950s marked the opening of the first two shopping centers anchored by branches of downtown department stores: Northgate, in Seattle, Washington, and Shoppers World, in Framingham, Massachusetts. This concept was refined further in Victor Gruen's Northland Center (1954) in Detroit, Michigan, with its cluster layout with a single anchor at the center, ringed by smaller stores and a parking lot completely surrounding the mall. In 1956, Gruen's Southdale Center, in Edina, Minnesota, was the world's first modern, completely enclosed multi-level regional mall. People drove there, reverted to pedestrians, if only temporarily, and then returned to their car and drove home.

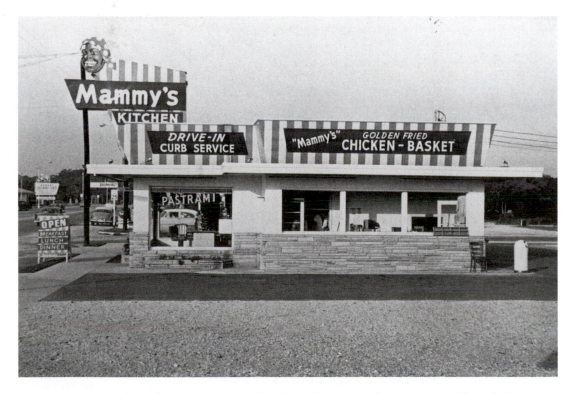

**FIGURE 2.4**  Mammy's Kitchen, Myrtle Beach, South Carolina, 1957. Photo courtesy of the Jack Thompson Photographic Trust

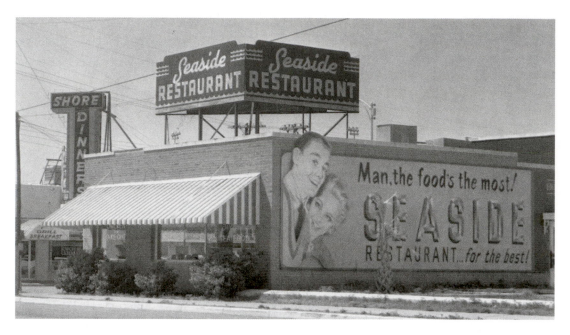

**FIGURE 2.5** Seaside Restaurant, Myrtle Beach, South Carolina, 1957. Photo courtesy of the Jack Thompson Photographic Trust

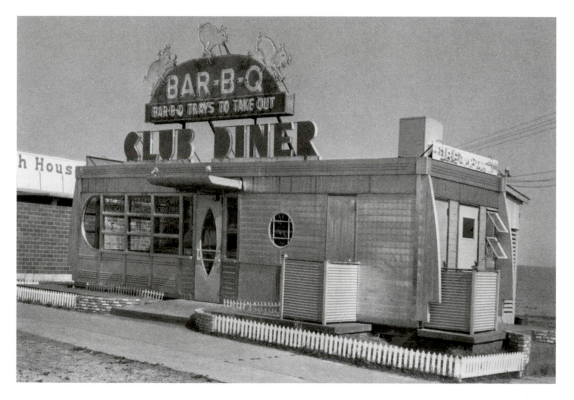

**FIGURE 2.6** Bar–B-Q Club Diner, Myrtle Beach, South Carolina, 1955. Photo Courtesy of the Jack Thompson Photographic Trust

In the 1950s, Victor Gruen and his followers passionately promoted the enclosed mall "shopping town."[22] Prior to this, malls were a risk because shoppers preferred to shop downtown in stores they knew and trusted. Born in Vienna in 1903, Gruen had fled to the U.S. from Nazi domination in 1938. By the mid–1950s he was firmly ensconced as the nation's preeminent mall architect. Gruen's Northland Center attracted more than 100,000 to its opening in 1954 and garnered praise in *Architectural Forum* magazine.[23] His avowed goal was to achieve a setting for informal human interaction in a safe, quasi–hermetic environment.[24] His malls turned inward, rejecting the indeterminacy and messiness of everyday urban life. In his words, cities "had permitted anarchy and ugliness to take over to such as degree that good architecture has no place to express itself." "We architects," he wrote, "have followed the merchants and commuters" to become "suburbanites and exurbanites." The enclosed mall was to be an idealized "middle ground" between city and country, between public and private realms.[25]

In 1962, Gruen's Randhurst Mall in suburban Chicago opened, complete with benches, and the first mall-based fast food court.[26] His malls pioneered the concept of multiple public entrances, to minimize needless walking.[27] As tax laws became ever more favorable to developers, they built malls at the intersections of major roadways.[28] The first U.S. Clean Air Act was enacted in 1963. By 1964 there were 7,600 shopping centers in the U.S.; most were strip centers serving nearby subdivisions while population growth fueled the thirst for more and bigger malls. By 1972, the number of strip centers and malls totaled 13,174. Regional mixed-use enclosed malls such as The Galleria (1974), in Houston, Texas, were built, setting a new standard for amenities, with interconnected hotels, office

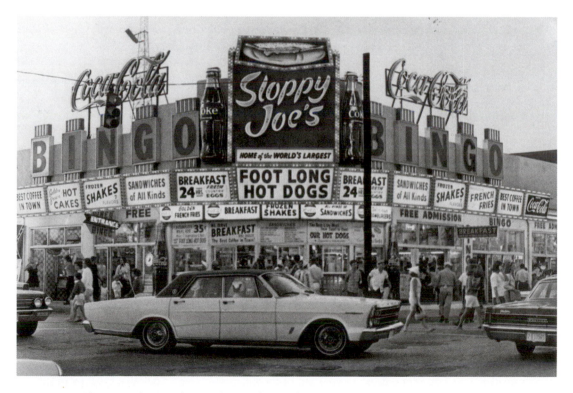

**FIGURE 2.7**   Sloppy Joe's, Myrtle Beach, South Carolina, 1965. Photo courtesy of the Jack Thompson Photographic Trust

towers, food court, and an ice skating rink. It was an immediate hit with local architects and with the public. Any health-related consequences of Houston's growing sedetarianism and extreme auto dependency remained unlinked with the city's mall-centered culture. The Galleria quickly became one of Houston's major tourist attractions.

Meanwhile, in 1955, Walt Disney had opened Disneyland, in Anaheim, California. Its spectacular success inspired Disney to plan his futuristic Experimental Prototype Community of Tomorrow, or EPCOT. EPCOT was to be a top-down and completely pre-planned utopian-cum-suburban community where everything was controlled, and all automobiles would be restricted to below-ground roadways. The horizontal surface plane would be devoted to pedestrians, trams, and people movers. It was to be radial in plan, inspired by his reading of Ebenezer Howard's *Garden Cities of To-Morrow*. It was to feature residential pods, a green belt for parks and recreational amenities, and high-density apartments for 20,000 inhabitants located at the periphery of the radial. There would be no private land ownership. EPCOT was to be increasingly decentralized further out from a dense urban-business core in the center of the radial. Apartments would be above the stores. Disney proclaimed the "pedestrian as king" and the original plan was for the entire EPCOT central business district (CBD) to be weather-enclosed, not unlike one of Gruen's recent regional shopping mall antecedents. Each family in EPCOT would have its own golf cart to drive around on the horizontal "habitability plane". There were to be no "slums" because there would be no crime allowed. Disney presented his fantastical, modernistic concept in a 1966 promotional film but died before it could be built as he had envisioned. Instead, his brother, Roy Disney, carried forward with the planning and a much-changed version of it opened in 1982 as a part of Walt Disney World, in Orlando, Florida. On part of the land originally intended for EPCOT, Celebration, Florida would be built some twenty years later. Celebration was laid out and its architecture designed according to New Urbanist precepts, in a near-total rejection of Disney's futuristic vision of EPCOT.

## 4. The Rise of the Megamall (1975–2000)

The shopping mall developers of the late 20th century were major beneficiaries of massive U.S. federal highway construction programs, commercial real estate tax subsidies, and local politicians' favors. Between 1955 and 1980, more than 22,000 suburban malls were built in America. The amount of land consumed by sprawl had increased exponentially by 1980, and this would grow by one-half again by 2000. Enclosed regional shopping malls ruled the day.[29] They were widely seen as mini-cities within the city, supposedly autonomous from racial and social inequities—protected civic safe houses. The more an aura of unreality was achieved the better: it was all highly calculated—an immersive experience.[30] By 1978, however, even Gruen himself voiced his disgust with the extent his utopian ideal had been bastardized and watered down by a generation of greed-obsessed developers blind to the perilous downsides of mass auto-dependency:

> What has happened to the shopping center itself in the twenty years since the pioneer centers opened?. . .the concept has been spread all over the world, but at the same time a tragic down-grading of quality has occurred. . .the environmental and humane ideals expressed in the original centers were not improved upon—they were completely forgotten. . .they have become a disastrous expression of mono-function. . .specialized ghettos have been built following the spread of Le Corbusier's ideas as expressed in the *Charter of Athens* and have resulted in serious malaise in many conurbations. The shopping center is an extreme, but by no means the only, example of substituting an artificial and therefore sterile order for naturally developed blends of

urban form. . .the public has woken to the dangers. . .among the reasons for growing concern are increasing air pollution, loss of landscape quality, loss of small local shops [downtown]—and the rising cost of car ownership. . .It is my personal view that the shopping center in its conventional form has no future at all. . .unmistakable signs of its downfall are already recognizable and will express themselves increasingly with every year that passes.[31]

Gruen had only promoted walking *within* his malls—but not to or from them. Yet the privately owned car had become the only fully socially acceptable mode of transport to and from the post-World War II American *megamall*. In 1962, in a small town in Arkansas, Sam Walton opened his first department store, Wal-Mart, with little fanfare. By the late 1990s there were 43,000 strip malls and shopping malls, including hundreds of immense, multi-level megamalls.[32] By 2000, Americans had constructed almost twice as much retail space per citizen than any other nation—more than 19 square feet per person, and nearly all of it was in malls. The Mall of America, in Bloomington, Minnesota (1992), personified the megamall as a retailing behemoth. It housed four massive anchors, 520 infill stores, fifty-one restaurants, eight nightclubs, and an amusement park. With 42.5 million visitors in its first year it became the region's most popular tourist draw.[33]

Megamalls in the U.S. were highly market-driven. In Newark, New Jersey, for instance, every one of its major stores abandoned the CBD for the suburbs between 1964 and 1992. Diverse social and ethic groups were no longer integrated in the CBD, having scattered to niche suburban markets, often geographically far from one another.[34] Because the malls and megamalls were owned by private corporations, growing concern soon emerged over the privatization of once-public urban space. To critics, it was anti-democratic.[35] Hospitals and related healthcare providers, for example, had migrated to suburbia *en masse* from central cities. After 1983, federal changes in U.S. healthcare policy forced a shift from hospital-based to outpatient services now housed in freestanding roadside strip centers and enclosed malls—signifying the *functional deconstruction* of the formerly highly centralized hospital.[36] Thousands of nondescript doc-in-a-box surgicenters were installed in strip malls right next door to the ubiquitous Chinese restaurant, coin-op laundermat, shoe repair shop, and Subway outlet. They cater more and more to aging suburbanites with their presence implying that if the mall itself was not dying, its clientele soon would—these sedentary patients had no option but to drive to and from these places because of the distance factor combined with the fact that sidewalks, bike lanes, and public transport options were usually nonexistent.

Architects who worked within these sprawl contexts were inadvertently dismissing the potential of natural landscape ecologies, community-based public health priorities, and their potential impact on both.[37] This differed little from the relationship of architects to sprawl, relative to public health, from back in the 1920s and 1930s. The more things changed the more they had stayed the same in this regard. Suburban architecture, from a contextual standpoint at least, was now all about accommodating the car, not pedestrians or cyclists. It was all about achieving maximum visibility for the passing motorist.[38] Legions of anonymous architects worked silently (and profitably) on their plentiful mall and roadside strip center commissions.

At this same time, postmodernism began to challenge the fifty-plus year reign of modernism and the International Style. A few daring firms, such as the iconoclastic firm SITE, critiqued the suburban milieu and the questionable underpinnings of American mass consumerism. SITE, founded in New York in 1970, at first aligned itself with a loosely defined group that included Hans Hollein, Emilo Ambasz, Ettore Sottsass, Archigram, Haus Rucker, Archizoom, and Superstudio. SITE's work questioned modernism, post-war sprawl, and the ambiguity between art and architecture in popular culture.[39] The firm designed a series of eight showrooms for BEST Products. SITE's clients sought to inject art into the everyday suburban milieu. SITE's big box retail outlets for BEST Products were infused with ironic, at times subversive, narratives critiquing their banal highway strip contexts. Disjunctive elements were fused with unorthodox, crumbling, twisting, dematerialized apertures, i.e. the Rainforest Showroom, in Florida (1979), via opaqueness and transparency, intentionally blurring the aforementioned disjunctions that existed in sprawl architecture between building and landscape.

The Indeterminate Façade (1975), also for BEST Products, was built in Houston as a semi-ruin, its façade in a relative state of advanced "decay" (Figure 2.8), a pessimistic statement on over-the-top American consumer culture. SITE's Notch Project (1977), also for BEST, was built in Sacramento, California. As in the Houston showroom, the generic aperture remained unaltered. However, unlike its predecessor the main entrance was a large, raw-edged gap that appears to have been ripped away from its generic box/aperture (Figure 2.9). This remnant itself becomes a sculptural element. The Tilt Showroom (1978), also for BEST, in Towson, Maryland, challenged formal disequilibrium as the generic box was here altered by a randomly displaced façade-plane appearing to be in a state of being pulled up away from its base in a direct challenge to the International Style's obsessive form follows function dictum, in this case its function is revealed by its "shop-lifted" façade (Figure 2.10).

SITE's Ghost Parking Lot (1978), in Hamden, Connecticut, was created for a national shopping center developer. It inverted conventions between the automobile and the ground, reappraising each within a single frame of reference. The paved ground plane critiques Americans' obsession with their cars by transforming them into grave-like, silhouetted artifacts. This outdoor civic art installation simultaneously critiqued suburban strip culture (Figure 2.11). SITE's prescient Forest Park project in Richmond, Virginia (1980), questioned fundamental precepts of sprawl machines and their relationship to landscape ecological health.[40]

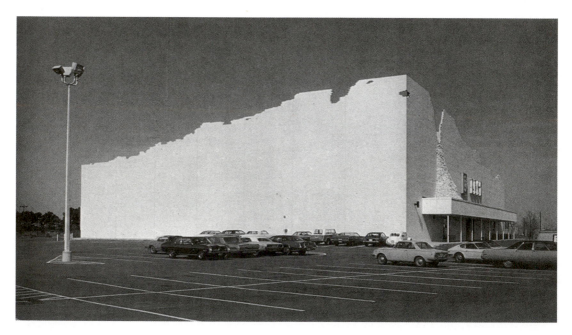

**FIGURE 2.8** SITE—Indeterminate Façade, Best Products, Houston. Photo courtesy of SITE—Architecture, Art & Design

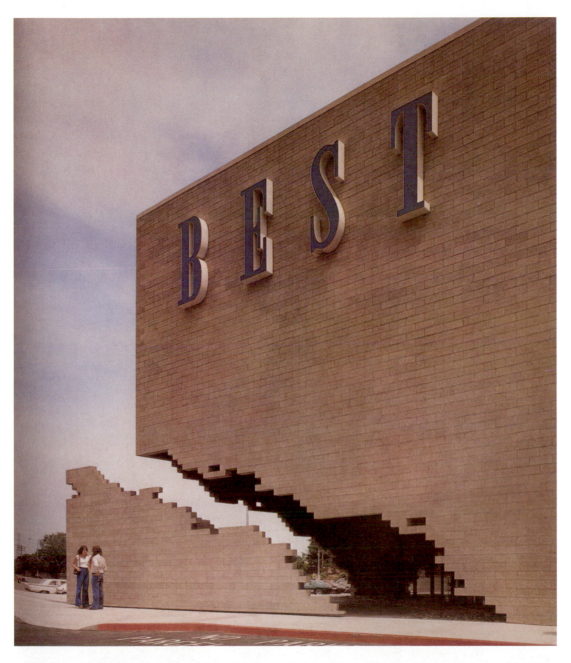

**FIGURE 2.9** SITE—Notch Project, Best Products, Sacramento, California. Photo courtesy of SITE—Architecture, Art & Design

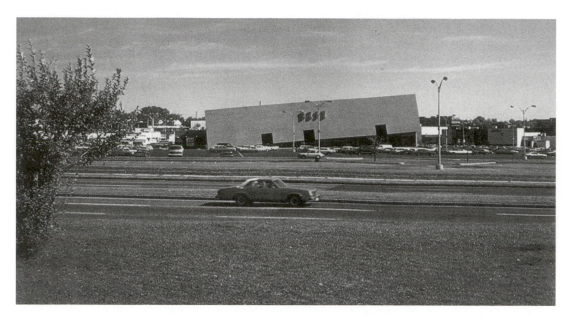

**FIGURE 2.10** SITE—Tilt Showroom, Best Products, Towson, Maryland. Photo courtesy of SITE—Architecture, Art & Design

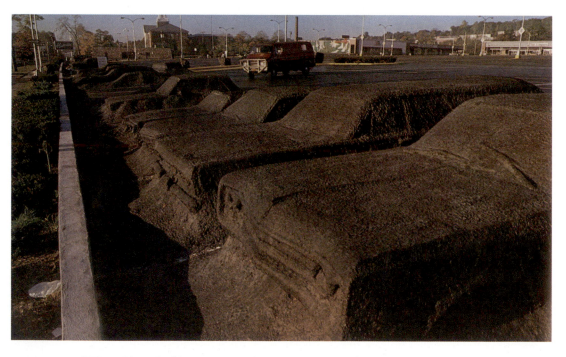

**FIGURE 2.11** SITE—Ghost Parking Lot, Hamden, Connecticut. Photo courtesy of SITE—Architecture, Art & Design

By 1990, the *malling* of America had reached a saturation point. Large malls were being built on the new suburban fringe—*exurbia*.[41] But it soon became clear that the megamall would experience a limited shelf life.[42] A cut-rate discount retail category was soon created whose express purpose was to put the regional megamall out of business—the big box store. Massive discount stores of 50,000–200,000 square feet would undercut the older generation of enclosed malls that once constituted the very heart of the sprawl machine. The rise of the largest of the big box global conglomerates, Wal-Mart, resulted in the downfall of long-established small businesses within any local community in which it operated. By 1999, Wal-Mart already had 900,000 employees in the U.S. alone. Other so-called "category killers" Toys-R-Us, Pet Smart, AutoZone, Staples, and Home Depot soon sought their own version of total niche domination. Wal-Mart's entry into a local market was the death knell for thousands of Main Street shopping districts across America. Architecturally disconnected from local vernacular precedents, or public health, Wal-Mart and other one-stop mega-box stores were soon clustered together in *power centers*.[43] Defenders of these global conglomerates argue that the public merely got what it asked for—rock-bottom prices of large quantities of nearly 100 percent Chinese-made goods.

In 1995, Bank of America Corporation commissioned its own report on sprawl, focusing soley on California. This report pronounced urban jobs to have decentralized to the suburbs, deep into agriculturally and environmentally sensitive areas as private auto use continued to rise, abated. The acceleration of sprawl had resulted in enormous cost burdens, as businesses suffered from higher infrastructural expenses, loss in worker productivity, and a corresponding disinvestment in older inner urban neighborhoods.[44] Sprawl and its consequences were by now an international concern and its dark side was being publicly revealed on a widespread basis.[45]

By 2010, America's malls and strip centers were overbuilt by one-third and the real estate interests who brokered on behalf of this industry were in a free fall.[46] Intense competition from lower-priced competitors such as Target and Wal-Mart were putting thousands of old-school regional megamalls on the ropes or out of business. Worse, home TV-based shopping channels and the Internet drew many younger consumers away from brick-and-mortar stores.[47] Bankruptcies and mergers ensued.[48] Dead and dying malls no longer served the targeted demographic niches they had been built to serve. As their customers leapfrogged further and further out towards exurbia and to edge cities beyond, older malls and strip centers were abandoned, left to wither and die. A "geography of nowhere" had been exacted with great precision across the American landscape.[49] Excess retail capacity resulted in thousands of *dead malls*.[50] These became the butt of jokes, such as the article "Ten clues your mall may be dying."[51] An Internet site, deadmalls.com, documented each one with photos and nostalgic narratives. The fact that only three enclosed malls were built in the ten-year period 2000–2010 in the U.S. proved that they had become dinosaurs. The City of Denver, as but one example, was forced to redevelop eight of its twelve dead or dying regional enclosed megamalls.[52] Dead and dying megamalls became symbols of a culture of rot brought on by stockholder-driven hypercapitalism and consumerism run amok. Not surprisingly, old school developers were at a loss as to how to cope with the new reality.[53] By 2010, big box power centers were also being shuttered by the hundreds. Architects were challenged by clients to find fiscally viable (and for the first time) more genuinely ecological, sustainable new uses for these abandoned carcasses.[54]

Mainstream architects in the U.S. turned to the New Urbanism. In the wake of the demise of many enclosed malls and power centers, open-air *lifestyles centers* were their response to the need for a new "product" type—really no more than old regional malls repackaged in new garb—as a supposedly more walkable and therefore more health-promoting alternative. They are mixed-use developments with residential, housing, office, and commercial functions, featuring multiplex cinemas, upscale restaurants, and greenspace "town squares." The lifestyle center excises the automobile from open plain sight (by hiding them in carparks underground or on roof decks). These places, inspired by a faux anti-suburbanist sentiment, are arranged as urban street grids. Their developers wish for the consumer to think he or she is really walking in an old-school Main Street shopping district. They are highly ironic places because they are being built smack in the middle of sprawl and sprawl remains their lifeblood in nearly every case. It is an illusion, in the end, roughly a surreal 21st-century equivalent to the pretenses that surrounded Gruen's 1950s "suburban downtown social centers." Notable examples of mixed-use lifestyle centers in the Southern U.S. include Atlantic Station (2007), in Atlanta, and Perkins Mill (2009), in Baton Rouge, Louisiana. They are contradictory places, because lifestyle centers really do little themselves to directly promote healthier lifestyles. People still have to drive to and from them. They are merely islands within the status quo of sprawl machines where, in this era of post-peak oil, gas prices are predicted by many informed specialists to rise to $20 per gallon by 2020.[55]

## 5. Ecological Architecture and Urbanism (2001–present)

By 2000, America had become a suburban nation. Albeit, the downtowns still boasted prominent civic institutions and entertainment venues but at the same time they were hemorrhaging corporate headquarters. In the burbs, ineffective land use controls resulted in banal, ugly landscapes devoid of either collective cultural memory or a genuine sense of place. The New Urbanism movement had originated back in the 1980s with an alternative vision. Andres Duany and Elizabeth Plater-Zyberk, both based in Miami, designed the newtown plans for Seaside, Florida and the aforementioned Celebration, Florida. This was the start of their crusade to recapture lost late 19th-century traditional town planning values. They founded the Congress for the New Urbanism (CNU) in 1993. This organization would grow into a formidable voice in American architecture and urbanism.[56] It championed the brand of time-tested urbanism as professed by Jane Jacobs, Christopher Alexander, and Leon Krier.[57] The form-based codes published by the CNU and field-tested by Duany and Plater-Zyberk in their firm DPZ spelled out the prescription.[58] Sensing a void at the time, they did not consciously seek any type of affirmation from well-established North American academic centers of architectural and urban theory, i.e. the Ivy League university-level design and planning schools.[59] Not coincidentally, the built work of DPZ and its allies would in time fall prey to harsh critiques for its neo-19th-century ethos, for sidestepping the complexities and contradictions of 21st-century life, and for what its harshest critics see as an attempt to throw architectural and urban theory into historical reverse gear.

Pragmatic from the outset, the CNU and its allies fought to rewrite land use and building codes. The *Smart Code*, developed and disseminated by the CNU, is a form-based code that incorporates *Smart Growth* precepts; this document also provided a basis for a CNU 2002 report on how to transform dead malls into viable mixed-use communities.[60] In 2003, the U.S. National Endowment for the Arts, in consort with the CNU, published *Sprawl and Public Space: Redressing the Mall*, on methods to ameliorate the proliferation of dead malls.[61] In 2005, the CNU together with the U.S. Environmental Protection Agency published *Malls into Mainstreets*.[62] In that same year, the book *Sprawl Costs* documented the vast resources consumed by unmitigated sprawl machines in the United States.[63] By 2009, Version 9.2 of the Smart Code had been released.[64] It addressed urban and suburban development at all scales of design from regional planning to the scale of building signage. It was based on an integrated spatial continuum, referred to by New Urbanists as the *transect*. By 2009 more than 100 U.S. municipalities and counties had adopted the Smart Code, or a close variant.[65] Also by this time, as a footnote, fresh produce in the U.S. traveled on average 1,500 miles from field to store, and to a significant extent due to the collective efforts of the CNU, *transit-oriented development* was experiencing a minor revival in the U.S (TOD-2).

Meanwhile, an alternative paradigm—*landscape urbanism*—was emerging. Its near-singular aim was to directly challenge the New Urbanism and its pragmatic, government-aimed Smart Codes. It was also about challenging the CNU's avowed goals and methods for the amelioration of sprawl. By contrast, landscape architecture's recent renaissance has largely been attributable to its focus on an ecological urbanism. At the same time, concern was increasing among architects that they might no longer function as the primary orchestrators to anywhere near the extent they had in the past. An intellectual and professional turf war was in the making. As Gwen Webber observed, if the lead 9/11 Ground Zero design commission in New York City were to be awarded today, would Michael Van Valkenburgh be a more likely candidate than Daniel Libeskind? She argued the probability of this would be high. A recent surge in prestigious commissions going to and being completed with landscape architects in the lead role, versus architects, who would have otherwise been in the lead orchestrator role in the past, immediately fueled a passionate discourse within academia over how (and by whom) built environments will be shaped in the future. In the past, the architect had been the self-styled "master builder," with the landscape designer typically serving in a support role.[66] The tables were turning.

Recent examples of this power shift include the redevelopment of Seattle's waterfront by Field Operations, Van Valkenburgh Associates' (MVVA) reinvigoration of Eero Saarinen's iconic Gateway Arch in St. Louis, and GroundLab's urban fabric project for Shenzhen, China. Landscape urbanists such as Charles Waldheim, head of the landscape architecture program at the Harvard Graduate School of Design, refers to these projects and MVVA's Lower Don Lands Inner Harbor project in Toronto as at once blurring traditional disciplinary boundaries and correspondingly increasing the focus on ecological urbanism. The Museum of Modern Art's 2010 exhibit "Rising Currents" further underscored this power shift by challenging a cadre of invited architects to respond to environmental catastrophe in the museum's call for "soft infrastructures," ecological design responses, and the drawing together of transdisciplinary teams of architects and specialists in ecological design, i.e. water and waste specialists, and climatologists, to join forces with landscape designers and others.[67] Architects were suddenly under unprecedented scrutiny as having been too narrowly educated in building-only concerns, and not in beyond-the-building ecological concerns. Landscape urbanism had presented itself at precisely the right moment.

Lars Lerup's seminal 1995 "Stim & dross" essay, where he did not chastise sprawl in good or bad (pro/anti) terms but from an alternative, apolitical perspective, inspired many landscape theorists to take action.[68] Using Houston as a case study, Lerup theorized over its vast expanse of urbanized landscape surface as a *holey plane* (with the holes being voids in the urban plane), dotted by a canopy of trees, and a network of highways criss-crossed by humans and vehicles. This plane captured the daily/momentary struggle between commerce and nature. *Dross* was defined as waste, as discarded, residualized spaces, artifacts, and related expendable byproducts of this process. Eschewing neither pro- or anti-sprawl rhetoric, Lerup suspended judgment on the formal merits of a sprawl-based horizontal city; a valueless condition he argued would hold enormous potential for the future, when society "woke up to the full potential of *stim* and *dross*" as opposed to always trashing sprawl as bad.[69] Alan Berger more recently has further rationalized the virtues of sprawl-based *drosscapes*, and has extended landscape urbanism's opposition to widely held negativity towards sprawl per se. He argued, "Why not protect the pre-existent waterways and wildlife habitats that were there before humans arrived?" "Why not reuse stormwater runoff to irrigate nearby suburban agriculture?"[70]

In the 20th century, a select few architects' proposals, notably Frank Lloyd Wright's Broadacre City (1934–1935), Ludwig Hilberseimer's New Regional Pattern (1945–1949), and Andrea Branzi's

Agronica (1993–1994) and Territory for the New Economy (1999), had each embraced the virtues of *horizontalism* and the critical role of natural ecological systems in suburban life. These precursors expressed a decentralized dissolution of the urban figure-ground relationship, thereby reinterpreting (recasting) the classical distinction that had separated city and countryside, replacing it with a conflation of suburb and region—*suburbanized regionalism*. Given the current reawakening of interest in urban agriculture (in some ways itself a reprise of the pre-industrial city, where urban dwellers could raise livestock in their sideyards, for instance), these propositions proffer a compelling reinterpretation of 21st century sprawl and its unhealthful byproducts.[71] Landscape urbanism views the horizontal plane and its residualized, even dead, parcels as potentially more ecologically productive, i.e. healing, than the mere insertion of conventional object–infill buildings could ever achieve in either suburban or inner urban contexts.[72] At the same time, architecture must remain a part of this reappraisal. For instance, roofscaping and vertical gardening are two architecturally based interventions of great interest both within the architectural avant-garde and also within ecological urbanism.[73]

Landscape urbanists attacked the both New Urbanism and the mainstream architectural profession as being frightfully and dangerously stuck on object-making. They also attacked mainstream urban planners, for having withdrawn from physical planning to focus instead on their obscure statistical analyses and reports versus any genuine focus on physical planning.[74] Now, the core dilemma for the traditionally trained architect was that of sole authorship, a condition perhaps better characterized as the dilemma of "autobiographical building." In sharp contrast, at the heart of the landscape urbanism agenda was the consensus that the core component of town planning and design is not the arrangement of any buildings, but the pre-existent natural landscape ecologies that predated when any and every single building was built. The site (with or without buildings) is viewed as a living ecosystem.[75] The challenge from here on out would appear to be the issue of how to equitably and ethically share credit, with the architect ceding sole authorship.[76]

The New Urbanists fought back by countering that landscape urbanism is an extreme school of thought that calls for the primacy of landscape and natural ecosystems at the expense of any and all conventional principles of town planning and design.[77] At the Harvard Graduate School of Design's 50th Anniversary Conference, held in November 2010, "Territories of Urbanism: Urban Design at 50," this intellectual turf war between the two camps erupted openly, turning into a very public and at times vitriolic debate.[78] Some months prior, the trenchant Duany had attacked the burgeoning academic discipline of landscape ecology in an essay published in *Metropolis* magazine.[79] In early 2011, Duany published a follow-up essay in *Metropolis*.[80] Duany's strongest point in his defense of the New Urbanism and the work of the CNU since 1993 centered on their actual built case studies (versus the largely unbuilt projects of the landscape urbanists). Second, Duany reminded his readership of how the CNU had pioneered the revelation of the failures of suburbia to a national and international audience. Third, he argued how the work of the CNU had directly extended and amplified the global healthy communities movement in public health, through the CNU's rejection of sprawl and the highly sedentary lifestyles it fosters, namely, obesity, and an array of attendant non-communicable diseases.[81] The CNU had aligned itself with the U.S. Centers for Disease Control and Prevention (CDC) a few years before, and with leading national public health specialists; in a joint call for the amelioration of the deleterious health outcomes resulting from sprawl, i.e. *bike share networks*. Non-New Urbanist architects, for their part, largely remained focused on having their buildings certified as LEED (Leadership through Energy-Efficient Environmental Design), which by 2011 had become global with 7,000 in-pipeline or built LEED projects in thirty countries.

Meanwhile, in 2003, the *American Journal of Public Health* and the *American Journal of Health Promotion* had each devoted special issues to the by-now hot topic of public health and the built environment.

Entire conferences were being devoted to this theme, and private philanthropic enterprises including the Robert Wood Johnson Foundation (RWJ) joined in by providing substantial start-up grant funding. In one published study, on the effects of urban sprawl on obesity rates between 1970 and 2000 in the U.S. (as a function of the expansion of the U.S. Interstate Highway System), a negative association was detected between population density and obesity. Restated, the decline in population density over this thirty-year period had resulted in a 13 percent increase in obesity rates, as measured by body-mass index (BMI) data among the residents of the communities examined.[82]

At this writing, landscape urbanists have achieved little to no formal link with the public health or healthcare design community (save for a presentation made in July 2011 in Boston at the Design & Health international conference. It was done in a way somewhat similar to what the CNU had done only a few years earlier). But any in-depth ventures that seek to join landscape urbanism and public health remain opaque, and it remained to be seen whether landscape urbanists would join in the call for compactness, alternatives to auto-dependency, and the healthful benefits of walkable, bike-friendly landscapes and communities. It also remained to be seen if ecological urbanism and existing federal government initiatives such as the CDC's Active Living Environments research program, its extensive online database (www.cdc.org/gov), or the promising discipline of *biophilia* would contribute to any extent to heightening physical activity levels outdoors in the everyday built environment. At the same time, additional published empirical studies, and especially those with a focus on suburban children and adolescents, continue to link sprawl to obesity and to numerous associated unhealthful outcomes.[83]

## 6. Ecological Architecture and Community-Based Public Health

Citizens expect and deserve the very best effort from those who plan and design the built environment. James Wines, founder of SITE, refers to the 21st century as the *Age of Ecology*, an era where architectural monument building is coming to a close and with it ends the architect's position of professional and intellectual primacy.[84] Wines has stated, "Architects who want to build a sculpture in the middle of physical space (apparently) live in an antiquated world of endless resources."[85] SITE's projects foreshadowed the regenerative possibilities of *architectural ecologies* far more than any mere act of object making could achieve. This broadened perspective of built form and nature will be essential in redefining the architectural discipline and profession to combat the deleterious health consequences of sprawl machines. Meanwhile, in a single year (2009), shopping mall owners in the U.S. lost a whopping 7.4 million square feet of paying tenants.[86] The economic turbulence that ransacked the global economy in 2008 offers a rare window of opportunity to reset the conventions of consumer culture as we now know it—to re-tool market capitalism into a greener, more socially conscious and, crucially, into a more profoundly personally satisfying proposition in everyday life.[87] The chronology of landmark events discussed in this chapter is re-presented here at the chapter's conclusion in a timeline-graphic (Figure 2.12), with the goal, is it hoped, to advance transdisciplinarianism in making the built environment a healthier place.

Designers, planners, and healthcare providers globally are increasingly being confronted with challenges with no immediate clear solutions, nor which neatly correspond to the usual traditional disciplinary parameters. More than ever, in the age of globalism (and growing anti-globalism), professionals must be able to see the bigger picture. The myriad challenges that lie ahead include pre- and post-disaster planning, the remediation of post-industrial landscapes and dying sprawl machines, adroit responses to public health epidemics and global pandemics, coping with water shortages and rising oceans due to global climate change, and coping with the innumerable other as

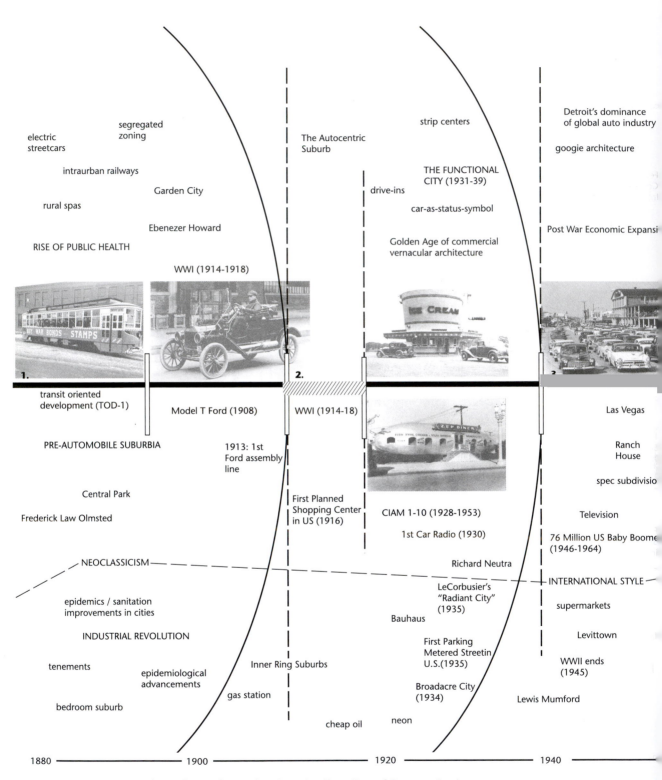

electric
streetcars

segregated
zoning

intraurban railways

Garden City

rural spas

Ebenezer Howard

RISE OF PUBLIC HEALTH

WWI (1914-1918)

The Autocentric
Suburb

drive-ins

strip centers

THE FUNCTIONAL
CITY (1931-39)

car-as-status-symbol

Golden Age of commercial
vernacular architecture

Detroit's dominance
of global auto industry

googie architecture

Post War Economic Expansi

**1.**

transit oriented
development (TOD-1)

Model T Ford (1908)

**2.**

WWI (1914-18)

Las Vegas

PRE-AUTOMOBILE SUBURBIA

1913: 1st
Ford assembly
line

Ranch
House

spec subdivisio

Central Park

Frederick Law Olmsted

First Planned
Shopping Center
in US (1916)

CIAM 1-10 (1928-1953)

1st Car Radio (1930)

Television

76 Million US Baby Boome
(1946-1964)

NEOCLASSICISM

Richard Neutra

INTERNATIONAL STYLE

epidemics / sanitation
improvements in cities

INDUSTRIAL REVOLUTION

tenements

epidemiological
advancements

bedroom suburb

LeCorbusier's
"Radiant City"
(1935)

Bauhaus

First Parking
Metered Streetin
U.S.(1935)

Broadacre City
(1934)

Inner Ring Suburbs

gas station

cheap oil

neon

supermarkets

Levittown

WWII ends
(1945)

Lewis Mumford

1880        1900        1920        1940

**FIGURE 2.12**  Chronology of Sprawl in America/Post–Sprawl Prognostications

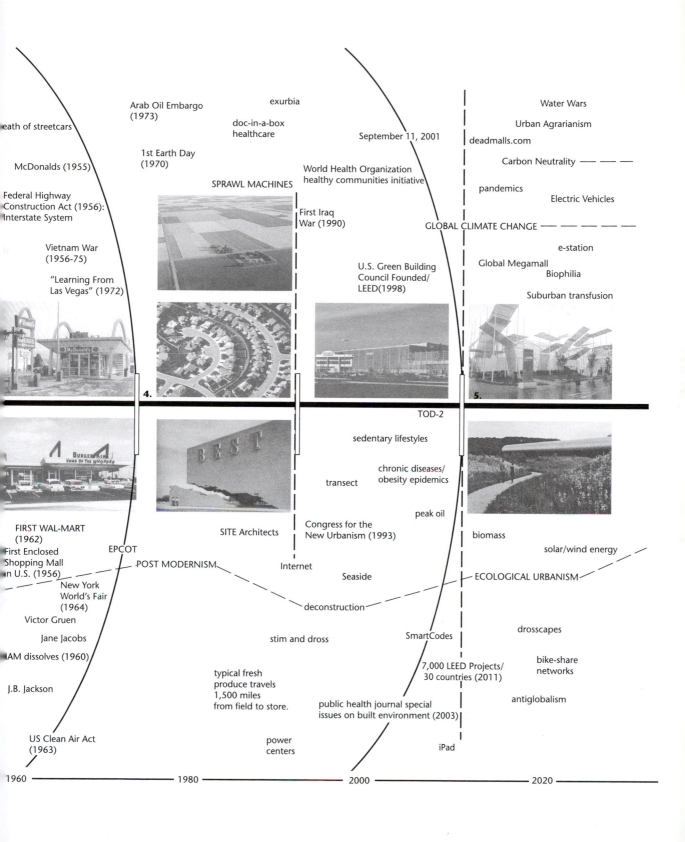

eath of streetcars

Arab Oil Embargo
(1973)

exurbia

Water Wars

Urban Agrarianism

doc-in-a-box
healthcare

September 11, 2001

deadmalls.com

McDonalds (1955)

1st Earth Day
(1970)

Carbon Neutrality — — —

Federal Highway
Construction Act
(1956):
Interstate System

SPRAWL MACHINES

World Health Organization
healthy communities initiative

pandemics

Electric Vehicles

First Iraq
War (1990)

GLOBAL CLIMATE CHANGE — — —

Vietnam War
(1956-75)

e-station

U.S. Green Building
Council Founded/
LEED(1998)

Global Megamall

Biophilia

"Learning From
Las Vegas" (1972)

Suburban transfusion

4.

5.

TOD-2

sedentary lifestyles

chronic diseases/
obesity epidemics

transect

FIRST WAL-MART
(1962)

First Enclosed
Shopping Mall
in U.S. (1956)

EPCOT

peak oil

SITE Architects

Congress for the
New Urbanism (1993)

biomass

POST MODERNISM

Internet

Seaside

ECOLOGICAL URBANISM

solar/wind energy

New York
World's Fair
(1964)

deconstruction

Victor Gruen

drosscapes

Jane Jacobs

stim and dross

SmartCodes

bike-share
networks

AM dissolves (1960)

typical fresh
produce travels
1,500 miles
from field to store.

7,000 LEED Projects/
30 countries (2011)

J.B. Jackson

antiglobalism

public health journal special
issues on built environment (2003)

US Clean Air Act
(1963)

power
centers

iPad

1960 —————————— 1980 —————————— 2000 —————————— 2020 ———

yet-unforeseen ramifications of global climate change at all scales in the built and natural environment. Architects, for their part, are justifiably concerned that landscape urbanism is out to supplant the traditional role of architecture as the focal point, and architects as the controlling orchestrators of what is built, why, and how. It also remains to be seen whether landscape urbanism is an open call for the mere continuance of suburbanization. The fields of community and epidemiological public health have, for their part, already awoken to the challenge. The actual attainment of their collective goal—healthier communities globally—remains in its infancy, however. Architects have long been responsible for the protection of the public's health and life safety at the scale of building-making. International and local building codes set forth stringent parameters to ensue that a building's anatomical systems function properly, provide full accessibility to the physically impaired, and are structurally sound and do not fail. This is not the issue. That's not what we're talking about. The profession—and discipline of architecture up to now has not fully awoken to the possibilities of ecological urbanism as expressed through an ecological architecture—transcending well-established instrumental life safety building code and accessibility responsibilities to achieve something much more.

## Notes

1 Le Corbusier (1935) *The Radiant City.* Trans. by Knight, Pamela, Levieux, Eleanor, and Coltman, Derek (1967). New York: Orion Press.
2 Egan, Timothy (2010) 'Slumburbia,' *The New York Times*, 10 February. Online. Available at www.opinionator.blogs.nytimes.com/2010/02/10/slumburbia?.html (accessed 12 February 2011).
3 Ibid., p. 3.
4 Leinberger, Christopher B. (2008) 'The next slum?' *The Atlantic*, March, pp. 44–51.
5 Verderber, Stephen (2003) 'Architecture for Health—2050: an international perspective,' *The Journal of Architecture*, 8(3): 281–302.
6 Hayden, Dolores (2004) *Building Suburbia: Green Fields and Urban Growth, 1820–2000.* New York: Vintage Books.
7 Farrelly, Elizabeth (2008) *Blubberland: The Dangers of Happiness.* Cambridge, MA and London: MIT Press.
8 Walters, David (2007) *Designing Community: Charrettes, Masterplans and Form-Based Codes.* Oxford, UK: Elsevier.
9 Howard, Ebenezer (1946 edition) *Garden Cities of To-Morrow.* London: Faber & Faber Ltd.
10 DeForest, Robert and Veiller, Lawrence (1903) *The Tenement House Problem: Report of the New York State Tenement House Commission of 1900.* Volume 1 (of 2 volumes). New York: Macmillan.
11 Hayden, *Building Suburbia*, p. 12.
12 Weiss, Marc (1987) *The Rise of the Community Builders: The American Real Estate Industry and Urban Land Planning.* New York: Columbia University Press.
13 Thomas, Bruce (2010) 'Nature and the city in 1920s America.' In Ballantyne, Andrew, ed., *Rural and Urban: Between Two Cultures.* London and New York: Routledge, pp. 134–144.
14 McKeever, J. Ross and Griffin, Nathaniel M. (1977) *Shopping Center Development Handbook.* Washington: Urban Land Institute.
15 Hayden *Building Suburbia*, pp. 92–97.
16 Longstreth, Richard (1999) *The Drive-in, the Supermarket, and the Transformation of Commercial Space in Los Angeles, 1914–1941.* Cambridge, MA, and London: MIT Press.
17 Horowitz, Helen L. (1998) 'J.B. Jackson as a critic of modern architecture,' *The Geographical Review*, 88(4): 465–473.
18 Heinmann, Jim (1985) *California Crazy and Beyond: Roadside Vernacular Architecture.* San Francisco: Chronicle Books. Also Liebs, Chester (1995) *Main Street to Miracle Mile.* Baltimore, MD: Johns Hopkins Press.
19 Mumford, Eric (2000) *The CIAM Discourse on Urbanism, 1928–1960.* Cambridge, MA: MIT Press.
20 Hess, Alan (2007) *Googie Redux: Ultramodern Roadside Architecture.* San Francisco: Chronicle Books.
21 Venturi, Robert, Scott Brown, Denise, and Izenour, Steven (1972) *Learning from Las Vegas.* Cambridge: MIT Press.

22 Gruen, Victor and Smith, Larry (1960) *Shopping Towns USA: The Planning of Shopping Centers*. New York: Reinhold.

23 Anon. (1954) 'Northland: A new yardstick for shopping center planning,' *Architectural Forum*, 10 (6): 102–119.

24 Gruen, Victor (1973) *Centers for the Urban Environment: Survival of the Cities*. New York: Reinhold.

25 Marx, Leo (1964) *The Machine and the Garden: Technology and the Pastoral Ideal in America*. New York and London: Oxford University Press.

26 Gillette, Howard, Jr. (1985) 'The evolution of the planned shopping center in suburb and city,' *APA Journal*, Autumn: 449–460.

27 Hardwick, M. Jeffrey (2004) *Mall Maker: Victor Gruen, Architect of an American Dream*. Philadelphia: University of Pennsylvania Press.

28 Hayden, *Building Suburbia*, p. 170. Also see Gottdiener, Mark (1977) *Planned Sprawl: Private and Public Interests in Suburbia*. Beverly Hills, CA: Sage.

29 Carlson, Harold J. (1991) 'The role of the shopping center in U.S. retailing,' *International Journal of Retail & Distribution Management*, 19(6): 47–60.

30 Cohen, Nancy E. (2002) *America's Marketplace: The History of Shopping Centers*. Lyme, CT: Greenwich Publishing Group.

31 Gruen, Victor (1978) 'The sad story of shopping centres,' *Town and Country Planning*, 44(4): 22–24.

32 Hayden, *Building Suburbia*, p. 170.

33 Hayden, *Building Suburbia*, pp. 171–172.

34 Anon. (1983) 'Closing of last department store stirs debate on downtown Trenton,' *Star-Ledger*, 5 June, p. A6.

35 Cohen, Elizabeth (1996) 'From town center to shopping center: The reconfiguration of community marketplaces in postwar America,' *American Historical Review*, 44(6): 1050–1081.

36 Sloane, David C. and Sloane, Beverlie C. (2003) *Medicine Moves to the Mall*. Baltimore and London: Johns Hopkins University Press.

37 Osmundson, Theodore (1999) *Roof Gardens: History, Design and Construction*. New York and London: W.W. Norton & Company.

38 Lamprecht, Barbara (2009) *Richard Neutra*. 2nd edition. Berlin and New York: Taschen.

39 Wines, James (2000) *Green Architecture*. Berlin and Los Angeles: Taschen.

40 Restany, Pierre, Zevi, Bruno, and SITE (1980). *SITE: Architecture as Art*. New York: St. Martin's Press.

41 Kowinski, William S. (1985) *The Malling of America*. New York: William Morrow & Company.

42 Lowry, James R. (1997) 'The life cycle of shopping centers,' *Business Horizons*, 40(1): 77–86.

43 Spector, Robert (2005) *Category Killers: The Retail Revolution and Its Impact on Consumer Culture*. Boston, MA: Harvard Business School Press.

44 Bank of America (1995) *Beyond Sprawl: New Patterns of Growth to Fit the New California*. San Francisco: Bank of America.

45 Jackson, Kenneth T. (1996) 'All the world's a mall: reflections on the social and economic consequences of the American shopping center,' *The American Historical Review*, 101(4): 1111–1121.

46 Ritzer, George (2004) *The McDonaldization of Society*. Revised New Century edition. Thousand Oaks, CA: Pine Forge Press.

47 Lueg, Jason E., Ponder, Nicole, Beatty, Sharon, and Capella, Michael L. (2006) 'Teenagers' use of alternate shopping channels: A consumer socialization perspective,' *Journal of Retailing*, 82(2): 137–153. Also see Rotem-Mindali, Orit and Salomon, Ilan (2007) 'The impacts of e-retail on the choice of shopping trips and delivery: Some preliminary findings,' *Transportation Research Part A*, 41(2): 176–189.

48 Lowry, James R. (1997) 'The life cycle of shopping centers,' *Business Horizons*, January–February: 77–86.

49 Kunstler, James Howard (1996) *Home from Nowhere: Remaking Our Everyday World for the 21st Century*. New York: Simon & Schuster. He has often said that suburban sprawl has been the most misguided investment in the history of recorded civilization.

50 Dobuzinskis, Caroline (2010) 'Dead malls,' *Core 77*, July. Online. Available at www.core77.com/reactor/deadmalls.asp.html (accessed 12 August 2010). This article reviewed the Los Angeles Forum's 2010 Dead Malls Competition.

51 Stumpf, Michael (2010) 'Ten clues your mall may be dying,' *San Francisco Examiner*, 12 January. Online. Available at www.examiner.com/x-16603-Economic-Development-Examiner~y2010m1d12.html (accessed 8 August 2010).

52 Calder, Chad (2010) 'Old spaces, new faces,' *The Advocate*, 29 August: A1–A8.

53 The Jerde Partnership and Barr, Vilma (2004) *Building Type Basics for Retail and Mixed-Use Facilities*. New York: Wiley.

54 Christensen, Julia (2008) *Big Box Reuse*. Cambridge, MA: MIT Press.

55 Steiner, Christopher (2009) *$20 Per Gallon: How the Inevitable Rise in the Price of Gasoline Will Change Our Lives for the Better*. New York: Grand Central Publishing.

56 Duany, Andres, Plater-Zyberk, Elizabeth, and Speck, Jeff (2000) *Suburban Nation: The Rise of Sprawl and the Decline of the American Dream*. New York: North Point Press.

57 Jacobs, Jane (1961) *The Death and Life of Great American Cities*. New York: Random House. Also Alexander, Christopher et al. (1977) *A Pattern Language: Towns, Buildings, Construction*. New York: Oxford University Press. Also Krier, Leon (2009) *The Architecture of Community*. New York: Island Press.

58 Neyfakh, Leon (2011) 'Green building,' *The Boston Globe*, 30 January. Online. Available at www.boston. com/yourtown/cambridge/articles/2011/01/30/green-building/?page=4.html (accessed 12 February 2011).

59 Benyis, Janine M. (2002) *Biomimicry: Innovation Inspired by Nature*. New York: Perennial.

60 Sobel, Lee, Greenberg, Ellen, and Bodzin, Steven (2002) *Greyfields into Goldfields: Dead Malls Become Living Neighborhoods*. Washington: Congress for the New Urbanism.

61 Smiley, David, ed. (2003) *Sprawl and Public Space: Redressing the Mall*. Washington, D.C.: National Endowment for the Arts.

62 Congress for the New Urbanism (2005) *Malls into Mainstreets: An In-Depth Guide to Transforming Dead Malls into Communities*. Washington, D.C.: Congress for the New Urbanism.

63 Burchell, Robert W., Downs, Anthony, McCann, Barbara, and Mukherji, Sahan (2005) *Sprawl Costs: Economic Impacts of Unchecked Development*. Washington, D.C.: Island Press.

64 The Smart Code—Version 9.2. (2009) Gaithersburg, MD: *The Town Paper*. Online. Available at www. smartcodecentral.org.html (accessed 10 January 2010). Also see Morris, Marya, ed. (2009) *Smart Codes: Model Land-Use Regulations*. Chicago: American Planning Association.

65 These are: T-1 Natural Zone; T-2 Rural Zone; T-3 Sub-Urban Zone; T-4 General Urban Zone; T-5 Urban Center Zone; T-6 Urban Core; and T-7 Civic Zone.

66 Webber, Gwen (2011) 'Contested ground,' *The Architect's Newspaper*, 26 March. Online. Available at www. thearchitectsnewspaper.com.html (accessed 30 March 2011).

67 Bergdoll, Barry (2010) 'In the wake of rising currents: The activist exhibition,' *Log 20*, Fall: 8–15.

68 Lerup, Lars (1995) 'Stim & dross: Rethinking the metropolis,' *Assemblage*, 25(2): 88–97. Also see Allen, Stan and McQuade, Marc, eds. (2011) *Landform Building: Architecture's New Terrain*. Baden, Switzerland: Lars Müller Publishers.

69 Lerup, 'Stim & dross,' p. 91.

70 Berger, Alan (2006) *Drosscape: Wasting Land in Urban America*. New York: Princeton Architectural Press.

71 Waldheim, Charles (2010) 'Notes toward a history of agrarian urbanism,' *Places: Design Observer*, 4 November. Online. Available at www.places.designobserver.com/feature/notes-toward-a-history-of-agrarian-urbanism/15518/html (accessed 14 March 2011).

72 White, Mason (2010) 'The productive surface,' *Places: Design Observer*, 1 November. Online. Available at www.places.designobserver.com/feature/the-productive-surface/14998/html (accessed 12 March 2011).

73 Belson, Ken (2009) 'The rooftop garden climbs down a wall,' *The New York Times*, 18 November. Online. Available at www.ntimes.com/2009/11/19/business/energy-environment/19WALLS.html (accessed 21 June 2010). Also see Venkataraman, Bina (2008) 'Country, the city version: farms in the sky gain new interest,' *The New York Times*, 15 July. Online. Available at www.nytimes.com/2008/07/15/science/15farm. html (accessed 21 June 2010).

74 Webber, 'Contested ground,' p. 3.

75 Neyfakh, 'Green building,' p. 3.

76 Webber, 'Contested ground.' Also see Anon. (2010) 'Professional practice: Combating climate change with landscape architecture,' *American Society of Landscape Architects*. Online. Available at www.asla.org/ ContentDetail.aspx?id=21910 (accessed 20 July 2011).

77 Garreau, Joel (1991) *Edge City: Life on the New Frontier*. New York: Random House.

78 Sherman, Genevieve (2010) 'GSD Throwdown: Battle for the intellectual territory of a sustainable urbanism,' *UrbanOmnibus*, 17 November. Online. Available at www.urbanomnibus.net/2010/gsd-throwdown-battle-for-the-intellectual-territory-of-a-sustainable-urbanism/html (accessed 12 March 2011).

79 Duany, Andres (2010) 'Duany vs Harvard GSD,' *Point of View: Metropolis*, 3 November. Online. Available at www.metropolismag.com/pov/20101103/duany-vs-harvard-gsd.html (accessed 19 August 2011). Also see Kreiger, Alex (2010) 'Krieger to Duany,' *Point of View: Metropolis*, 8 November. Online. Available at www.metropolismag.com/pov/01101108/krieger-to-duany.html (accessed 19 August 2011).

80  Duany, Andres (2010) 'New Urbanism: The case for looking beyond style,' *Metropolis*, 14 April. Online. Available at www.metropolismag.com/story/20110414/new-urbanism-the-case-forlooking-beyond-style.html (accessed 21 April 2011).

81  Ibid., p. 4. Also see Michael Mehaffy's essay 'The landscape urbanism: Sprawl in a pretty green dress,' *Planetizen*, 4 October 2010. Online. Available at www.planetizen.com/node/46262.html (accessed 20 July 2011).

82  Zhao, Zhenxiang and Kaestner, Robert (2010) 'Effects of urban sprawl on obesity,' *Journal of Health Economics*, 29(6): 779–787.

83  Patnode, Carrie D., Lytle, Leslie A., Erickson, Darin J., Sirard, John R., Barr-Anderson, Daheia J., and Story, Mary (2011) 'Physical activity and sedentary activity patterns among children and adolescents: A latent class analysis approach,' *Journal of Physical Activity & Health*, 8(4): 457–467.

84  Wines, *Green Architecture*, pp. 226–237.

85  Webber, 'Contested ground,' p. 4.

86  Pein, Corey (2009) 'Mall-Aise,' *Santa Fe Reporter*, 21 April. Online. Available at www.sfreporter.com/santafe/article-4459-mall-aise.html (accessed 7 July 2010).

87  Dery, Mark (2009) 'Dawn of the dead mall,' *Places/The Design Observer*, 9 November. Online. Available at www.designobserver.com/changeobserver/entry.html (accessed 12 January 2010).

# 3

# GLOBAL SPRAWL MACHINES

We can't solve problems by using the same kind of thinking that created them.

*Albert Einstein*

For the first time in history, more people live in cities than in rural locations.[1] The number of cars on our plant has surpassed 1 billion. As developing nations become wealthier, the waistlines of their citizens are expanding. Rising levels of obesity and related chronic non-communicable diseases (NCDs) is indeed unfortunate news with respect to the healthcare budgets of nations. It is a trend that correlates with rising per capita levels of median income. A recent article in *The Lancet* reports obesity was already a worldwide phenomenon by 1980. By 2008, the "rich world" had itself expanded, geographically, bringing obesity to countries previously considered too poor, such as Brazil and South Africa, and previously thought outside the scope of this epidemic. During this period, the occurrence rate of obesity among men doubled to nearly 10 percent in these places. Congo is currently the "thinnest" country in the world, and Nauru, the heaviest.[2] The encroaching wave of Western fast food conglomerates is having an equally adverse effect on sprawling parts of Latin America, the Middle East, and Sub-Saharan Africa.

As of 2011, KFC, Inc. alone had built an estimated $3.4 billion empire, with its 3,000 fried chicken restaurant outlets earning in that year more revenue than its corporate parent's entire network of KFC, Pizza Hut, and Taco Bell outlets combined. In China, KFC, Inc. opens a new location every eighteen hours, and the food generally has far more calories than the locals are traditionally used to consuming in their daily diet.[3] Russia is similarly developing a desire for the suburban comforts of America and other wealthy countries in the West. A middle-class consumer culture there has arisen since the fall of communism in 1990. Gated communities on the edge of Moscow are named Linden Park and Greenfield, names straight out of America or the U.K., built in architectural styles that would be warmly received by any Western striver. Moscow has expanded to four times its "planned size" in the post-Soviet era. McDonalds and Starbuck outlets continue to proliferate, as well as *Amway*, that American bastion of living-room consumerism.[4]

Company towns used to be common in the West. The Cadburys and Rowntrees built them in England, as did William Hesketh Lever, founder of what is now Unilever. At their peak, the U.S. had more than 3,000 such places but they have long since disappeared. As so often occurs, what dies in the West survives and booms in the developing world. In Jamshedpur, India, the corporate headquarters of Tata Steel continues to outdo itself. Jamshedpur was founded at the turn of the 20th century to solve a practical problem. The resources needed to make steel—coal, iron ore, and running water—were stuck in the middle of an isolated forest. Jamsetji Tata, the founder of both the town and what became the Tata Group, dreamed of constructing an industrial jewel, with wide avenues, good schools, and sports facilities. Recently, the company expanded the town horizontally, and independent from what is generally viewed locally as an incompetent state government. Tata Steel now runs a newly-built 900-bed hospital and medical center on what was once farmland. Tata's Victorian vision lives on as it continues to acquire land and sprawl outward with low-density development.[5]

In India, many are curious when they hear cautionary tales from Westerners about the perils of unchecked urban growth. For the first forty years of independence, entrepreneurs in India were looked down upon. India had lost confidence in its ability to compete, so it opted for protectionist foreign polices. By the 1990s, when the government was nearly bankrupt, however, the technology sector advocated creating a new high tech sector. It has flourished since, yet has brought with it concomitant issues, i.e. unmitigated sprawl, air pollution, and environmental degradation. It appears that the "American Dream," for better or worse, has been imported to India.[6] For India's newly rich farmers, upward mobility pressures place strains on the status quo:

> Bhisham Singh Yadav, father of the groom, is stressed. His rented Lexus got stuck behind a bullock cart. He has hired a truck to blast Hindi pop, but it is too big to maneuver through the village. At least his grandest gesture, evidence of his upward mobility, is circling overhead. The helicopter has arrived. Mr. Yadav, a wheat farmer, has never flown, nor has anyone else in the family. And this will only be a short trip: delivering his son less than two miles to the village of the bride. But like many families in this expanding suburb of New Delhi, the Yadavs have come into money, and they want everyone to know it. . .they are members of a new economic caste in India: nouveau riche farmers. Land acquisition for expanding cities and industry is one of the most bitterly contentious issues in India, rife with corruption and violent protests. Yet in some areas it has created pockets of overnight wealth, especially in the outlying regions of the capital, New Delhi. By Western standards, few of these farmers are truly rich. But in India, where the annual per capita income is about $1,000 and where roughly 800 million people live on less than $2 a day, some farmers have gotten windfalls by selling land. . .in [recent] years, more than 50,000 acres of farmland have been purchased as Noida has evolved into a sprawling suburb of 300,000 people with shopping malls and office parks.[7]

This new wealth has fueled social competitiveness with the upper economic castes, conspicuous consumption of high-end exotic cars, and lavish vacations. Many of India's key industries—auto manufacturing, software, and entertainment—are establishing themselves in its once relatively obscure cities of Bangladore, Ahmedabad, and Chennai.

At the present time, developing countries such as India have no incentive to seek international funding to help prevent the spread of NCDs, and it is the invisible poor who are typically left behind.[8] Health ministers in these places continue to cling to the myth that NCDs are the bane of affluent societies only, as they continue to focus nearly singularly on battling infectious diseases.

The transition from desert to sprawl machine is a major undertaking. In Dubai, lines of traffic stretch as far as the eye can see, with impatient drivers pounding their horns as cars stop cold in the middle of the road, blocking the lane while families slowly pile out into the searing desert sun. It is just another day at the Middle East's largest mega shopping center, Mall of the Emirates (MoE). On average, this mall attracts between 70,000 and 80,000 visitors a day during the week and between 100,000 and 110,000 on weekends.[9] With soaring temperatures outside, a fourteen-screen cinema, gaming casino, performing arts theatre, and its thoroughly impressive indoor ski slope, the MoE expects to expand further, but has since been eclipsed in size by the Dubai Mall and the gargantuan Mall of Arabia. The Dubai Mall's aquarium has 41,000 fish. Sprawl is increasing not only across the BRIC nations—Brazil, Russia, India, and China—but also in the Middle East, the Czech Republic, and other former Soviet Block countries. In 2005, heart disease, stroke, and diabetes caused an estimated loss of national income of $9 billion (U.S.) in India and $3 billion in Brazil.[10]

The situation does not seem to be improving anytime soon in the U.S., either. Since 2000, Raleigh, North Carolina, has amassed numerous accolades as among the best places to live, work, play, start a small business, and relocate to in the U.S.[11] The result: Raleigh's population has ballooned faster than nearly any other major American city in the past decade. This mostly unmitigated growth has resulted in a less desirable moniker—Sprawleigh. In 2010, a report by CEOs for Cities identified Raleigh as one of the most sprawling cities in America, where residents can spend as much as 240 hours per year in traffic due to their distorted commuting distances. In response, the city did some soul searching. What kind of place did it want to be "when it grew up?" It concluded it did not want to be like Atlanta or Charlotte. Raleigh had grown recently with little forethought as people relocated from colder northern climates, and this rapidity of expansion proved overwhelming for the city's infrastructure. Prior to the Great Recession of 2008 and the U.S. housing bubble's subsequent implosion, not having to build vertically meant horizontalism ruled the day.[12] From 1950 to 2000, Raleigh's land use grew 1,670 percent, 3.5 times faster than the population, which increased by 480 percent to more than 400,000. This created a massive problem: in a 2002 study by U.S. national advocacy group Smart Growth America, the city was ranked third worst, based on measures of low density, non-mixed land uses, lack of a sense of place, and road disjointedness.[13]

## Time is Running Short

In 2005, the World Bank published a report on the dynamics of global urban expansion and the acute dilemma posed by unmitigated sprawl. The population in developing-country cities is expected to double in the next thirty years, from some 2 billion in 2000 to almost 4 billion in 2030.[14] Cities with populations in excess of 100,000 contained 1.7 billion people in 2000, and their total built-up land area, at average densities of 12,875 persons per square mile, was nearly 124,280 square miles at that time. If average densities continue to decline due to sprawl at the annual rate of 1.7 percent—as they have during the past decade—the built-up area of developing country cities will increase to more than 600,000 square kilometers or 372,822 square miles by 2030. In other words, by 2030 these cities can be expected to triple their land area, with every new resident converting, on average, approximately 160 square meters of non-urban land, or 525 square feet of non-urban land, to urban land during this period. Globally, cities are now expected to expand 2.5 times in land area by 2030, consuming more than 1 million square kilometers, or 1.1 percent of the total land area of countries, or more than 620 square miles. In some places this may be as high as 5 to 7 percent of the total arable land.[15]

The ongoing debate over the virtues of uncontrolled and minimally controlled expansion, versus strict geographic containment, has been raging for centuries. At the one extreme, special interests fight to severely limit the growth of footprints while at the other extreme other special interests fight for expansion on the justification that it is the best way to expand economic opportunities, i.e. jobs.[16]

Without question, the proliferation of sprawl machines globally is a complex and contradictory, even paradoxical, proposition: it commands attention in the West, but the opposite is often the case elsewhere. In most of these places, little genuine attention, by comparison, appears to be devoted to the crisis at this time.[17]

The morphology of expansion unfolds in substantially different ways in different places. It can occur within identical densities as those which prevail in existing, developed areas, at higher densities, or at reduced densities. It can occur vis-à-vis the infill of remaining open spaces at higher densities, or through new greenfield development that either is contiguous with existing built-up areas or it leapfrogs outward away from dense urban cores, skipping or circumventing already-built-up districts, i.e. parks, industrial zones, natural boundaries such as rivers and lakes, and/or residential neighborhoods. Expansion can encroach upon sensitive environmental ecosystems, including farmland, fields, and forests. It can ultimately maintain or increase the amount of total open space. However, precise patterns of expansion are dependent upon the degree this expansion is controlled. Complicating matters, expansion can yield a higher, equal, or lower percentage of new employment opportunities and can be orderly or chaotic in how it happens, leaving little space for adequate roads, rail transport, or for cycling and pedestrian amenities.

Additional variables include whether the expansion is legally sanctioned, or unsanctioned. Illegal modes of uncontrolled growth and infill in a given place may include squatter encampments, informal land subdivisions, the outright non-compliance with local zoning ordinances, or new construction that occurs on steep slopes or in flood plains subject to mudslides and/or inundation by flooding.[18] Regardless of the mechanics of its permutations, sprawl is now empirically linked with NCDs and higher greenhouse gas emission levels associated with higher levels of auto travel necessitated in expanding low-density contexts.[19] The authors of World Bank report articulated six key variables: the effects of the natural environment; the effects of demographics; the effects of the local and regional economy; the effects of the public transport systems in place (or not in place); consumer preferences for close proximity to jobs and services; and the efficacy of government at all levels.[20] The report concluded that population growth within any given urban/suburban area is predicated on:

> Its own natural birth and death rates and on its attractiveness to those who perceive opportunity and promise there. Successful cities, where economic growth is robust, employment is plentiful, urban services are adequate, and the quality of life is high, attract people. These cities naturally grow faster than other cities in the country where economic opportunities are few and the promise of a better life is less than convincing. It is hard to imagine, therefore, that the residents or the policy makers of a successful city will agree to curtail its economic growth or to reduce either its level of urban services or its quality of life so as to prevent people or firms from moving in.[21]

Many governments have, as of late, sought to control the inward urban migration levels, but most if not all such attempts have been failures[22] In China, one of the very few places where people are still required to possess residence permits (*Hukou*) to live in a given city, a floating population of between 18 and 20 million resided in Chinese cities illegally in 2000, just to be there, presumably to seek opportunities unavailable in the rural areas regardless of the associated potential health risks incurred in urban life.[23] Meanwhile, the World Bank reported in 2007 that China is expected to lose roughly $558 billion in national income between 2005 and 2015 due to the effects of NCDs that result in premature deaths.[24]

## China: Constructing Unhealthful Sprawl Machines as Fast as Possible

China has 1.3 billion citizens. The Communist Central Government hopes to spur consumer demand in the nation's undeveloped rural provinces—which will, it is hoped, spur the need for new roads, gas stations, motels, restaurants, and so on in close proximity to these new roads. In short, sprawl is needed and wanted, Western style. Up to now, there were only a miniscule number of private autos per every 1,000 people in China, as compared to per every 1,000 people in the U.S. In 2009 alone, 12 million light vehicles were purchased as the Chinese auto industry expanded by 50 percent, versus only 10.3 million purchased in the U.S. China's sales were predicted to rise by 25 percent annually in each of the next five years. In 2010, 26,000 newly registered light vehicles were placed on China's roads each day. Most experts conclude the U.S. auto industry will never surpass China's again.[25]

If we want to anticipate the future of global sprawl machines, China presents the perfect case study. It is urbanizing at a rate unprecedented in history. Between now and 2030, according to a 2009 McKinsey Global Institute report, Chinese cities are expected to add more than 350 million people, swelling to an urban population of more than 1 billion. By then, China will have more than 220 cities with a population of more than 1 million. By comparison, Europe has only thirty-five cities with 1 million or more inhabitants, and twenty-four *megacities* with more than 5 million inhabitants each.[26] China will build more than 50,000 skyscrapers, 170 completely new mass transit systems, and as many as 7,000 hospitals and clinics during this period.[27]

On the potential for disaster:

> Already, China is teetering on the edge of ecological catastrophe. It suffers from some of the worst air pollution in the world. For instance, Hong Kong's air quality meets the bare minimum *World Health Organization* standards on average of only 41 days a year. . .*The World Bank* says that 16 of 20 most polluted cities in the world are in China, and 400,000 people a year die as a result of poor air quality. The picture only worsens if we look at the broader picture. China is suffering rapid desertification. . .Chinese waterways are more than twice as degraded as previously reported. . .[with] two-thirds of [its] rivers and lakes dangerously polluted [cancer rates are extraordinarily high in riverside cities in China]; the Yangtze River is now biologically dead. . .and more than 340 million Chinese have no access at all to safe drinking water. The natural systems China's people depend on for the basics of life are unraveling at astonishing speed.[28]

In China, expenses from strokes alone have pushed 37 percent of patients and their families below the poverty line. Research from the International Diabetes Federation in 2009 found that of 2,300 persons with Type 2 diabetes, one in six could not work because of their health, where the average annual income level is less than $2,000. Organizations, including Partners in Health (PIH) and Family Health International (FHI), argue that unless rapid action is taken in fast developing parts of the world, the financial burden of treating NCDs will reach levels that are beyond the capacity to cope. As the world's largest emitter of greenhouse gasses, China must quickly implement carbon neutral policies.[29]

More than half of the world's population now lives in metropolitan areas, as mentioned at the outset. However, there have never been so many concurrently hyper-expanding cities in history.[30] When *Forbes* magazine published its 2010 list of the world's fastest growing cities, it intentionally eschewed the most likely mainstream suspects, i.e. New York, London, Paris, Hong Kong,

Tokyo—cities which have dominated mainstream rankings for a generation. It also passed over cities that achieved global prominence within the past twenty years, such as Seoul, Shanghai, Singapore, Beijing, Delhi, Sydney, Toronto, Houston, and Dallas-Fort Worth. Nor did it include the well-known massive yet largely dysfunctional megacities—Mumbai, Mexico City, Dhaka, Bangladesh—that are among the world's most populous today. Rather, its list focused on emerging places such as Chonqing, China (population: 9 million), in the middle of the world's most significant region for mandated hyper-sprawling cities—interior China. These new cities are prefabricated and "pre-designed" to provide a more viable alternative to the extremely dense older, established cities of the Eastern provinces, with their crime, pollution, congestion, increasingly wide class disparities, and increasing public and personal health risks.[31] It is a risk-filled venture in social engineering on a massive scale. China's risky, bold, de-densification central government policies hinge on the construction of hundreds of completely new sprawl machines.[32]

To say that China is overbuilding is an extreme understatement. In 2010, approximately one of every four square feet of feasible commercial office space in Beijing sat empty (about 100 million square feet). Tall buildings are built that sit virtually empty, awaiting their new occupants. In Eastern Beijing, officials doubled the size of its CBD, although vacancy rates were above 35 percent there already. Entire new towns currently sit empty. The new-town sprawl suburb of Huariou is a mock alpine village, with a 200-foot clock tower that rises at the center of a generic suburban district near yet another "industrial suburb."[33] It is a replica of Hallstatt, in Austria, and was built at a cost of $9 billion in 2006 in an attempt at horizontal decentralization. Today it is filled with empty shops, almost no residents, unused roads and an artificial lake that attracts few tourists; it feels like the set of the 1998 Jim Carrey film *The Truman Show*.[34] This and many similar ghost sprawl machines feature expensive, State-sanctioned public artworks, vacant museums, and vast public squares. On the surface, it may appear to be vibrant economic growth, but in reality it is merely *zombie growth*.

## Sprawl Machine Ghost Towns

The Chinese border outpost of Erenhot is part boomtown, part ghost town. Residents are few and far between in this part of the Gobi Desert, where little that is green grows on its own. Tons of sand frequently blow from this region, turning Beijing's sky bright orange, a harsh reminder of the country's expanding deserts.[35] Since 2000, scores of empty strip malls and apartment buildings have been built here. It is an eerie skyline visible for miles across the desert. And yet economists rave about China's double-digit annual growth in its GDP, even as much of the rest of the world struggles through a deep recession. But China's hyper-expansionism is not at all about so-called unrestricted "free market" economics. It is all about strict top-down authoritarian rule by decree: the enormous engine of the State drives China's GDP at the expense of everything else:

> China's obsession with economic metrics harkens back to the Mao days, when industrial production stats took center stage. Nowadays, careers of Chinese bureaucrats hinge on two things—growth and lack of social unrest—often in conflict. Pollution has been a major cause of dissent, as the poor struggle with rising costs, especially in healthcare and education. . .despite this, the country has entombed its new wealth in concrete and steel. You can see it in Dongguan, in Guangdong province, where the world's largest mall stands empty, save for a few hamburger chain outlets. . .in cities like Erenhot, where the relentless construction continues, oblivious to a dearth of demand. . .the place feels like a video game backdrop.[36]

## Ordos City

China's new-town ghost towns are basically empty, with the poster child being the "visionary" development in Ordos, a completely new city built for 500,000 west of Beijing. It includes a compound of luxury villas in the Ordos desert of Inner Mongolia and a 1,000 acre theme park replica of the old Imperial Summer Palace, which was destroyed by British and French troops in the 19th century. Its newest sector, Kangbashi, is has a capacity for 300,000 residents. But by some measures this resource-rich city in northern China is a major success.[37] It has large reserves of coal and natural gas, and a property market so hot that virtually every dwelling unit built is immediately sold, as people invest here in real estate as a way to store cash, with many investors stockpiling multiple units of every size and type in the hope of turning a profit later by "flipping" them.[38] Yet the single most glaring missing ingredient is the absence of inhabitants. Ordos proper has 1.5 million residents although the sprawl of Kangbashi, built from scratch on immense acreage 15 miles south of the old city, sits all but deserted:

> Broad boulevards are unimpeded by traffic in the new district, called Kangbashi New Area. Office buildings stand vacant. Pedestrians are in short supply, and weeds are beginning to sprout up in luxury villa developments devoid of residents. . .(and yet) cranes are every-where. . .including a $450 million financial district. . .with six high rise office towers. Last year, housing sales in Ordos reached $2.4 billion, up from $100 million in 2004. . .during that span, the average square foot price of real estate rose by 260 percent, to $53 per square foot. "This is a city of the future," Li Hong, a government official, said, during a recent tour. . ."We are going to build this into a center of politics, culture and technology. That is our dream." But the future has not yet arrived. . .the vacant amenities surrounding the [new-town's] square include a theater, an opera house and an art museum. . .formerly impoverished, the region boasts a growing number of coal billionaires and the nation's highest GDP per capita ($19,679), with Land Rovers a leading symbol of Ordos's newfound affluence. . .In 2004. . .city officials drew up a bold expansion plan to create Kangbashi, a 30-minute drive south of the old city center on land adjacent to one of the region's few reservoirs. Because land auctions are a major source of fiscal income in China, part of the plan's allure was the prospect of elevating the value of property in an undeveloped area. In the ensuing building spree, home buyers could not get enough of residential developments with names like Exquisite Silk Village, Kanghe Elysees, and Imperial Academic Gardens.[39]

Writing in *Time* magazine, Bill Powell explains the immense economic risks associated with building speculative sprawl machines on this scale in China:

> No question keeps more economists, investors, hedge-fund managers and bankers up at night than this one: Is China's property market a bubble? The reason for their angst is clear: A prop-erty meltdown in China would imperil the whole world's fledging economic recovery. Throughout the most severe global economic downturn in decades, China's economic growth has remained remarkably buoyant. . .and nothing has driven China's growth more than real estate investment. Last year, fixed-asset investment accounted for more than 90 percent of China's overall growth, and residential and commercial real estate investment made up nearly a quarter of that. For years, regional governments across China have been building massive real estate projects that have attracted both private and corporate buyers. As prices have continued

to rise. . .more [speculators] have bought brand-new properties with the sole intention of flipping them. . .But many analysts fear a replay in China [of the U.S. housing bust] could prove disastrous. Indeed, evidence of property oversupply is everywhere. . .throughout the Chinese interior, there are eerie monuments as entire cities built for millions of inhabitants stand all but empty. . .only a handful of cars drive down Kangbashi's multilane highways. . .and an occasional pedestrian, appearing like a hallucination, can be seen trudging down a sidewalk, like a lone survivor of some horror-movie apocalypse. When bubbles burst, they tend to do so with a bang. . .authorities in Beijing—and Ordos, for that matter—are hoping they can deflate their housing bubble without a pop. And it's not just the Chinese who should be praying that they can pull it off.[40]

## The South China Mall

The world's largest shopping mall sits almost entirely empty. It is an impressive place: a 7 million square foot retail and entertainment behemoth in the heart of China's Pearl River Delta. It is the wealthiest region within the world's fastest expanding economy. Now China can boast it has the world's largest mall, largest airport, and golf resort. Visitors to this megamall have many options for spending their time. The mall features a replica of the Bell Tower of St. Mark's in Venice, a replica of a street in Old San Francisco, and a 1,650-foot indoor–outdoor roller coaster known as Kuayue Shi Kong (translation: Moving Through Time and Space). The few people there are awash in zombie space:

> The South China Mall, which opened with great fanfare in 2005, is not just the world's largest. With fewer than a dozen stores scattered throughout a space designed to house 1,500 it is also the world's emptiest. . .what sets this mall apart, besides its mind-numbing size, is that it never went into decline. The tenants never jumped ship (as in the case of dead U.S. malls) because they never came on board in the first place. This mall entered the world pre-ruined. . .a spectacular real estate failure and yet. . .a strangely beautiful monument to the big dreams that China inspires. . .Just before it opened it was featured on the front page of the New York Times as a symbol of China's astonishing new consumer culture. . .its developers expected more than 70,000 visitors a day.[41]

Its failure appears to be a classic case of the chicken and egg conundrum. Did it fail due to lack of stores, or the lack of customers? Nonetheless, it appears that financing remains available to build just about anything these days without having to submit a business feasibility plan, or without any pre-leasing tenant commitments. This is now known within China as "cowboy development."[42] At present, fewer than 10 percent of China's 1.3 billion inhabitants have enough discretionary income to be considered middle class although nearly 500 new malls have been built in China since 2003. Government officials hope this preordained new middle class will materialize soon so the country can quickly take its place among the world's super-materialistic powers.[43]

## Shanghai

As a key goal in the 12th Five-year Plan (2011–2015) for Shanghai, local provincial governments have elected to focus on constructing new and extending existing sprawl machines into seven new *satellite cities*. It is seeking to rapidly suburbanize the Yangtze River Delta. The Shanghai Municipal Planning,

Land and Resources Administration claims this initiative will improve the infrastructure of the entire region. These seven new "cities" will include Lingang New City in Pudong New Area, Qingpu New City, and Jinshan New City. They are being created as core industrial centers for advanced manufacturing and new service industries, in coordination with neighboring Kunshan and Suzhou. The intent is to reduce the density of the Shanghai urban core by encouraging people to relocate to these suburbs. Talk about repeating the zombie-like mistakes of the West! According to Li Tianhua, a registered urban planner for the Shanghai Urban Planning and Design Research Institute:

> The urban plan for new cities in the suburbs of Shanghai fits in the structure well by having resources divided reasonably to relieve the crowded city center by encouraging people to live in the suburbs.[44]

The goal for the Songjiang New City, the biggest among these seven *supersuburbs*, is to entice as many as 1.1 million new residents to the area by 2020. The quality of life in these places will purportedly be as good as that in the traditional urban center of Shanghai, with the provision of public services, hospitals, and transport, and smart land use planning and building design amenities.[45] However, not all agree that this massive resettlement plan will work, as critics question whether enough jobs will be created to attract enough workers and their families to the new supersuburbs.

## Southern China

City planners in South China have laid out similarly ambitious plans to merge the nine principal cities geographically situated within the Pearl River Delta.[46] This new megacity will cover a large part of China's manufacturing heartland stretching from Guangzhou to Shenzhen and will include Foshan, Dongguan, Zhongshan, Zhuhai, Jiangmen, Huizhou, and Zhaoqing. Together, they account for nearly a tenth of the entire Chinese economy, and contain 42 million inhabitants. More than 150 major infrastructure projects are underway to link transport, energy, water, and telecommunication networks of these nine cities together, at a cost of more than 2 trillion yuan. A new express high-speed rail line will connect its core hub with nearby Hong Kong. Cultural amenities and social services are being connected so that residents can freely commute to different areas within this network by public transit. Curiously, this aggregation as of yet remains nameless, although it is destined to become the world's largest sprawl machine (because it will not be named after any one of its nine constituent urban areas). The public policy intent is to evenly distribute jobs and economic opportunities across the entire aggregation. Universal annual rail passes will make it possible for people to use public transport anytime to get virtually anywhere via the twenty-nine new rail lines being constructed. The government's goal is for no one-way rail commute longer than one hour.[47]

The intent of the South China sprawl machine is to compete with the sprawling megacities of Beijing and Shanghai. By 2020, the central government plans to have relocated 50–100 million people into various "small-scale" sprawl machines, each of 10–25 million inhabitants.[48] Meanwhile, in the north, around Beijing and Tianjin, the megacity is being ringed with a network of high-speed rail lines to be known as the Bohai Economic Rim, serving a population of as many as 260 million inhabitants. It is a monumental undertaking, by any metric, and not without monumental risks.[49] The Chinese public's uproar (as silently expressed on Internet blogs) over a high-speed rail accident that killed 39 and seriously inured more than 200 in July of 2011 is a case in point of the delicate issue of government censorship.[50]

All this begs the question. What about building upward—vertically—more compactly, versus chronic continued low-density horizontalism? It appears inevitable that more than 1 billion people will inhabit China's cities by 2030. This presents the central Communist government with a unique opportunity to create and develop cities that at least aspire to eco-humanism and environmental sustainability. In building taller, fire safety concerns indeed exist, as the public service infrastructure continues to lag behind the accelerated pace of the construction boom.[51] Even at the present rate, however, China annually could continue to build 1,000-plus buildings that are more than thirty floors tall, equivalent to a new Chicago every year, resulting in more than 950 sprawl machines by 2030.[52] The inherent environmental and public health risks in all this will be extremely high. Regardless, foreign planers and urban designers argue that greater densities, if not too dense, can yield a more appropriate, sustainable balance than to overemphasize horizontalism. One example of this approach is the 108-story ICC tower in Hong Kong, built in the heart of the city's Central District, on reclaimed industrial land. It made use of innovative construction technologies to minimize its carbon footprint.[53] Such strategies can yield additional green space—an increasingly rare amenity in rapidly expanding sprawl machines globally. All societies, democratic or otherwise, need urban civic spaces that function as repositories, reinforcers, and arbiters of collective cultural memory.[54]

Samuel Becket once said, "Try again. Fail again. Fail better." Ultimately, for China's existing and coming wave of new sprawl machines, this will come down to issues of economics, auto-centricity versus pedestrianism, the challenges of environmental stewardship, the power of collective cultural memory, technology, and the orderly and equitable transfer of land use rights.

In contemporary China one always hears this: "The business of the country is business."[55] In the South, journalist Peter Hessler wrote of how factory development is occurring extremely rapidly in Lishui, a previously sleepy small city whose leaders are determined to increase wealth and employment through advanced manufacturing. Most Chinese manufacturing cities specialize in a single product. In Lishui, that product is a small ring used in the assembly of bras. A Western observer may wonder how accelerated expansion can occur in a culture so different from Western capitalism.[56] In fact, the answer lies beneath the surface and centers on land use rights, and how they are transferred from rural to urban/suburban uses. In the Chinese countryside, all land is collective, and farmers have no right to sell off their plots and homes on the open market. Instead, the village handles all land use transactions, and the village per se has little bargaining power if a nearby city decides to expand and expropriate its rural farmland.[57] After the sale is finalized, and the farmers have been forced to move off the land, the city then constructs basic infrastructure and reclassifies the land as "urban." Then, urban land use rights are auctioned off at prevailing market rates to the highest bidder. It is a type of arbitrage, buying rural land and reinventing it as urban.[58]

As for the intertwined problems of the growing volume of auto usage and traffic congestion, the situation is worsening daily. New roads can't be built fast enough to meet the growing daily demands of the 35 million light vehicles purchased since 2000. It has been a period of mass catch-up consumerism. Worse, the government has had a very hard time controlling the sheer number of vehicles on the road, when they are operated, and where. In Shanghai, a city of more than 20 million, new car registrations are restricted to 6,000 per month, while typical traffic speeds are no greater than 6–10 miles per hour in the city, well under the speed of a bicycle. In 2011, Beijing launched a lottery to restrict the number of new cars in the city to 240,000 in 2011.[59] In 2010, 700,000 private autos were sold in the city. But the measure backfired because 20,000 rushed to buy their car the day before the lottery went into effect. Now, such events as the ten-day, 60-mile traffic jam on the outskirts of Beijing in 2010 will become commonplace. This, although only 20 percent of all daily trips in

Shanghai and Beijing currently are by auto, compared to 80 percent in most U.S. cities. Yet for those who opt to walk or bike, this means breathing in a large amount of fouled air. Even so, there are still only eighteen private autos for every 1,000 Chinese citizens, (equivalent to what it was in the U.S. in the 1920s), versus 740 private autos for every 1,000 Americans.[60]

The average citizen in China travels only 600 miles per year by bus, train, car or plane, compared to 15,000 motorized miles per capita in the U.S., and yet China is now the number one in the sales volume auto market on the planet. In 2010, General Motors sold more cars in China than in the U.S., as did BMW. It is predicted that China will have four times the number of private autos by 2020.[61] The plethora of mass transit systems currently being built must convince people not to drive their newly purchased cars. But as people become more emotionally attached to their cars, sprawl machines will further engulf the Chinese countryside. Recent experience from Bangkok, Jakarta, and Manila suggests that recovering from unmitigated sprawl and its unhealthful public health effects will be extremely difficult. Traffic planners in the West fear that China does not have the time at this point to do anything but to blindly import past mistakes from the U.S. and elsewhere, even if they have already proven as serious failures in their countries of origin.[62]

Suffice to say, unmitigated sprawl in developed countries needs to become a hot topic. The West dominates the discourse, as most of the quantified data have focused mainly on sprawl in rich countries. Because of this geographic and socio-economic bias, it is a risk to cavalierly export do's and don'ts as pre-packaged "solutions" to developing places without fully considering the implications for NCDs and related epidemiological issues. As such, health and urban planning ministers should view any such activity with skepticism. It is critical within this discourse to compare/contrast the on-the-ground realities between often strikingly different cultural contexts. China is now repeating many of the same urban planning mistakes made in the U.S. forty to fifty years ago, as well as Brasilia in the 1950s and 1960s, in the post-World War II communist architecture of the Soviet bloc during the halcyon years of the International Style, and most recently in Dubai. Regardless, China, for its faults, engages in far longer-term planning horizons in terms of its infrastructure than does the U.S. at this time.[63] China's unfortunate mistake is its segregated land-use zoning, which results in excessive U.S. style auto-dependency.[64] Has anyone stopped to think of whether its new middle class really wants to live just like suburban Americans—having to drive everywhere to do everything?

## Global Villages and Our Endangered Public Health

Global sprawl machines consume tremendous human and capital resources. Now they can be studied more openly than ever before. Today, within seconds, millions of empowered citizens can potentially access vast information about them in relation to their own personal health. The ubiquitous Google Earth, fused with geographic information systems (GIS), have become mainstream geospatial mapping tools for people everywhere to examine interdependencies between built form and public health outcomes.[65] In the case of Google Earth, anyone can now access its rich database, anywhere, anytime, from the scale of an individual building and its streetscape, to an entire region. The technology itself will, it is hoped, remain a-political, because as Wilson et al. (2003) rightly argue, no universally accepted definition of sprawl yet exists. The danger exists that these and related databases can be manipulated or skewed to mislead or distort the facts.[66] This threat was proven in the weeks after Hurricane Katrina, when the blue tarp-dominated satellite photos of the ruined city were mysteriously replaced with the pre-storm satellite imagery. This unethical breach on the part of Google Earth was detected right away, and was immediately rectified. In the developing world, the main problem until now has been one of extremely poor coordination between various planning agencies in cities such as New Delhi. There, disparate municipal planning agencies poorly coordinate with public health and medical agencies and providers, e.g. a primary care clinic's power is shut off on its busiest clinic days due to an adjacent street being excavated often, many times over, often unnecessarily.[67] China now has 430 million bikes and it is by far the world's largest fleet. As its cities continue to hyper-expand will bike use precipitously fall in favor of auto usage?[68] What are the public health risks associated with a lower bike ridership rate? Would this correlate with increased urban air pollution levels? What are the ecological and human public health costs associated with the growing amount of unlimited free parking being built right now in China and elsewhere?[69] More than 90 percent of the U.S. workforce commutes to work by car and 90 percent of those commuters park for free.[70]

In the developing world, the risk is real that the same mistakes made by developed countries are being repeated verbatim. But the inner profundities of sprawl machines and their anti-salutogenetic public health consequences are by no means limited to developing countries. The City of Barcelona has a population of over 1.5 million inhabitants. The metro area has a population of nearly 4.4 million and rural land consumption at the periphery has been accelerating.[71] Urban ecologists are now investigating horizontalism in relation to global climate change and its impact on human ecosystems.[72] The twenty largest U.S. cities each year currently contribute more $CO_2$ into the global atmosphere than the entire land area of continental U.S. can absorb. Metaphors are being utilized to help understand and analogize sprawl as a biological organism that takes in "food," consumes it, and then releases its harmful wastes into the physical ecosystem.[73] Finally, conceptions of *electronic space* will be of importance within the broad context of the ever shifting, contested geographies of sprawl machines in relation to global public health. A new geographical discipline of centrality/marginality is emerging—it focuses on the redistribution of wealth from urban centers to peripheral sprawl zones, and vice versa.[74] Morphologic, socio-cultural, and (compressed versus elongated) electronic space–time–distance relationships between the poor and the wealthy are at risk of becoming ever more polarized. Why? Physical space as well as electronic cyberspace is increasingly being commoditized and privatized globally. Disadvantaged suburbs are at more risk than ever before of disproportionate marginalization (and therefore becoming even less healthy places than now) with wealthier suburbs becoming disproportionately favored even more than now, becoming evermore healthier. This troubling pattern is reprised in the following chapters.

## Notes

1  United Nations, Department of Economic and Social Affairs, Population Division (2009) *World Urbanization Prospects: The 2009 Revision*. New York: United Nations. Online. Available at www.unpopulation.org.html (accessed 14 July 2011).

2  Anand, Sonia S. and Yusef, Salim (2011) 'Stemming the global tsunami of cardiovascular disease,' *The Lancet*, 377(9765): 529–532. One country has stubbornly resisted this trend, however. For all its dynamism since India opened up its economy in 1990, its men on average have become thinner in recent decades.

3  Hatton, Celia (2011) 'KFC's finger-lickin' success in China,' *CBS News*, 6 March. Online. Available at www.cbsnews.com/stories/2011/03/06/sunday/main20039783.shtml (accessed 7 March 2011).

4  Levy, Clifford, J. (2010) 'Time to wake up, sleeper spy,' *The New York Times*, 9 July. Online. Available at www.nytimes.com/2010/07/11weekinreview.html (accessed 16 July 2011).

5  Schumpeter, Jan (2011) 'The universal provider,' *The Economist*, 19 January. Online. Available at www.economist.com/blogs/schumpeter/2011/01/company_towns.html (accessed 12 February 2011).

6  Friedman, Thomas (2010) 'India chases the American Dream,' *The Times-Picayune*, 2 November, p. B5.

7  Yardley, Jim (2010) 'For India's newly rich farmers, Limos won't do,' *The New York Times*, 19 March, pp. A8–A9.

8  Agarwal, Siddarth (2011) 'The invisible poor,' *World Health Design*, July, pp. 20–26.

9  Anon. (2008) 'Mall carves out space as parking problems mount,' *The National*, 3 July. Online. Available at www.thenational.ae/apps/pbcs.d11/article?AID=/20080703/national/935736461/1042.html (accessed 19 August 2010).

10  World Health Organization (2008) *2008–2013 Action Plan for the Global Strategy for the Prevention and Control of Non-communicable Diseases*. Geneva. Online. Available at www.whqlibdoc.who.int/publications/2009/9789241597418_eng.pdf.html (accessed 20 July 2011). Also see Boutayeb, A and Boutayeb, S. (2005) 'The burden of non-communicable diseases in developing countries,' *International Journal of Equity in Health*, 4(2). Online. Available at www.ncbi.nlm.nih.gov/pmc/articles/PMC546417/html (accessed 18 July 2011).

11  Anon. (2009) 'Best cities: It's all about jobs,' *Kiplinger*, July. Online. Available at www.kiplinger.com/magazine/archives/2009/07html (accessed 29 July 2011).

12  Chase, Carolyn (2010) 'Sprawling America,' *San Diego Earth Times*, February. Online. Available at www.sdearthtimes.com/cut_to_the_chase.ctc_44.html (accessed 29 July 2011).

13  Goldberg, Steve (2011) 'Reigning in Sprawleigh,' *Time*, 25 March. Online. Available at www.time.com/time/specials/packages/article.html (accessed 12 June 2011). Also see Head, Peter (2011) 'Healthy cities in an ecological age,' *World Health Design*, July, pp. 10–14.

14  Buckley, Robert, Chabaeva, Anna, Gitlin, Lucy, Kraley, Alison, Parent, Jason, and Perlin, Micah (2005) *The Dynamics of Global Urban Expansion*. Washington, D.C.: Transport and Urban Development Department, World Bank.

15  United Nations (2004) *World Urbanization Prospects—the 2003 Revision*. New York: United Nations.

16  Lai, Richard Tseng-Yu (1988) *Law in Urban Design and Planning*. New York: Van Nostrand, pp. 27–33.

17  Buckley et al., *The Dynamics of Global Urban Expansion*, p 3.

18  Ibid., p. 5.

19  Ibid., p. 6.

20  Ibid., p. 8.

21  Ibid., p. 10.

22  Windrow, Hayden and Guha, Anik (2005) 'The Hukou System, migrant workers, and state power in the People's Republic of China,' *Northwestern University Journal of International Human Rights*, 3(3): 1–10. Online. Available at www.law.northwestern.edu/jpurnals/jihr/v3/3.html (accessed 28 July 2011).

23  Anon. (2000) 'China begins massive census,' *BBC News*, 31 October. Online. Available at www.bbc.co.uk/1/hi/world/asia-pacific/1000357.html (accessed 12 June 2010).

24  World Bank (2007) *Cost of Pollution in China: Economic Estimates of Physical Damages*. Washington and Beijing: World Bank.

25  Chu, Kathy and MacLeod, Calvin (2010) 'Car sales rocket as China tries to boost consumer spending,' *USA Today*, 4 March. Online. Available at www.usatoday.com/money/autos/2010-03-04.html (accessed 12 March 2010).

26  McKinsey Global Institute (2009) *Preparing for China's Urban Billion—City Profiles: 14 City Case Studies*. Shanghai: McKinsey & Company. Also see Devan, Janamitra, Negri, Stefano, and Woetzel, Jonathan R. (2010) 'Meeting the challenges of China's growing cities,' *The McKinsey Quarterly*, June. Online. Available at www.solutions.mckinsey.com/insightchina/_SiteNote/WWWhtml (accessed 29 July 2010).

27  World Bank, *Cost of Pollution in China*, p. 6.

28  Steffen, Alex (2010) 'A Climate-Neutral China,' *Worldchanging*, 28 June. Online. Available at www.world-changing.com/archives/011075.html (accessed 12 February 2011).

29  French, Maddy (2011) 'Why non-communicable diseases hit the developing world so hard,' *The Guardian*. Online. Available at www.guardian.co.uk/journalismcompetition/html (accessed 22 July 2011).

30  Capon, Anthony (2011) 'The view from the city,' *World Health Design*. July, pp. 6–9.

31  World Health Organization and UN-HABITAT (2010) *Hidden Cities: Unmasking and Overcoming Health Inequalities in Urban Settings*. Kobe: The WHO Center for Health Development.

32  Kotkin, Joel (2010) 'The world's fastest-growing cities,' *Forbes*, 7 October. Online. Available at www.forbes.com/2010/10/07.html (accessed 20 December 2010).

33  Bonner, Bill (2010) 'China's Zombie Growth,' *The Christian Science Monitor*, 8 March. Online. Available at www.csmonitor.com/business/the-daily-reconing/2010/0308/html (accessed 19 August 2010).

34  Anon. (1999) 'The meaning of The Truman Show,' *Transparencynow*. Online. Available at www.transparencynow.com/trusig.htm (accessed 12 July 2011).

35  China's expanding deserts now cover one-third of the country because of overgrazing, deforestation, urban sprawl, and drought.

36  Rabkin, April (2010) 'China's Potemkin cities,' *Mother Jones*, 18 August. Online. Available at www. motherjones.com/politics/2010/04/china-ghost-mall.html (accessed 19 August 2010). Also see the website sponsored by the Chinese central government, '10 years of China's Western Development,' for detailed profiles of the nation's hyper-expansionist economic policies and monumental sprawl machine construction initiatives.

37  Caploe, David (2011) 'China housing inequality: Ordos—Wealthy Mongolian ghost town,' *Economy Watch*, 30 July. Online. Available at www.ceonomywatch.com/economy-business-and-finance-news.html (accessed 4 August 2011).

38  Ibid., p. 2.

39  Barboza, David (2010) 'Chinese city has many buildings, but few people,' *The New York Times*, 19 October. Online. Available at www.nytimes.com/2010/10/20/business/global/20ghost.html (accessed 12 November 2010).

40  Powell, Bill (2010) 'Ghost City,' *Time*, 5 April, pp. 40–44.

41  Donohue, Michael (2008) 'Mall of misfortune,' *The National*, 12 June. Online. Available at www. thenational.ae/article/20080612/review/206990272/1042.html (accessed 12 June 2011).

42  Ibid., p. 4.

43  Doctoroff, Thomas (2010) 'China's new middle class: constants and variables,' *Huffpost Business*, 29 May. Online. Available at www.huffingtonpost.com/tom-doctoroff/chinas-new-middle-class.html (accessed 28 July 2011).

44  Ran, Yu (2011) 'Shanghai unveils plan for 7 new satellite cities,' *China Daily*, 30 June. Online. Available at www.chinadaily.com.cn/china/2011-06/30/content_12805181.html (accessed 15 July 2011).

45  Doctoroff, 'China's new middle class: constants and variables.'

46  Anon. (2011) 'China's state council OKs urban planning of key city in Pearl River Delta,' *Latest China/ China News*, 17 May. Online. Available at www.latestchina.com/article/?rid=36786.html (accessed 29 July 2011).

47  Pierson, David (2011) 'China feeling like No. 1 with a bullet train,' *The Los Angeles Times,* 30 June. Online. Available at www.aericles.laimes.com/2011/un/30/world/la-fg-china-train-20110701.html (accessed 1 August 2011).

48  Foster, Peter (2011) 'China to create largest megacity in the world with 42 million people,' *The Telegraph*, 24 January. Online. Available at www.telegraph.co.uk/ournalists/peter-foster/html (accessed 14 March 2011).

49  Ibid., p. 3. Also see Lei, Qi and Lu, Bin (2008) 'Urban sprawl: A case study in Shenzhen, China.' Paper presented at the 44th ISOCARP Congress, 2008.

50  Shank, Megan and Wasserstrom, Jeffrey (2011) 'China's high-speed crash leads to legitimacy crisis,' *Miller-McCune*, 29 July 2011. Online. Available at www.miller-mccune.com/politics/chinas-high-speed-rail-crash/html (accessed 30 July 2011).

51  Yin, Cao and Yinan, Zhao (2011) 'Fire risk rising as cities grow taller,' *China Daily*, 30 June. Online. Available at www.chinadaily.com.cn/china/2011-06/30/content_12805031.html (accessed 1 August 2011).

52  Woetzel, Jonathan (2011) *China's cities in the sky*. 'What Matters,' 7 January. Online. Available at www. whatmatters.mckinseydigital.com/cities/china.html (accessed 15 February 2011).

53  Gluckman, Ron (2011) 'Skyscraper, moneymaker,' *The New York Times*, 12 April, p. D6.

54  Goldhagen, Sarah Williams (2010) 'Democracies need physical spaces,' *The Dirt*, 22 October. Online. Available at www.dirt.asla.org/2010/10/22/goldhagen-democracies-need-physical-spaces-in-cities.html (accessed 1 January 2011).

55  Ma, Xiulian (2006) 'Foreign direct investment, urban sprawl, and coastal states in China.' Paper presented at the American Sociological Association Annual Meeting, Montreal, August. Online. Available at www. allacademia.com//meta/p_mla_apa_research.html (accessed 12 February 2011).

56  Goodson, Teddy (2010) 'China facts we should consider when thinking ahead (if we do),' *Blue Virginia*, 6 August. Online. Available at www.bluevirginia.us/user/Teddy%20Goodson.html (accessed 12 August 2010).

57  Batson, Andrew (2008) 'China to create market for land rights in effort to boost farmers' prosperity,' *The Wall Street Journal*, 20 October. Online. Available at www.online.wsj.com/article/SB12244598532148351. html (accessed 27 July 2011).

58  Hessler, Peter (2011) *Country Driving: A Journey Through China from Farm to Factory*. New York: Harper.

59  Anon. (2011) 'Car purchase lottery starts in traffic clogged Beijing,' *People's Daily Online (English)*, 26 January. Online. Available at www.english.peopledaily.com.cn/90001/09776/90882/7273516. html (accessed 29 July 2011).

60 Burns, Melinda (2011) 'Can China avoid getting stuck in traffic?' *Miller-McCune*, 6 February. Online. Available at www.miller-mccune.com/environment/ca-china-avoid-getting-stuck-in-traffic-27997/html (accessed 8 March 2011).

61 Ibid., p. 3.

62 Khawarzad, Aurash (2011) 'Urban freeways: A negative pattern being exported to China,' *Pattern Cities*, 12 January. Online. Available at www.patterncities.com/archives/302.html (accessed 8 March 2011).

63 Tse, Edward (2010) 'The China challenge,' *Strategy+Business*, Spring: 34–43. Online. Available at www.strategy-business.com.html (accessed 12 February 2011).

64 Praendl-Zika, Veronica (2006) *Urban Sprawl in China: Land Use Change at the Transition from Village to Town. Technical Report.* Oikodrom—The Vienna Institute for Urban Sustainability. Online. Available at www.holcimfoundation.org/portals/1/docs.html (accessed 12 February 2011).

65 Malhotra, Shriya (2009) 'Conflating boundaries to envision urban public health,' *Parsons Journal for Information Mapping*, 1(3): 1–27.

66 Wilson, E.H. (2003) 'Development of a geospatial model to quantify, describe and map urban growth,' *Remote Sensing of Environments*, 86(3): 275–285.

67 Vir Gupta, Pankaj (2011) 'Urban journal: mapping the city,' *Indiarealtime*, 8 March. Online. Available at www.indiarealtime/2011/03/08/urban-journal-mapping-the-city/html (accessed 8 August 2010).

68 Brown, Lester R. (2010) 'The return of the bicycle,' *IPS News*, 10 July. Online. Available at www.ipsnews.net/interna.asp?idnews+52066.html (accessed 24 August 2010).

69 Shoup, Donald C. (2005) *The High Cost of Free Parking*. Washington, D.C: American Planning Association. The average auto in the U.S. is parked 95 percent of the time.

70 Motavalli, Jim (2005) 'Commentary: The high cost of free parking,' *E-magazine*. Online. Available at www.emagazine.com/view/?2418.html (accessed 10 August 2010).

71 Roca, J., Burns, M.C., and Carreras, J.M. (2008) 'Monitoring urban sprawl around Barcelona's metropolitan area with the aid of satellite imagery.' Paper presented at the 35th ISPRS Congress. Online. Available at www.isprs.org/proceedings/XXXV/congress/comm1/papers/53.pdf.html (accessed 12 March 2011).

72 Grimm, Nancy B., Faeth, Stanley H., Golubiewski, Nancy E., Redman, Charles L. Wu, Jianquo, Bai, Xuemei, and Briggs, John M. (2008) 'Global change and the ecology of cities,' *Science*, 8 February, 319(7): 756–760.

73 Fischer-Kowalski, Marina (1998) 'Society's metabolism: The intellectual history of materials flow analysis, Part I, 1860–1970,' *Journal of Industrial Ecology*, 2(1): 61–78.

74 Sassen, Saskia (2000) 'The global city: Strategic site/New frontier,' *American Studies*, 41(2/3): 79–95.

# 4

# TRANSFUSION: DESIGN CONSIDERATIONS

Sprawl is a complex system of systems. In the aggregate, it is about competing geographic, socio-economic, political, and cultural influences, each competing for attention and dominance. A rare opportunity exists at this moment to fundamentally reappraise, deconstruct, and reinvent. As has been discussed in the previous chapters, many signature aspects of sprawl machines are universal—reproducible—exhibited across board geographic and cultural landscapes. It would be dangerous and even naïve to postulate any single monolithic criterion that alone would be adequate to take on the complex inner profundities associated with remediating unmitigated sprawl. In other words, no single sprawl remediation method exists, given current geopolitical realities. The ubiquity of sprawl machines requires the simultaneous application of multiple remediation measures, measures implemented by diverse individuals and groups at scales spanning macro to micro levels of intervention. *Suburban transfusion*—a process involving the removal of dysfunctional tissue and its replacement with new tissue—offers promise as but one method to remediate sprawl and its deleterious public health consequences. It is proposed here as a process not unlike an organ transplant or blood transfusion in a human being. It is about the injection of a new sensibility in the suburban landscape. Suburban transfusion is iterative and it builds upon itself. Recent attempts to put forth so-called comprehensive remedies such as the New Urbanists' handbook, the *Smart Growth Manual*, miss the mark because they are too prescriptive and clinical in tone, content, and format.[1] Its step-by-step "how to" format (as evidenced in the book's title) comes off, unfortunately, too much like a car repair manual—the built environment is exponentially more complex than changing the spark plugs in your Volvo. Sprawl mitigation from a public health perspective requires:

- Taking cognizance of indigenous cultural traditions, demographic trends, and the health history of the community
- Articulating community aspirations with regards to disease prevention and health promotion
- Identifying obstacles to healthier lifestyles and behaviors
- Reinventing building codes and zoning regulations as needed to achieve successful transfusion
- Creating and sustaining strong grassroots support for the promotion of community public health and environmental stewardship
- Establishing sustainable public–private partnerships from the very beginning

- Obtaining the needed resources to reinvent existing physical infrastructure
- Modifying cultural attitudes to achieve healthier, more active lifestyles
- Developing metrics to define and assess progress and in making in-progress adjustments during implementation
- Exceeding expectations in the replacement of dead and dying built form (tissue) and infrastructures within suburban communities

A compendium of seventy-five transdisciplinary design considerations has been structured into five categories:

A.   Infrastructure (A1–A27)
B.   Ecological Architecture (B1–B20)
C.   Mall Transfusion (C1–C14)
D.   Suburban Agrarianism (D1–D7)
E.   Implementation (E1–E7)

This compendium of health-based design considerations is intended to be broadly interpreted and expanded upon by designers, planners, engineers, sustainability specialists, public healthcare providers, evidence-based health researchers, community activists, philanthropic foundations, politicians, governmental agencies, and, perhaps most importantly, by individual citizens and their grassroots neighborhood-based organizations. They are evidence-based, that is, based upon case studies and recent empirical research. The intent is for them to be revised and reshaped in response to new research findings. It is hoped this baseline lexicon is not misconstrued as prescriptive or didactic in tone, presentation format, or content because no less than a fundamental re-imagination of what is possible in the everyday built environment is needed at this time.

## A. Infrastructure

**Public Health in the Everyday Milieu (A1)**—Sprawl machines are unhealthy. They foster sedentary lifestyles. They foster environmental degradation and threaten natural ecologies. Health, in the broadest sense—physical, spiritual, social, personal, and environmental—should not be compartmentalized into small corners of our lives or small corners of the built environment. Equally so, health should be the basis of our entire existence and the continued existence of a healthier planet. Chronic health conditions, whether human-based or ecologically based, place needless limitations on the lives of tens of millions around the globe. Heart disease, cancer, and diabetes are the leading causes of death and disability in the U.S., and in many other developed nations; in the U.S. alone they account for 70 percent of all deaths (1.7 million each year). These diseases cause major limitations and put serious restrictions on daily living for almost one in ten Americans, nearly 25 million people. Children and the aged are two groups who are particularly susceptible. In suburbia, less than 40 percent of older adults in the U.S. obtain regular routine vaccinations. Much more can be done to encourage self-health promotion in the everyday landscape. One such initiative is called SPARC (Sickness Prevention Achieved through Regional Collaboration), co-sponsored on a pilot basis by the U.S. Centers for Disease Control and Prevention (CDC). It has yielded success in broadening the use of recommended preventive services among older adults. A field evaluation by the CDC found increases in immunizations for influenza and pneumococcal disease, and more screening for breast, cervical, and colo-rectal cancers as well as for cholesterol and high blood pressure among participants.

SPARC's operative approach is to establish collaboration and coordination across a wide array of community agencies and organizations, i.e. local health departments, area agencies on aging, and local healthcare providers with a vested interest in health promotion among the aged. An innovative feature has been Vote & Vax, a strategy that makes vaccines and appointments for cancer screenings available at neighborhood polling places on election days.[2] Endeavor to establish wellness centers and primary care clinics in formerly dead malls and other vacant buildings. Provide healthcare services, particularly geared to the aged, children, and to medically underserved members of historically disadvantaged groups. Promote wellness through education on how a healthier lifestyle through physical activity in the outdoor and indoor built environment can improve one's long-term quality of life (Figure 4.1).

**Competing Discourses (A2)**—The New Urbanism is paradoxical. To its critics, it is a what-once-was-old-is-new-again interpretive excursion in urban and regional planning and architecture discourse, drawing its core inspirations almost exclusively from 19th-century town planning precepts. In response, they argue back it is in fact a highly progressive movement insofar as it rejects mindless sprawl and its unchecked deleterious consequences. Indeed, sprawl does promote social isolation and unhealthy lifestyles: it inhibits face-to-face social intercourse in the public realm, inhibits the drawing together of diverse groups of people, inhibits engagement in healthful physical activity in the outdoor realm, and is environmentally unsustainable. It is a risk, however, to buy into New Urbanism's attacks and its proposed solutions to sprawl's inner profundities without a more thoughtful analysis of sprawl's broader socio-cultural, economic, political, aesthetic, and landscape infrastructural under-pinnings. Will the obese, for instance, simply switch from their fossil fuel to their new non-fossil fuel

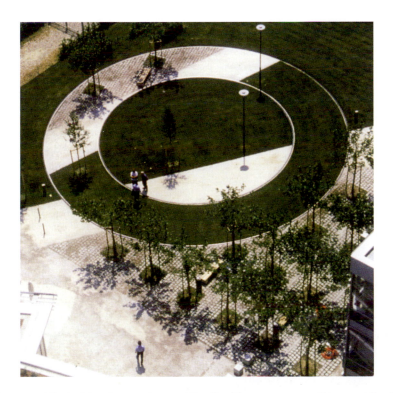

**FIGURE 4.1**   Courtyard Park, New Jersey, Acconci Studio. Photo courtesy of Acconci Studio

car? As for the socio-cultural parameters of the New Urbanism, its critics argue it is elitist, neo-romantic, nostalgic—a call for density and compactness at any cost. In the age of globalization we face challenges that will require pluralistic responses, with no single built environment theoretical discourse fully "equipped" to respond alone. Yet this is precisely what New Urbanism seeks to do at this moment in history—to establish itself as the standard of excellence. It runs real risk of becoming dominant in places such as post-Katrina New Orleans, in post-earthquake Haiti, in India and now in seeking to extend its reach into China's burgeoning metropolises. The danger does exist that its singular reinterpretation of history will have, in retrospect, been misinterpreted both in terms of where we were a century ago as much as where we need to go in the future. It is therefore healthy for competing theoretical discourses to co-exist and learn from one another as long as the public's health and the ecological health of the planet remain of utmost priority. It would be rather unhealthy for any singular perspective, New Urbanism or otherwise, to attain hegemony in seeking to express the *zeitgeist*. In the 21st century, blended, plural, hybrid, non-hegemonistic infrastructuralities are needed. It is time for both/and rather than either/or theoretical discourses.

**Sprawl and the Medically Underserved (A3)**—Thousands of dead and near-dead malls in the U.S. are located within or on the edge of lower-middle- and low-income communities. Many of the residents who reside in these neighborhoods are among the 47 million Americans who lack comprehensive medical insurance protection. Individuals and families with partial coverage fall into the category of the medically underinsured, while individuals and families without any insurance whatsoever are referred to as medically uninsured. These places are medically underserved communities. Their vulnerable populations are at risk of adverse health effects by circumstances involving such factors as lack of income, homelessness, developmental or mental health disability, and racial and ethnic discrimination. They lack the functional healthcare infrastructure, i.e. hospitals, clinics, and allied healthcare services essential to the provision of a safety net of preventative care. As a result, many persons do not receive care and become sicker than would otherwise be the case and they then have no option but to seek out far costlier hospital emergency care as the option of last resort. The opportunity exists to transform dead and dying buildings within sprawl machines, including dead/dying malls and strip centers, into viable, valued resources for community and personal health and wellness. The definition of what constitutes a community's public health infra-structure must expand. Work for radical change in medically underserved communities, turning them into centers for the elevation of the public's health. In so doing, the immediate neighborhood as well as the entire city's quality of life will have been elevated. The elimination of medically under-served neighborhoods will uplift everyone and provide common ground for persons of all ages to congregate and interact together in a far more health-supportive manner (Figure 4.2).

**Food Deserts and Sprawl (A4)**—Many neighborhoods in America's inner cities and poorer inner suburbs lack the nutritional infrastructure for their residents to maintain a proper diet. A food desert is an area that provides little or no access to the foods needed to maintain a healthy diet and that is served instead by a disproportionate number of fast-food franchise restaurants and convenience stores. The large food chains long ago abandoned these places and in their place the residents are left with a corner convenience store that nearly exclusively sells unhealthy food. This food is high in carbohydrates, saturated fat, sugar and artificial preservatives, and there is a near complete absence of fruit and vegetables. These food establishments cater to people with few options because many do not have private transportation to make the long drive to the nearest suburban supermarket. More than fifty studies have examined the unequal distribution of food resources, as measured by proximity to commercial food outlets. More than 6.5 million U.S. children

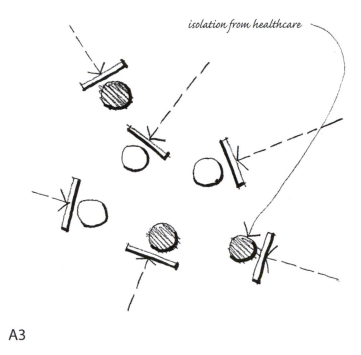

A3

**FIGURE 4.2** Eliminate Medically Underserved Neighborhoods

live in communities without supermarkets, and agricultural and food distribution polices have been set at the national level with little or no concern for these communities. The U.S. Centers for Disease Control and Prevention (CDC) Healthy Communities Program provides grants to cities to develop methods to counter the deleterious health outcomes associated with residents struggling to cope with being trapped within urban and suburban food deserts.[3] Some positive changes are underway to ameliorate the underlying conditions that have resulted in food desertification. Large and small food retailers in many U.S. cities are starting to build smaller stores within mixed-use centers in neighborhoods that previously did not have any full service grocery store. These markets are increasingly within walking distance, and near public transport routes. Recent examples include three new Safeway's in Washington, D.C., and the New Season Market, in Portland, Oregon.[4]

**Children, the Aged, and Sprawl (A5)**—Children who grow up in sprawl machines often lack viable places to exercise outdoors. Their neighborhood may not have sidewalks or bike paths, parks, or places to play sports that are within close proximity to home or school. Additionally, social networking sites such as Facebook and high-tech video games exert an increasingly inhibiting effect on young people's engagement in alternative outdoor physical activities. These devices function as electronic pacifiers, as magnets, with the net effect of contributing to keeping children and adolescents indoors when in the past they would have often likely been engaged in non-sedentary recreational activities outdoors. It is a pity, as young people can benefit in myriad ways from sustained/sustainable exposure to the outdoors and to nature. Regular physical activity has many important health benefits for children, including aerobic capacity, weight maintenance, and the psychological benefits that accompany physical fitness among one's peers. Regular physical activity as a child can reduce one's chances of developing chronic disease as an adult. Diseases such as heart disease and osteoporosis have their origins in early life. Obese children often suffer from elevated blood pressure, hypertension, orthopedic abnormalities, discrimination, and, in females, menstrual abnormalities. Once overweight, a child tends to suffer this condition throughout life.[5] Physical inactivity is the single biggest threat to healthfulness among children and adolescents. The distance from home to school often is too far to walk. Parental fear of unsafe traffic in the immediate vicinity also contributes to overreliance on the auto for daily transport. A 1999 CDC study asked parents if their children faced obstacles getting to school on foot or on bicycle. Distance from school was the biggest obstacle (cited by 55 percent of respondents), followed by traffic dangers (40 percent). Only 16 percent indicated no present dangers.[6] Similarly, for the aged who are stranded due to their inaccessibility to public transport, sprawl machines ostensibly created to provide safe play spaces for young people yielded large *superblocks* disconnected from one another. Major traffic arteries separating the quilt work of subdivisions from one another are, hence, too congested, lacking sidewalks or bike lanes; these barriers restrict walking or bicycling even within one's subdivision. Worse, public parks are often few and far between, the result of speculative homebuilding without adequate set-aside provisions for public health.

**Reverse Infrastructural Decline (A6)**—Sprawl machines are perpetuated in the name of economic expansion—job creation, to be more specific—or as a symbol of a developing nation having arrived at some level of parity with the West. As a result, citizens too often foot the bill for poorly planned or otherwise misguided public infrastructural "improvements" put forth by officials and/or private developers in the name of progress. In the U.S., the Troubled Asset Relief Program (TARP) resulted in the infusion of billions of federal stimulus funds in 2008–2010 for the purpose of upgrading the nation's degraded public infrastructure of decayed bridges, roads, and civic facilities, but has to date yielded widely varying results. In Easley, South Carolina, for instance, $13.5 million in public funds, including $6 million in federal TARP stimulus funds, paid for the construction of a new bridge that replaced a two-lane bridge built over sixty years ago. The new four-lane bridge involved creating an expanded intersection, with two dedicated left turn lanes. This new intersection and bridge were elevated 10 feet higher on earthen berms and a completely new roadbed was constructed in both approaching directions for an adjacent state highway that parallels the train tracks. The project was justified on the basis that the old bridge was too low and therefore posed a hazard to passing trains. It proved to be no more than a thinly disguised enticement for Wal-Mart to build a new superstore on an open parcel directly across the tracks. Wal-Mart abandoned its older, existing store on the other side of town only because of this new bridge and politicians' promise of the upgraded access roads. Immediately afterwards, Wal-Mart opened its mammoth superstore.[7] The adjacent parcels were subdivided for mini big box outlets on the stipulation the developer build a number of other new structures at this site, although (to date) the slow economy has resulted in newly built yet mostly empty storefronts. It is nearly impossible to walk or cycle there because there are no paths or sidewalks along the primary access roads. Taxpayer funds paid for nearly the entire fiasco (Figure 4.3). This is no way to redirect resources in order to combat the deleterious public health effects of auto dependency in suburbia.

**Landtrusting (A7)**—Government-sponsored, private philanthropic, and joint public-private coalitions are a promising solution to this unfortunate condition. A *land trust*, or *conservancy*, is a private, non-profit organization that actively works to conserve land by undertaking or assisting land acquisition and stewardship activities. It typically consists of an agreement whereby a trustee agrees to hold ownership of a parcel of property for the benefit of another party. In the U.S., the Washington, D.C.-based Land Trust Alliance was formed in 1982 (then called the Land Trust Exchange) as a national conservation organization, and it currently represents more than 1,700 land

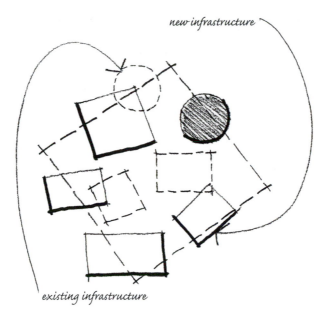

*new infrastructure*

*existing infrastructure*

**FIGURE 4.3**   Reverse Infrastructural Decline

trusts nationwide. It strives to advance favorable tax polices, best practices, and foster further land trusting in the face of continued threats. As of 2010, its membership represented 37 million acres. Land trusts have existed since Roman times but their most direct lineage dates from the reign of Henry VIII in England. In the U.S., lands trusts date from the late 19th century, in Illinois, and the 1891 Trustees of Reservations, and currently operate in all fifty states and in many other parts of the world. Over 300 new local land trusts were formed in the period from 1998 to 2003, and 173 in California alone. The goal is to preserve sensitive natural areas, farmland, ranchland, water sources, cultural resources, and notable landmarks forever. Private-sector initiatives overlaid with federal policies of using "stimulus" or similar funds can foster economic competitiveness, environmental sustainability, and social inclusiveness.[8] Another source of financial support consists of private equity markets. In this scenario, a portion of the acquired land entrusted would become permanent green-fields, restored as wetlands, or parkland. The Spanish firm ecosistema urbano designed such a place for the outskirts of Maribor, Slovenia, a former municipal landfill site in the process of ecological as well as economic recovery. The multi-phased aspects of this infrastructural conversion will occur over a period of ten years (Figure 4.4).[9] At present, scant funds exist for the transformation of dead malls, subdivisions, and industrial sites and their related infrastructures into redeveloped natural ecologies within the suburban milieu. In the U.S. it would be prudent at this time to establish legislation such as a National Anti-Sprawl Act or a Dead Mall Conversion Act, with the principal aim at increasing the rate of land trusts dedicated to reverting seas of pavement to parks and related ecologically sensitive infrastructural redevelopment for the public's benefit. Suffice to say, myriad long-term challenges remain, with the largest challenge quite possibly continuing the sheer lack of a national commitment to promote its cultural legacies or public health in this manner.

**Cyburbia (A8)**—The concept of *intelligent cities* has become an uppermost policy priority to those who plan and design built environment infrastructural systems. It expresses in many ways the essence of applying 21st-century person–environment digital technologies in our daily life. Handheld devices

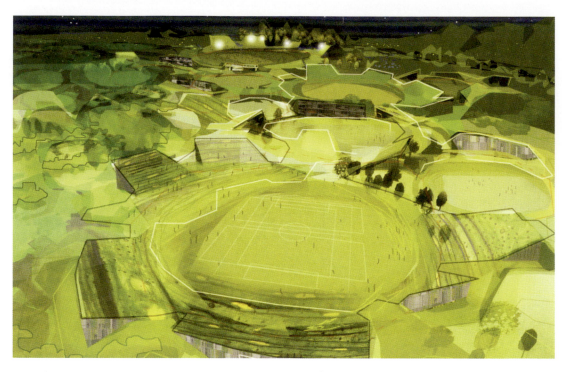

**FIGURE 4.4** Landfill Reclamation, Maribor, Slovenia, ecosistema urbano. Photo courtesy of ecosistema urbano

provide information on a 24/7 basis about when and how many people cross a given street, road congestion data, or the peak use periods at a given restaurant, grocery store, or transit station. Soon, these devices may be implanted on our clothing, or bodies. Handheld software informs commuters of available parking slots in a parking deck, optimal routes there and back any given time, day or night, or whether the public transit route closest in proximity to one's destination is running on time. This trend reflects *smart growth*: an extension of smart growth infrastructural planning precepts. As smart growth's emphasis on density and compactness has become mainstream public policy in many communities, cyberurbanism (cyburbia) has gained traction through the backing of environmentalists and large corporations such as IBM, Siemens, Phillips, and Cisco. The term cyberurbanism appears to have first been used in 1997.[10] Digital software apps and hardware technologies now enable people to interact synchronously with the built environment on multiple levels of engagement. This technology will, if properly channeled, spark citizen engagement with respect to infrastructural management and quality of life issues of public health concern from the scale of the private residence, workplace, to the civic scale. The challenge will be to harness and make sense of the immense volumes of data now available at our fingertips. Technologies are meshing to enable the sculpting of new, collaged networks so that an individual can in effect *design* one's hourly and daily transactions with/within the built and natural environment. It is possible to link personal health indicators, such as obesity rates in a given neighborhood with, for example, physical attributes such as the quality and condition of sidewalks, type of available housing options in the search for an apartment, local public transport amenities, whether bike lanes exist, the caloric content of food served at the local restaurants, as well as walking distance times to the nearest public transit stop. Public access Wi-Fi networks quickly gave rise to cyburbanism. For persons currently living amid sprawl, it can function to attract them back to denser infill neighborhoods if they know that density per se need not be feared and can be far more intelligently navigated than before. Cyberurbanism need not be geographically tethered solely to urban centers; it is a universal model for everyday life. During periods of economic expansion (or otherwise) smart growth management, if cogently applied, seamlessly, with cyburbanism, will help to guide and shape intelligent infrastructural reinvestment.

**Smart Grids (A9)**—As population densities increase in metropolitan areas around the globe, unrestricted sprawl machines further burden already stretched municipal infrastructures. Many systems are already buckling through decades of expanded user demand, deferred maintenance, disinvestment, and political indifference (utility grids don't vote). One answer is for our infra-structures to perform *smarter* than they do today. Suburban transfusion calls for integrating electrical, water, sewerage, gas and solid waste systems, security, and emergency response infrastructure, transport, and other related systems into coordinated networks. A transparent coordination of municipal utilities, ERP (enterprise resource planning), and financial systems can yield less energy consumption. The Pecan Street initiative in Austin, Texas, seeks to do precisely this. The pilot program compares conventional housing with recently built "green houses" in the study of consumer energy consumption patterns. Smart energy grids collect data at fifteen-minute intervals (or greater) for all customers within the network's geographic reach. Individual smart grid consumer-customers can monitor their energy consumption online at these same fifteen-minute intervals. By contrast, non-smart grids at present typically collect only monthly readings of energy usage. Large-scale smart grids are currently being developed in Dubai's Internet City, Kochi, in India, and in Guangzhou, China. Post-World War II sprawl communities in the U.S. will increasingly see the benefits of mustering the civic will and the requisite financial resources to develop smart grids in their communities. But this will be an uphill struggle in existing suburbs. In a trailer park in a walkable, pedestrian-scaled older section of Santa Monica, California, mobile homes constructed entirely of formaldehyde-free materials, and with 2kW solar photovoltaic panels on their roofs, send energy back to the grid. The status quo is hard to break because it is far more expedient and cheaper to implement smart grid technologies in newly built, greenfield site contexts. In older communities there is also often the natural tendency of citizens to be deeply distrustful of any "big brother" inter-ventions perceived as a threat to their personal liberties.[11] This is understandable to a certain extent, although it is self-defeating, ultimately. Intelligently built and operated smart grid infrastructural networks in transfused suburbs require "smart meters" or *smartometers* placed on every structure within the geographic grid. New educational programs and public polices will need to be structured to notify consumers of the optimal times to draw, and when not to draw down, energy from the local smart grid (Figure 4.5).

**Subterranean Utilities (A10)**—A majority of rights-of-ways (ROW) and associated utility systems within the mid-20th-century precincts of sprawl machines remain a rough, frayed patch-work, the result of generations of incremental revisions and repairs. The aging, ubiquitous above-ground network of utility wires and poles that dominate many urban and suburban streetscapes often detract much. Their presence detracts aesthetically because in the majority of instances the tangle of poles, wires, and junction boxes overshadow a streetscape's overall image. They are often intrusive, unnecessary infrastructural components. It is counterintuitive to retain these elements as aboveground amenities in suburban communities undergoing reinvestment and redevelopment and yet it is far easier for politicians to gain votes by proposing aboveground public taxpayer infra-structural investments versus belowground investments in infrastructure. One is seen by all, the other

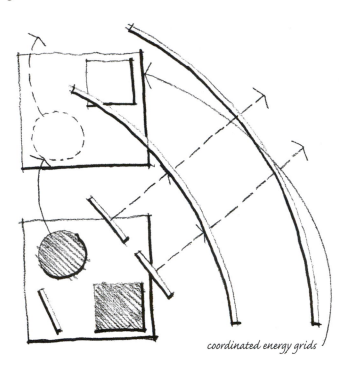

*coordinated energy grids*

**FIGURE 4.5**    Construct Smart Grids

is invisible. The adage "out of sight, out of mind" is apropos. Strategies are needed to reverse this unfortunate bias on the part of the general public, for it does it a major disservice in both the short and long term. This is of particular concern in older, inner suburban settings where gangly overhead wires stand out awkwardly, conflated by streetscapes characterized by excessively low densities between buildings, further compounded by the absence of trees or other types of vegetation. Utility location is the process of identifying and labeling public utility mains which are underground. These mains may include lines for telephones, electrical distribution, natural gas, cable television, fiber optics, traffic lights, streetlights, storm drains, water mains, and wastewater lines. Utility color codes are used in the U.S. for identifying underground utilities. The American Public Works Association (APWA) Uniform Color Codes consists of nine colors and is an aid to better coordinate location and interfacing between types of below-grade infrastructural utility systems. Integrated subterranean strategies are called for that consider the below-grade infrastructure as being of equal importance to all above-grade improvements such as new and renovated buildings, green spaces, and the like. It is integral to an ecological architecture: encompassing all rights-of-ways and related, complex utility systems above and belowground. Coordinated rights-of-ways (ROWs) afford much potential for improved integration of services. Significant economic and environmental benefits are accruable through integration of all underground utility support systems in support of above-ground public transport, water, sewer, lighting, and power grids serving carbon neutral buildings and recreational amenities.[12]

**TOADS and Sprawl (A11)**—A dead mall is a a temporary, obsolete, abandoned, or derelict site (TOAD). The aforementioned Internet site deadmalls.com is filled with descriptions of scores of dead and dying shopping malls across the U.S. The TOAD phenomenon owes its existence to the rapid construction, consumption, abandonment, and discarding of land parcels and their structures; a trend occurring in the wake of hyper-intense overexpansion.[13] The current economic system is structured to foster massive overdevelopment. Abandoned malls, big boxes, strip centers, shuttered industrial sites, abandoned landfills—often are brownfield sites with tattered histories of environmental mismanagement and degradation. Forest Park Mall was once a 400,000 square foot enclosed mall in a south Chicago suburb. It was built on the site of a World War II naval torpedo plant. After that, it was used as a naval training site. Currently, the Living World Christian Center occupies a part of the dead mall. Chicago's' granddaddy dead mall, however, is the Dixie Square Mall, in Harvey, Illinois, in another nearby suburb. It was prominently featured in the 1980 film *The Blues Brothers* and was already closed for a year before filming began. Since then it has been subjected to various questionable redevelopment proposals for its rebirth, but none has come to fruition. The mall has been vacant for more than thirty years, and has been condemned for public health and safety concerns. In 2010, a $4 million federal grant was awarded for its demolition. Believe it or not the plan is to redevelop the site for *shopping* (presumably big box outlets in a power center configuration), but this time with light industry and affordable housing included.[14] An important activity of local grassroots neighborhood organizations is to identify all TOADs within their local community and to analyze each site/building relative to its unique strengths, challenges, and opportunities for redevelopment.

**LULUs and Sprawl (A12)**—Unmitigated sprawl produces undesirable land uses and development patterns and yet much of such development is deemed essential, at least at the outset, i.e. schools, branch libraries, hospitals, and malls for the jobs they generate and so on. In time, however, these come to yield undesirable outcomes. A locally unwanted land use (LULU) is planning jargon for a specific land use deemed useful to society-at-large yet found to be objectionable to its immediate neighbors. It is perceived as posing a dilemma for surrounding communities due to the way it may look, smell, sound, or pollute the environment. The term was coined in 1981 and includes, in the U.S., public housing, homeless shelters, shelters for victims of domestic violence, fire stations, national guard training facilities, landfills, industrial sites, refineries, distribution centers, even educational institutions, medical centers, correctional centers, and prisons. Society agrees that each entity in its own right is important yet no one wants one of them in his or her own backyard. The attitude often is "Better it were in someone else's neighborhood." Historically, LULU sites were typically mandated from the top-down, independent of input from local grassroots organizations and local politics.[15] A related dilemma swirls around the myriad issues associated with *environmental racism*—racial disparities imposed across a range of actions and policies in both the public and private sectors. It is premised on patterns of land use whereby poor communities are exposed to pollution and exploitation largely created and perpetrated for the benefit of wealthier communities elsewhere. For example, LULUs often foster leapfrog development patterns because, in accord with NIMBYism (not in my back yard) they end up being built at the suburban fringe and spawn new roads and related infrastructural "improvements" that extend further the boundaries of sprawl. This occurred in Louisiana's once rural but increasingly suburban "cancer corridor" that stretches up the Mississippi River from New Orleans to Baton Rouge. It is a nettlesome challenge to ameliorate the effects of these development patterns, after the fact. For these reasons, local organizations need to strive to anticipate *a priori* the full ramifications of LULUs so their many negative impacts are abated outright.

**Cell Tower Epidemic (A13)**—The ubiquitous cell tower and its associated side effects—*cell-toweritis*—has become an integral component of sprawl machines. These intrusive transmission towers have been constructed all across the American landscape and elsewhere since about 1990 and have become a virtual high-tech plague on the landscape. The visual blight caused by this development pattern is spreading globally. In populated areas, masts are typically sited 1–2 miles apart, and in dense urban areas are sited only one fourth to one half mile apart. Their owners often resort to clandestine tactics in order to get them built. More and more, cell masts are being camouflaged as *stealth sites*—as telephone poles, light poles, as ornamentation (such as a striped red–white candy cane at holiday time)—even as religious *crosses*, including the 100-foot tall white cross erected at Epiphany Lutheran Church in Lake Worth, Florida. Some stealth masts express biomorphic aspirations, disguised to resemble palm trees and pine trees. The U.S. Federal Telecommunications Act of 1996, Section 704, guaranteed corporations the right to erect innumerable cell towers, overriding local zoning laws, although many public health questions remain unresolved because human response to electromagnetic fields remains poorly understood. In spite of this, more than 154 million Americas acquired cell phones between 1992 and 2004, resulting in the proliferation of thousands of ungainly towers. As with billboards, land speculators frequently acquire permits to erect towers and tower farms well in advance of demand.[16] A *tower farm* consists of a cluster of broadcast towers, such as the grove of cell towers perched atop Paris Mountain in Greenville, South Carolina. The suburban mast is perhaps the most insidious type, however, because it is sneaked in behind parking lots, at the edges of strip malls, public parks, along roadsides, and next to churches. At street level, they are often sequestered behind fences "invisibly" to the extent possible, although they are anything but invisible. It remains curious that the New Urbanists, other advocates for smart growth, and health advocates do not directly address the ubiquity of these towers or their potential long term public health consequences. Regardless, local communities should remain highly skeptical of requests to approve cell towers in their neighborhood until more is known of their effects on the public's health.

**Greenfielding (A14)**—Cities continually evolve. It remains axiomatic that some flourish while others wither. A major event such as an earthquake, hurricane, or a severe economic tsunami can result in massive change and the reasons are many and well documented. When a once flourishing urban center or sprawl agglomeration experiences a period of rapid downward change, it often occurs through a combination of internal as well as external determinants. This remains the situation facing cities such as Detroit, Michigan. Longtime observers, current and former residents, and various civic boosters of Detroit within the city and elsewhere are attempting to stem the hemorrhaging. The same has happened in other cites fallen on difficult economic times in recent years (Figure 4.6). In Detroit, the controversial conversion of once economically and culturally vibrant neighborhoods into urban farms is being proposed as an alternative to urban blight. In the New Orleans Katrina-devastated Lower Ninth Ward neighborhood, the Ford Foundation in 2010 awarded the Greater New Orleans Foundation (GNOF) a $1.3 million grant to explore and implement a locally controversial land trust program to help resuscitate its severely depopulated post-flood neighborhoods. Prior to Katrina in 2005, more than 18,000 persons lived in this area of the city. As of 2011, however, this number had shriveled to approximately 2,800.[17] Auto travel had been required for most aspects of daily life in these neighborhoods, while they de-evolved from medium density residential enclaves to a virtual urban prairie.[18] In conducting due diligence studies of the costs/benefits of urban greenfielding—converting once inhabited, economically sustainable but now blighted areas into green space—it remains prudent to explore all the options and ramifications of doing so. Increasingly, suburban communities too are forced to confront these same challenges to ensure their continued viability.

**Redfielding (A15)**—In the jargon of redevelopment, the terms greenfield, brownfield, and grayfield are now joined by *redfield*, as applied to a building/site that is drowning in red ink or has fallen into foreclosure. It generally denotes an underperforming or underwater property, i.e. the amount

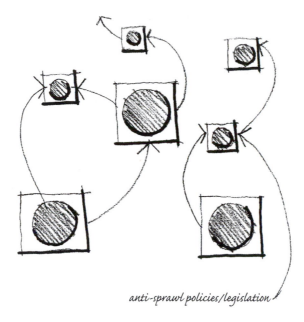

*anti-sprawl policies/legislation*

**FIGURE 4.6**   Greenfielding

owed on its financing is greater than the property's current market value, or foreclosed-upon properties. In the past it has generally been seen as a financial condition, not a development strategy per se but recently it has taken on a redevelopment dimension, in relation to sprawl. A brownfield or grayfield site can also be a redfield site, along with any distressed, outmoded, or undesirable built landscapes, i.e. a failed apartment complex, dead mall, abandoned in-ruin steel mill, commercial strip, big box store, or an unfinished subdivision fallen victim to the Great Recession.[19] A redfield-to-greenfield program is an initiative aimed at reducing the oversupply of near-dead and dead properties in a given market while seeking to reinvigorate the immediate site environs. One strategy that has gained momentum in recent few years involves the systematic acquisition of underperforming and/or vacant properties, clearing the land, then transforming them and restoring the site to its pre-development state as green open space and/or as land conservation zones. Such landscape restorations can be permanent civic interventions or held in land-banked status and viewed as temporal interventions, held in a trust until the local real estate market recovers. Support for such public-private initiatives is being provided in the U.S. by the City Parks Alliance, a national advocacy coalition of parks professionals, environmental groups, and citizen organizations. The first case study was implemented in 2010 in Atlanta and is currently centered at the Georgia Institute of Technology. To date, parallel feasibility studies have been completed in Cleveland, Denver, Houston, Los Angeles, Phoenix, and the Savannah-Hilton Head area. In this scenario, a dead shopping mall can be reverted back into a wetlands conservation zone, with adjacent dead properties equally benefitting in the process as a valuable parcel of nature now exists that did not before, and with regards to adjacent infill sites that can greatly benefit from the adjoining redfielding intervention. There is, however, the risk that a redfielding program could be launched and then midstream become undermined by rising land values, thereby placing pressure on land reclamation developers to delete the land conservation component and/or set-aside landscape restoration provisos. In distressed markets this practice is particularly well suited to declining or dead suburban commercial zones although it is considered unsuitable to apply to currently greenfield or agricultural land at the suburban fringe in situations where stable land values prevail.

**Water and Sprawl (A16)**—Water is a life sustaining resource that pervades the atmosphere as clouds, rain, humidity, haze, hail, sleet, snow, rainbows, and vapor. In terms of its conservation and consumption, a full reappraisal of its many environmental and human benefits has been underway for some time. Wastewater discharge ecologies are often in direct conflict with the consumption of land for profit-making purposes: namely, subdivisions. Water is by no means an infinitely available, low-cost resource as if always present for endless consumption. Rainwater flows across driveways, parking lots, roadways, and other impervious surfaces, draining away the accumulated wastes of sprawl machines— including oil and related toxic chemicals discharged from fossil fuel powered vehicles.[20] For millennia, water has been valued, celebrated, and ritualized in everyday life and in religious ceremonies. The ancient Roman baths were places of prominence in local civic life. Sadly, the post-World War II suburb relegates water to low status, as of functional necessity only. Rainwater is treated as mere waste, to be eliminated quickly, routed through gutters and storm sewers and catch basins prior to discharge into lakes, streams, and wetlands. It is often concealed, hidden underground, resurfacing only to sustain our daily hygiene needs then immediately flushed out of sight. Water conservation ecologies will be central to smart growth within salutogenetic public health discourses centered on global climate change: rising seas, natural disasters, atmospheric pollution, and water wars fought in drought-stricken areas and areas suffering from aquifer depletion. It will become an ever higher status resource because it covers 70 percent of the earth's surface. Suburbia must rethink its relationship to water, its role in landscape reclamation and conservation, and develop appropriate stewardship protocols honoring and valuing its presence (and potential absence), and the hardships inflicted upon natural and human-built environment ecologies. Landscape reclamation will entail, in part, deconstructing massive expanses of underutilized, impervious pavement, with the aim of restoring natural hydrological processes.

**Water Typologies (A17)**—Over the past century, civil engineering prowess has defeated and devalued the naturalistic role of water. Engineers harness water in reservoirs, behind dams, in wells, in sewerage and storm drain systems, behind levees, in cisterns, and in potable water distribution systems. Water is of critical necessity to the cellular structure of living organisms and is the unifying element of natural ecologies which support life (Figure 4.7). Saltwater comprises 97 percent of all water on earth. Of the remaining 3 percent, most is in (melting) glaciers, the polar icecaps, and in non-circulating groundwater systems. The *biophilics* of water have been described as a typology comprised of nine constructs: *dominionistic* (the triumph of mastering a wild river or a long downhill ski run); *humanistic* (direct person-environment transactions); *naturalistic* (hiking a challenging, remote trail in a forest); *negativistic* (the fear of water, including floods, drowning, falling through ice, being swept away in a riptide, severe weather, and waterborne disease); *aesthetic* (a rainbow, deep blue ocean, sunset over water, sound of the surf, a mountain waterfall, rain, the rhythm of a thunderstorm, and the taste of freshwater); *moralistic* (ethics and conservation, equitable sharing, religious uses); *scientific* (aquatic chemistry, ecology, biology, hydraulics, groundwater transport); *symbolic* (communicative functions, ebb and flow patterns, force and restraint); and *utilitarian* (transportation, recreation, agriculture, aquaculture, waste disposal, hydropower, and nuclear power).[21] Suburban transfusion can benefit greatly from applying this typology to stormwater integration, water treatment for landscaping and for graywater functions, and in visible water features and systems. The buildings and landscape design elements within the Potsdamer Platz in Berlin integrate roof collection, downspouts, underground storage, retention ponds, and hydrologic connections with a nearby open canal and as such express many dimensions of the aforementioned biophilic typology.[22]

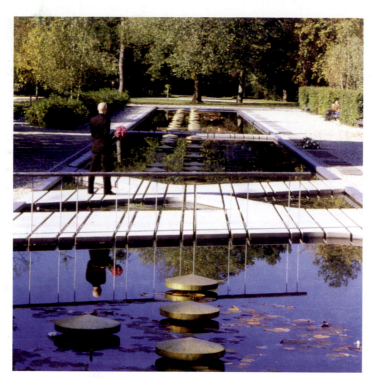

**FIGURE 4.7**    Zig Zag Watergarden, The Netherlands. Photo courtesy of Jeroen Musch/Karres en Brands Landschapsarchitecten

**Transform Water Edges (A18)**—Urban waterfronts in many parts of the globe are being transformed from their former shipping and related industrial land uses, and this is especially occurring in places where the prior commercial functions and land uses are no longer economically viable. The decline of land values adjacent to these bodies of water represents a tremendous opportunity to reinvent the adjoining water resource itself, i.e. ocean, river, or lakefront, the adjoining land, and to reaffirm the civic role and significance of both it and the adjacent land in terms of collective cultural memory, placemaking, visibility, and in the reappraisal of their combined importance to future generations. The reappraisal of water sites and their adjoining environs require viewing each as both a passive and active resource. Together, they can be restored/reclaimed to function as a single landscape ecology possessing diverse, deeply interconnected functional and aesthetic qualities. Endeavor to restore disused and underused shoreline landscapes with parks and wetlands, and retention ponds, lagoons, and wetland conservation zones where water can be seen and appreciated, and employed in a manner that promotes the community's public health. Similarly, bike and pedestrian paths that embrace these elements as one and link them to the larger neighborhood and beyond are significant contributions in public health promotion and more active living patterns. Explore hydro mimicry and naturally contoured forms versus highly rigid, anachronistic, regimented civil engineering solutions. Engineers tend to think in straight lines whereas the natural forms created by water are anything but straight lines. Employ ecological solutions and geometries found in nature, including biomorphic forms in harmony and not in opposition to the intrinsic aesthetics of the natural environment (Figure 4.8). Frederick Law Olmsted believed that naturally configured water elements in urban as well as

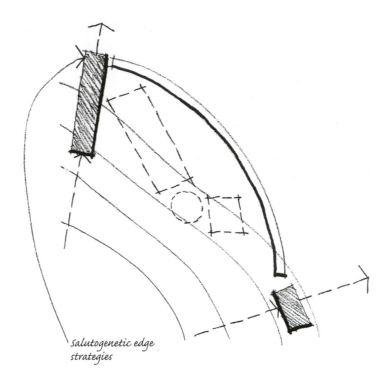

Salutogenetic edge
strategies

**FIGURE 4.8**   Transform Water Edges

inner ring suburban contexts function as magnets for human physical activity, and provide therapeutic respite to persons of all ages. Views of lagoons, people boating, geese, benches to sit and rest,
waterline paths, vistas, and shade trees contribute to a positive, therapeutic experience. Such experiences are absent within most sprawl machines because water was seen as a mere functional necessity
rather than a progenitor of a higher quality of life.[23]

**Recycle Stormwater (A19)**—The recycling of stormwater runoff is an overlooked opportunity
to reclaim a renewable natural resource that otherwise too quickly disappears from sight and from
reclamation measures and which afford Salutogenetic public health benefits to a community. This
can occur in many ways, such as a local organization adopting and restoring a long-abused creek that
for decades traversed a neighborhood, allowing polluted runoff to flow unabated off-site into underground canals and stormwater systems, later fouling the groundwater table in the process. A small
creek may be a perennial stream or a land configuration wet only after a storm event. Swales, and
linear vegetated depressions that retain stormwater are landscape design interventions that retain and
hold stormwater in a manner that simultaneously promotes natural infiltration cycles. These landscape interventions are far preferable alternatives to the conventional practice of the construction of
hundreds of miles of concrete curbs and storm drains. Rain gardens and human-made retention
pond/wetlands hold stormwater rather than disposing of the water for dispersal into the nearest
watercourse. The water that is retained on the surface can then be absorbed by vegetation through
natural infiltration. The standing water remains visible for some time after the rain event although it
now supports natural hydraulic ecologies. Buildings and bridges are in need of reappraisal in this
regard as they can be designed to be wholly integrated with adjacent surface stormwater retention

elements while simultaneously affording a positive aesthetic experience. Biologically active tanks, cells, cisterns, and related structures are capable of reprocessing and purifying wastewater on-site; such vessels contain plants, algae, microorganisms, bacteria, and fish.[24] Bio-remediation landscape elements are capable of breaking down organic contaminants in the blackwater or graywater waste stream. Retention vessels can be housed in a greenhouse or similar structure, extendable in size to several acres in outdoor site configurations. The purified water can then be discharged into a nearby wetland or recycled for use for non-drinking water purposes.[25]

**Brownfields as Energy Farms (A20)**—Numerous American cities are launching incentive programs to transform abandoned brownfield sites into large solar farms. Chicago's massive City Solar project is co-sponsoring the largest urban solar farm in the U.S., with 32,000 photovoltaic (PV) panels, providing 10 megawatts (MW) of energy, enough for 1,500 local homes. In addition, the farm's GPS tracking systems guide moveable heliotropic panels to capture the maximum amount of solar energy. Heavily contaminated brownfield sites can cost up to $150,000 per acre to remediate. The West Pullman site for City Solar would have cost $20 million alone to remediate. Instead, the corporate partner simply placed solar panels on the surface of the site, leaving contaminated subsurface soils relatively undisturbed. Similar programs have been launched in Philadelphia on a number of city-owned sites. In New York City, SPEED, a searchable database for heavily contaminated brownfield properties, has attracted much interest from private developers, as they peruse more than 3,150 vacant commercial and industrial sites dispersed throughout the city's five boroughs. To attract investment, local government created a $9 million reinvestment fund whereby a developer can receive upfront 60,000–140,000 to redevelop a given brownfield or grayfield site for solar farming or a closely related alternative energy source use. New York City also recently established a Green Property Certification program, which can provide online documented verification relative to a given site's potential for its intended new use.[26] Tens of thousands of dead shopping mall parking lots are available across the U.S. for similar adaptation to solar and/or wind farms. It is the responsibility of inventive local governments working together with the private sector to enact similar programs to attract reinvestment in alternate future energy sources within densely populated communities. Solar farms, in particular, are quiet neighbors, though it remains to be seen if they will in time be viewed as TOADs or subjected to NIMBYism (Figure 4.9).

**Sidewalks and Sprawl (A21)**—A telltale story unfolded in Elmhurst, Illinois, a suburb of Chicago, on the evolving role of the sidewalk in suburbia. On Gladys Avenue a new sidewalk was built in 2010 that ran intentionally only halfway down the block. That was because the residents on the street could not agree on whether there should be one at all. Local's government's compromise was to build only half of the sidewalk's total length, while the other side of the street remained without any sidewalk whatsoever.[27] Claude Pagacz, a retired carpenter and longtime resident, successfully opposed the construction of the sidewalk on his side of the street. "What concrete adds to the value of my house," he said, "I have no idea." Meanwhile, his neighbor Brian Cahill, a father of three young children, could count the ways citing how sidewalks make it possible for his children to walk to school, ride their bikes, make friends with other kids. "There have been more young families moving in," he said. "We are the future of this community." As it is, this issue divides neighbors in subdivisions elsewhere built without sidewalks. The tension between the haves and have-nots has intensified as young families seek to make their communities more healthful and safer, perhaps in an effort to make them more like the older cities and suburbs their parents and grandparents were raised in. This welcome trend is being overshadowed, unfortunately, by shrinking local municipal budgets and arguments over who should pay when public funds are scarce—developers, local municipal government, or the homeowners themselves. The growing counterargument is *Build it—and they will*

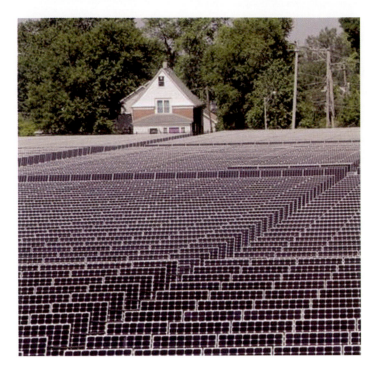

**FIGURE 4.9** Energy Farming, Chicago. Source unknown

*walk*. More and more sprawl communities are mandating full service streetscapes that meet the needs of automobiles as much as pedestrians, cyclists, and public transport lines all within close proximity to home and work. Pulte Homes, one of America's largest perpetrators of sprawl machines, remains hesitant, however, to install sidewalks in its new suburban subdivisions. Such policies continue to discriminate against the elderly, against move-up buyers with young children, against multi-family housing occupants, and against first time homebuyers. Ironically, the children and adolescents themselves usually have no say whatsoever in a community's decision whether to build a sidewalk in front of their homes. Nonetheless, suburbs everywhere must grapple with trade-offs centered on costs–benefits, and their attractiveness as places to live, work, and raise a family.

**Pedestrians (A22)**—During the 18th and 19th centuries, *pedestrianism*, the athletic counterpart to contemporary walking behaviors in the everyday environment, was a popular spectator sport in the U.K. Interestingly, it remains an Olympic sport, as its athletes typically walk timed distances on behalf of charitable causes. At the present time, the competitive aspect of walking remains but one stream of a growing international movement to plan and build places that promote the healthful aspects of walking. It is specifically centered on the many health-promoting benefits of walking in the everyday built environment. It is equally centered on creating incentives for people to walk instead of routinely driving their private auto everywhere, especially on short trips in the immediate vicinity that could easily otherwise be accomplished by walking (Figure 4.10).[28] Pedestrianism flourishes in places where local cultural values support the provision of pedestrian amenities for use on a 24/7 basis by persons of all ages and levels of functional ability. Unfortunately, most sprawl machines inhibit walking because the distances between destination points are typically

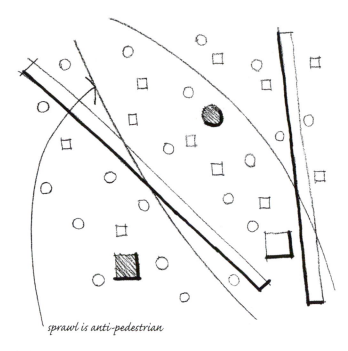

*sprawl is anti-pedestrian*

**FIGURE 4.10** Pedestrianism

deemed too far or the route too difficult to negotiate, needlessly perpetuating this overreliance on autos. A prerequisite is for local infrastructural systems to be in place to support salutogenetic walking behaviors in the everyday environment as the option of first choice, with cycling made an equally strong, attractive, alterative to always driving. Dysfunctional sidewalks are those that pose difficult-to-negotiate physical barriers such as high curb obstructions, walking surfaces in poor condition, poor lighting, irregular surfaces, and episodic and discontinuous walking surfaces. By contrast, high tech sidewalk networks provide multi-sensory support for users such as auditory cues for the blind. The latter infrastructural component interweaves threaded ramps at intersections, audio assistance devices, proper lighting, and handrails.

**Street Furniture (A23)**—Commodious street furniture judiciously positioned along sidewalks and at other key nodes provides salutogenetic support for the essential activities of everyday life. If an aged person knows, for instance, that there is a place to stop and rest along the route from destination point A to destination point B, he or she will be that much more inclined to venture outdoors and engage in the healthful activity of walking. In New Orleans's Jackson Square, in the heart of the city's Vieux Carré district, each morning, artists and fortune tellers set up their folding tables and chairs and proceed to ply their craft. Tourists and curious passersby stop to partake or merely to gawk. Numerous long cast iron benches augment these portable street furnishings. These amenities are non-moveable and yet they allow for persons to hold a conversation without necessarily having to sit too close to one another—thereby maintaining the "at arms length" interpersonal spacing that makes such seating successful in urban spaces globally. Long rows of parallel benches of this type do not promote social conversation among friends and acquaintances, however. This is why a mixture of fixed and non-fixed tables and chairs and benches should be provided wherever possible. The ability to create informal spatial groupings creates what Jan Gehl refers to as a *talkscape*.[29] A pair of benches can be set up in an L-configuration with a small table in front of them so people can talk and simultaneously use the table. The angle and positioning of benches should allow for people to remain alone or to engage in conversation. Iconic talkscapes exist in the centers of great cities and urban spaces, such as the example cited in New Orleans. The great sidewalk cafes of Paris also come to mind and the concept of establishing talkscapes along the streetscape exists in very old as well as in new places. It is not advisable to provide a backless, flat plinth, as this does not allow for sufficient physical comfort. Provide open spaces that can accommodate artists, the exhibit of their works, impromptu musical performances, and various public events. Street furnishings should not be an afterthought but an integral element of any effort to transfuse a dead or dying sprawl machine through the provision of these health-promoting amenities.

**Bike Culture (A24)**—Unfortunately, it remains rather difficult to envision Americans in large numbers ever abandoning their beloved private automobile for bicycle, to any significant degree, unless jolted out of their complacency. It is pure folly to think that this would ever occur unless a very dramatic set of transformative events should transpire to render it too costly or too dangerous to drive. Americans view their private auto as some sort of inalienable, god-given human right. Although the average number of autos owned by the typical American family continues to rise, it is entirely possible, however, that a decade from now it may likely own fewer fossil-fueled cars, with more family members opting to use their bikes for far more daily trips. The trusty fossil fuel vehicle will remain on standby for essential trips, such as interurban excursions, or trips that require the transport of items too voluminous to transport via bike, or for use in inclement weather. The propensity of people to drive will change dramatically depending on affordability, availability, and safety factors. In most parts of the globe, biking is deeply woven into the cultural fabric of daily life and cycling is as integral to everyday existence as is eating, sleeping, and sex. It is accepted as more than a means of getting from point A to point B (Figure 4.11). A significant amount of money remains in a local community when a bike replaces an auto. Local businesses reap the benefits. A Portland, Oregon, 2008 study found that bike-centric commerce contributed $90 million to the local economy annually. Annual commuting expenses can be reduced by 75 percent or more. Bike tourism is an additional benefit to a local economy.[30] Bicycle traffic in Europe has been seamlessly woven into the total transport network, where certain rail cars provide space for bikes onboard, as well as in the subway, or as placed on a rack on a bus or even taxi. Whenever this is possible, travel options can be greatly enhanced. A bike-share cycling exchange can lower a family's healthcare costs, reduce a business's need to build and maintain large parking lots, and stimulate a denser and more geographically compact local economy. Bike-share depots are one way to transform the bicycle into a mass-use mode of public transport. Washington, D.C. was the first large American city to launch a bike share program, named SmartBike, and has rapidly expanded its successful program to more than 50 miles of bike lanes, with 1,100 bikes available at 114 stations throughout the District and in next-door Arlington County, Virginia. Annual counts conducted in key bike-share cycling corridors show rush-hour bicycle trips increased by 82 percent in 2007–2010 in twenty such corridors.[31] The economic and health benefits accrued from biking are undeniable, as has been proven repeatedly in cites in many parts of the globe. This alone should validate bike-share and similar health-promotion initiatives as an essential part of salutogenetic public health policies.[32] Provide amenities for bikes, cyclists, the storage and retrieval of their bikes, and for bike repair and maintenance.

**Social Media Parks (A25)**—The widely held conception of parks as places to spend time outdoors—interacting with natural ecologies, engaging in health promoting physical activity—is fast

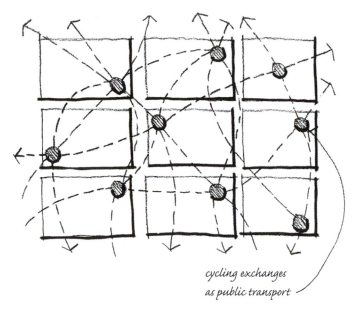

*cycling exchanges
as public transport*

**FIGURE 4.11**    Cycling Culture

fading from relevance to a generation now accustomed to a sedentary lifestyle increasingly centered on passively sitting in front of a computer screen. The lure of interactive media such as Facebook and related sophisticated video games has fixated the attention of a generation that now considers it "quaint" to spend any time outdoors after school or on weekends. It appears to be seen as more stimulating to proponents of video games to sit motionless, silently, in front of a laptop screen, indoors, for hours on end. The cumulative effects of Vitamin D deficiencies are yet to be documented by nutritionists and epidemiologists although the early warning signs of sedentarianism are clearly discernable. To critics, it symbolizes a dystrophic worldview diametrically opposed to the 19th- and early 20th-century conception of making an excursion to an urban park because it afforded many social and health advantages. In the classic Olmstedian view, the urban park functioned as a social, recreational, and intellectual anchor of a community in a way that the typical suburban enclosed mall could never match. The neighborhood park functioned to draw people together to commune with nature, not disconnected from it. The opportunity exists at this time, especially with the advent of technologies such as fiber optics and lasers, and interactive *video walls*, to reinvent the suburban/urban park to fuse a classically designed park's traditional components with these types of high tech attractors, and being able to walk or bike to an interactive media park. Interactive media parks can include sit down spaces as well as options for physical exercise, sports, and related activity. Media parks offer promise to ameliorate the acute social isolation currently experienced by many children and adolescents—a subculture that is rapidly becoming less and less comfortable with face-to-face social interactions. The laptop, iPad, or handheld LED screen need not become a permanent substitute for human interaction and health promoting activity outdoors. A local social media park can function as a key infrastructural magnet for health promotion.

**Light Rail/Intermodal Transit (A26)**—The reinvention of sprawl machines will require a paradigmatic shift from auto-centric to multi-nodal transportation infrastructures. Light rail transit generally has a lower capacity and lower speed than heavy rail, though a higher speed and transport volume capacity than traditional street bus and tram-based transport. Light rail can operate on dedicated rights of way with auto/truck street traffic. The U.S. Urban Mass Transportation Administration (UMTA) introduced the term *light rail* in 1972. It is similar to the British light rail system. S*treetcars* are often mixed interchangeably with light rail transport systems although streetcars operate nearly exclusively on conventional city thoroughfares whereas light rail systems tend to have dedicated rights-of-ways. Originating in the 19th century, nearly all such systems vanished by the 1960s. Electric-powered light rail vehicles (LRVs) are distinguished from rapid rail transit (RRT) vehicles. Many communities are reintroducing light rail and are in the process of constructing or expanding the necessary infrastructure. These include New Orleans, Houston, San Diego, Austin, New York City, Fort Lauderdale, Norfolk, Detroit, and Sydney, Australia. With *transit oriented development* (TOD) in mind, transport stations and stops are coordinated with existing infrastructural street grids, pedestrian and cycling networks, and redevelopment. Strategies include an intermodal mix of heavy rail, light rail, rail stops, intermodal stations, bus rapid transit routes, tram/circulator bus routes, and pedestrian and bike paths. A ¼ mile *pedestrian shed* (defined in this context as the ability to walk from destination Point A to Point B within a ¼ mile radius) should be coordinated with a shuttle bus stop every ⅛–¼ mile, and/or a tram/circulator bus stop every ½ mile. A ½ mile pedestrian shed should be coordinated with a light rail stop at every mile interval, and with a heavy rail line stop every two miles. Prerequisites in the planning process include analyzing all existing thoroughfares and transit networks, the identification of new interconnections and thoroughfares with multimodality based on utilization and on highest-volume destination points, and the assessment of its performance on an ongoing basis (Figure 4.12).[33]

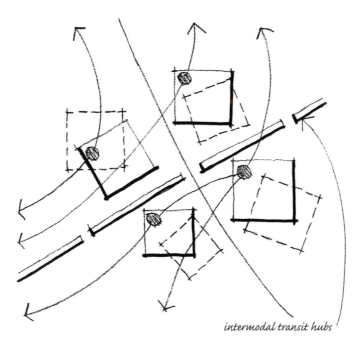

*intermodal transit hubs*

**FIGURE 4.12** Intermodalism

**Celebrate Health Achievements (A27)**—A bicycle path can accommodate five times more traffic than a single auto lane. A sidewalk has space for twenty times more travelers than a single auto lane. Copenhagen's bicycles save more than 90,000 tons of $CO_2$ every year, where a brightly colored balloon is placed on display in a civic plaza to illustrate the volume of each ton of $CO_2$ conserved annually. Promoting cycling through celebrating those who take up the activity and proceed to improve their health status can serve as an inspiration to others. Another strategy is the vertical farm created at the center of a plaza in the suburban outskirts of Madrid, created by a Madrid design firm; this structure is called the *ecosistema urbano Ecoboulevard*—an urban recycling intervention where its three pavilions function as virtual "trees" situated within an open grid frame aperture built to accommodate the planting and harvesting of plant species "farmed" by the local residents. This *air tree* is a lightweight structure, easily dismantled, and is carbon neutral (Figure 4.13). It celebrates what a community can accomplish when it bands together for a common cause that fuses environmental activism with public health activism. It can be a cost effective public health policy strategy to create carbon neutral public spaces such as this that function as stages for the proclamation and celebration of individual as well as collective public health improvements. Such achievements can include a neighborhood's collective reduction in its obesity rates, chronic diseases, and associated deleterious health outcomes that would otherwise have been associated with sedentary, auto-centric lifestyles. Such achievements can also be proclaimed through works of art (such as the aforementioned orange-balloon example), the installation of large video screens in public spaces, interactive kiosks, mobile clinics-on-wheels that roam throughout the suburban milieu, and through interactive social media, i.e. flash mobs.[34] Perhaps an *anti-obesity kiosk* or interactive art installation can depict

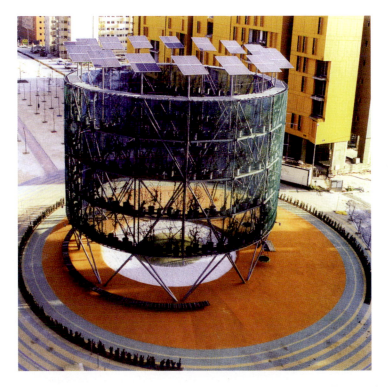

**FIGURE 4.13**  Pavilion for Urban Agriculture, Madrid, Spain, ecosistema urbano. Photo courtesy of ecosistema urbano

the faces (with before–after images) of local citizens who overcame the adverse health effects of their sedentary suburban lifestyles, and specifically their fight against obesity, chronic disease, fatigue, and stress.

## B. Ecological Architecture

**Modernism and Public Health (B1)**—In the hands of the 20th century's most influential architects, the automobile was a machine that symbolized an unprecedented degree of personal freedom for their clients. The automobile had a profound impact on modernism, from the "machine for living" accommodation of the private auto's carport vis-à-vis the pilotis of Le Corbusier's iconic Villa Savoye, to the decentralized, semi-agrarianist sprawl envisioned by Frank Lloyd Wright in his visionary Broadacre City proposal of 1934. Amid this manifold of concerns, auto-dependence was by no means to be considered a bad thing during the halcyon decades of the International Style. It was not of priority (nor up until remarkably recently for many architects) to take full cognizance of the interdependencies between auto-dependence and human health. In architecture, the rise of sedentary lifestyles and a given buildings relationship to its neighborhoods street, and urban context have not been viewed until only recently as being of potentially negative contributing impact on building inhabitants' unhealthfulness (Figure 4.14). Prior to the advent of elevators, escalators, and people movers, the staircase was the option of first and last resort. The design of stairs, inlieu of ramps and elevators, is now being reappraised for their reconfiguration, visibility, and location within a building in such a manner as to invite staircase usage as the option of first choice. Examples

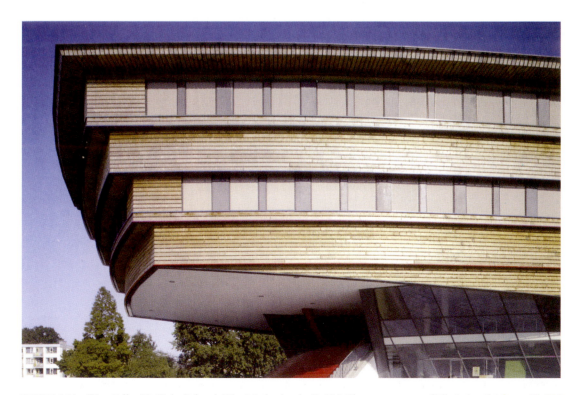

**FIGURE 4.14**   Piter Jelles YnSicht School, The Netherlands, RAU. Photo courtesy of Christian Richters/RAU

include museum staircases and ramps that encourage their usage as the first option during art viewing, allowing works of art to be viewed while one circulates internally. Frank Lloyd Wright's iconic Guggenheim Museum (1958) in New York City is one well-known example of this circulation design strategy. Its circular ramp fuses health promoting physical activity, aesthetics, and ambient spatial attributes.[35] Throughout history, a building of high navigational amenity allowed the individual to circulate in a way that encouraged walking as the primary means of experiencing its interior and the relationship of its interior to the exterior world. Architects' reappraisal of walking behaviors within buildings, and stair usage, can be facilitated through the provision of health education (motivational cues) informational signage placed at key decision points where one must decide between taking the stairs versus taking the elevator or escalator. Locate *stair prompts* where they are most visible. These should be multilingual, providing information, for example, on the amount of calories expended per trip through usage of a staircase versus the other available means of vertical or horizontal circulation.[36]

**Ruins and Selective Entropy (B2)**—Sites of former importance provide opportunities for their redevelopment through the creative harnessing of entropic forces vis-à-vis landscape urbanism reclamation strategies. Reoccupation of an abandoned, reclaimed former steel mill in Pittsburgh can be part of a deliberate strategy to reclaim, selectively, portions of in-ruin sites in a phased manner.[37] Decay can be interwoven with selective erasure to allow new uses to flourish within old ones. The selective reclamation of a dead mall may allow for a part of it to become a garden or water element. A "ruin" thereby becomes a civic space in its own right, a catalyst. The Sylvan Slough Natural Area is a private/public partnership to convert a contaminated, long-dormant brownfield industrial site into a public park along the edge of the Mississippi River in Rock Island, Illinois. It is now a 7.5-acre public amenity within a formerly dead manufacturing zone. Partial deconstruction retain selected remnants of its 19th-century historic industrial structures; these were incorporated into the park, thereby reducing substantial demolition and site remediation costs that would otherwise have been necessary. Foundations, walls, and pavements were selectively reconditioned, transformed into bird viewing platforms, walkways, and a small amphitheatre. On-site concrete remnants were crushed and recycled as a parking lot's sub-base and as pathway surfacing material. The site includes bioswales, native landscape restoration, porous pavements, and rain gardens.[38] Resurrection of a lost post-industrial landscape involves rediscovering a once prosperous but now degraded place. Conservation of such places will remain financially challenging until stimulated by innovative reinvestment incentives established at the local, regional, and national level. Sports fields and a wide range of recreational amenities can be incorporated to promote health and contribute, therefore, to placemaking in this regard.[39] Search, therefore, for ways to reclaim these lost landscapes fallen into disuse and ruin. Deconstruct, and reinvent entropic landscapes to attract and promote human activity and exercise outdoors, and particularly dead mall sites and big box carcasses as new building types through the injection of landscape, i.e. SITE's unbuilt Forrest Building proposal (1978–1980) for Richmond, Virginia, for BEST Products (Figure 4.15).[40]

**Reprise the Community Center (B3)**—Sprawl machines tend to dismiss the cultural and health promoting of neighborhoods. A neighborhoods heart and soul often centers on social interaction. Ubiquitous high-speed mass multimedia is now deliverable to every private home and business and, combined with the impact of central air conditioning, causes people to have fewer reasons to spend time out of doors socializing, walking, and connecting with those around them. Neighbors seek interaction with other neighbors while structures are sited in close proximity to one another as opposed to the typical subdivision today. Mixed-use streetscapes were traditionally composed of closely sited dwellings, businesses, and civic institutions. The drug store, movie theater,

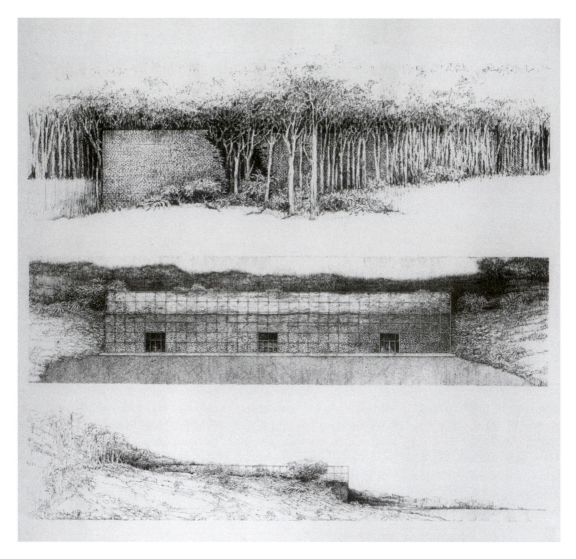

**FIGURE 4.15** SITE—Forest/Terrarium Building (Proposal), Richmond, Virginia. Drawing courtesy of SITE—Architecture, Art & Design

public library, schools, town hall, county courthouse, and commercial businesses were usually within close walking or cycling distance from home or work. These destination points attracted people to the outdoor realm—in stark contrast to today's highly sedentary lifestyles. The local church in particular served this predilection, with its community multipurpose room available for activities programmed across a wide spectrum of age and interest groups—from bingo nights, to a proving ground for neophyte rock bands who performed on "teen nights" on the weekends (Figure 4.16). These community centers were genuine and evolved over time—versus the ubiquitous, dull, instant "activity room" or "party room" that sprawl developers provide in a small nondescript building place at the center of a generic suburban subdivision. These generic "party rooms" are an inauthentic facsimile, usually a mono-use building and not near at all to any generic

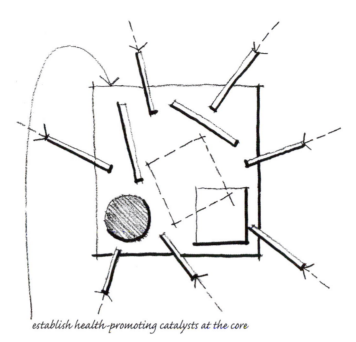

*establish health-promoting catalysts at the core*

**FIGURE 4.16**   Reinvent Suburban Centers

town center. It looks and feels inauthentic, nor well integrated. Ironically, the developers of gated communities often include precisely this type of "activity building" and it is sometimes combined with a swimming pool, tennis courts, golf course, and perhaps, in wealthier subdivisions and gated enclaves, a snack bar or restaurant—all housed in a "clubhouse." Yet these places tend to be artificial and too often do not contribute to anything resembling a genuinely interactive, socially or ethnically diverse experience. In response, take the opposite approach from that exhibited throughout much of suburbia—start with a community center at the physical center of the neighborhood—as a gathering place for all ages and multiple uses. Include an adjacent outdoor space and stage. Locate the community center so that it does not cause undue disturbance to nearby neighborhoods and link it directly with a network of bike and pedestrian paths. This will nurture the cultural as well as physical health of the community.

**Nomadic Healthcare (B4)**—Underperforming shopping malls in the U.S. and elsewhere are currently suffering substantial vacancy rates and foreclosures. The Great Recession has forced many national "storefront" big box megachains and their smaller counterparts into bankruptcy. For multi-site businesses that find a way to avoid bankruptcy, systemic contraction often occurs in the number of outlets that remain within their national networks as they search for viable options to combat the severe economic downturn. A number of national chains have in the past few years opened temporary outlets in vacated spaces in underperforming malls. These operations, known as *pop up stores*, are commercial businesses open for only a few months at a time, perhaps seasonally, or even for only a few weeks. From the standpoint of the distressed mall or strip center, pop ups fill otherwise empty commercial storefronts, inject a modicum of vibrancy, and provide much-needed cash flow. Why can't this concept work with regards to pop up outpatient community health and wellness centers? Why not pop up primary care clinics and wellness centers in storefronts and vacant spaces in distressed malls? During peak flu season, and when children are in need of immunizations just prior to the start of the school year, specialty pop ups serving their needs can be opened on a temporary basis. They are nomadic, redeployable rotatable from location to location as patient needs change, and can be relocated to adjust to seasonal ebbs and flow in the demand of healthcare services within a given neighborhood. Themed pop up sickness prevention and wellness centers can be tailored to optometry, podiatry, cancer screening, orthopedics (particularly during peak summer sports season), and mental health care, such as for the treatment of depression, eating disorders and seasonal affective disorder (SAD). Locate pop up clinics in vacant existing commercial storefronts that provide direct, walkable and bikeable, and public transport links, with adjoining streets linked to the local community. These places are embedded within existing buildings, or installed as freestanding autonomous, transportable clinics-on-wheels—able to be easily redeployed on short notice to new sites as needs shift from month to month, seasonally, or annually, or deployed as adjuncts to fixed-site healthcare provider sites such as the local hospital, outpatient community primary care, fitness center, or nutritional health education center.[41]

**Modular Infill Buildings (B5)**—Intermodal shipping containers (ISCs) and other variations of standard international shipping containers are increasingly being reclaimed as building modules. They offer tremendous potential as ecologically responsive infill structures for a variety of functions in otherwise dead sprawl zones—*cargotecture*. This term was coined in 2003 by the ecological archite-cure firm HyBrid Architecture. Its prototypes consist of reusable ISCs as homes, apartments, offices, stores, emergency shelters, libraries, police substations, small outpatient-based health centers, well-ness centers, and schools. ISCs and their derivatives are manufactured in standardized sizes, typically 20, 30 or 40 feet in length, 8 feet wide, and 8 or 10 feet in height. They provide pre-engineered systems for site-specific installation, are low-cost, prefabricated, easily transportable, environmen-tally sustainable, and stackable in close-packing configurations. They can be assembled in small groups of a few containers to numbering into the thousands.[42] Over 7,000 double-stacked ISCs comprise the 3,200-foot-long Dordoy Bazaar in Kyrgyzstan, one of Asia's largest marketplaces. Employing more than 20,000 people, it is jammed with a spectrum of goods and its "architecture" is nearly 100 percent reclaimed. The Seventh Kilometer market, in Odessa, Ukraine, covers more than 170 acres and consists of tens of thousands of ISCs. Other examples include the Freitag Retail Store-tower in Zurich, consisting of seventeen rusty, recycled ISCs. It can be disassembled at any time. HyBrid Architecture designed Seattle's first ISC-based building, which currently houses 7,000 square feet of office space and a retail showroom. Its ISC modules reduced construction costs by 20–40 percent while requiring only four hours to assemble in place with a crane. At Utrecht University in The Netherlands, ISCs are stacked three levels in height in a student dormitory painted in four complementary colors (deep red, sky blue, yellow, and pale green) and close-packed as two "build-ings" with a courtyard in between. This colorfully collaged composition features entry portals at its rear. Keetwonen Container City is a university student housing complex in Amsterdam and the largest ISC-based aggregate building constructed to date in Europe, with 1,000 apartments. Each modular unit is 40 feet in length with one wall comprised entirely of glass. Each unit has a private balcony. The units are arranged in "blocks" around small courtyards. The complex contains a café, food market, and offices.[43] Intermodal shipping containers adapted as ecological architecture hold promise as small and midrise infill buildings on mid-block and corner sites. Mondragon, designed by Acconci Studio, in the Basque country of Spain, features geothermal-powered ISC modules that consume 90 percent less energy than conventional housing of equivalent size (Figure 4.17 and Figure 4.18). From a health promotion perspective, they are eco-friendly, compact, affordable, and can be significant contributors to pedestrian-centered communities.[44]

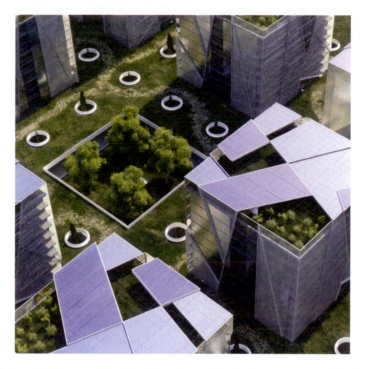

**FIGURE 4.17**    Redeployable Housing Modules, Mondragón, Spain. Photo courtesy of Studio Luis de Garrido

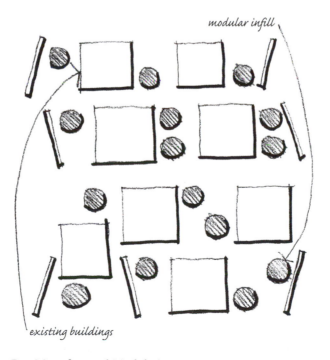

**FIGURE 4.18**    Embrace Pre-Manufactured Modularity

**Civic Space at the Heart (B6)**—Innovative land trust initiatives and reclamation strategies can transform once-vacant shopping malls into active, vibrant civic places at the heart of reborn suburban districts. Reinventing long dormant, residualized parcels such as malls and their expansive dead parking lots presents unprecedented opportunities at this time. Reclaimed dead land and buildings at the heart of declining sprawl machines can restore a community's health when health promoting amenities are created in their place—plazas, public squares, commercial, educational, heath-related functions, religious and recreational functions—in the spirit of the great plazas of the world and their surrounding buildings, such as the Piazza del Campo in Sienna, Italy. Expropriating dead and dying malls and their constituent parts, particularly parking lots, can take years, however, without effective reclamation protocols and implementation strategies. Provide microclimate immersions, i.e. incorporate innovative material, color palettes, textures, light and sounds in reclaimed places to create unique, multisensory experiences and establish sense of place.[45] Aim to create something of enduring value and legitimacy, grounded in local vernacular building traditions and architectural precedents. Short-term economic paybacks are tempting yet need not overshadow longer-term priorities. This must be of high priority in this type of infrastructural reinvestment. Unfortunately, most current suburban zoning laws are completely obsolete. Most local land use ordinances, written more than fifty years ago are anachronistic and often difficult to amend without a protracted political and/or legal fight on a case-by-case basis, which can, as mentioned, take years to resolve. Invent proactive, transformative zoning policies and protective covenants as a mechanism to transform hundreds of dying and dead malls in the U.S. and elsewhere into viable, vibrant centers of suburban civic life. The challenge is to meaningfully weave together the carcasses, especially those left behind when a megachain constructs a larger big box store nearby, as is the standard practice of Wal-Mart.[46]

**Walkability (B7)**—In the U.S., prior to the Surgeon-General's 1996 report *Physical Activity and Health*, it was thought sufficient to devote twenty minutes per day to intensive aerobic-level activity, as this was the recommended best type of daily exercise. The poor, of course, are unable to go to the local private health club to exercise on a regular basis to stay fit, and the choices available to residents in food deserts are of poor quality, as previously discussed. The 1996 report instead called for a far broader, more inclusive approach to health promotion, advocating the great health benefits obtainable through moderate daily activities such as walking and cycling.[47] Everyone can do this. Walking and cycling are activities that the poor engage in out of necessity if not by design, as they are very often unable to afford a car. Yet for the poor this may place jobs and shopping far out of reach. How can a suburb become more walkable and bikeable? To traditionalists, walkability tends to be viewed in elitist terms, in neighborhoods of discernibly upscale character, with neo-traditionalist central commercial districts, architectural landmarks, and appealing, safe public squares, parks, and plazas. The New Urbanists have argued for compactness as the prerequisite condition, defining a walkable neighborhood as one sufficiently dense and compact for local businesses to flourish, with housing and workplaces located nearby, affording easily accessible public transport connections and alternatives to always having to drive everywhere in suburbia. The utopian ideal of the New Urbanism has been for job opportunities to naturally arise for individuals and families of all income levels and age strata living side by side in compact communities—the young, midlife adults, and the elderly—across the socio-economic, ethnic, and racial spectrum. Businesses, i.e. jobs, can be plugged into small mixed-use structures and as part of larger aggregations, along with residences and workplaces. Jobs, presumably, are created in small businesses near to where one lives. Vibrant streetscapes and public spaces are to define the character of these egalitarian places. It follows that its intrinsic urban amenity and upscale appeal thereby promotes its walkability and it is such qualities that trend spotter Richard Florida refers to as core amenities that attract an educated, innovative *creative class* to a city. This is extremely elitist. How can walkable places be created *for all* and not just for the well-off? Why are New Urbanist communities in nearly every case so expensive to live in? The New Urbanism does not yet have an answer to the question of how walkability can become the province of everyone, equitably and especially for the acutely medically underserved who live in sprawl machines.

**Architectural Legibility (B8)**—It is all too easy to become disoriented in a sprawl machine. It's stressful to be lost, searching for a particular address on a street in a subdivision where all the houses look the same. At night, the problem of disorientation and illegibility on a street becomes far worse when the only distinguishing feature marking one house in the subdivision from another may be the color of its curbside mailbox, the garage door, the color of the roof, or the shape of the front porch light. Sprawl machines are notoriously difficult to navigate from a wayfinding perspective due to the layout of the streets, poor lighting, repetitive street configurations, poor signage, and absence of people outdoors (because there often are no sidewalks). The lack of pedestrians makes it nearly impossible to ask anyone for directions. Making matters worse, the streets are deserted because there is nowhere interesting to walk to within close distance: it is harder to catch the attention of a passing motorist for directions than it is a pedestrian. Cars speed by, slowing only for the proverbial traffic-calming device—the subdivision street's beloved speed bump (speed bumps are parental aids where there are no sidewalks). Street names are often named similarly, and this is a particular problem in gated communities—Sparrow Way, Sparrow Trail, and Sparrow Boulevard—all may be parallel streets to one another within the same subdivision. Allow the various buildings along a street to express their unique individuality and each its own imagery. Imagery, materials, formal composition, color, siting, are all variables that when expressed on a building-by-building basis along streetscapes can yield a diverse yet cohesive overall effect. Similarly, coordinate the configuration of streets, intersections, sidewalks, and outdoor seating areas, and focal points, with diverse, legible and differentiated architecture as a means to establish a more navigable, and aesthetically interesting neighborhood. The use of landmarks can be particularly effective, for example the Swedish firm Gora art&landscape's Bubble is an iconic greenhouse/landmark sited within a neighborhood in Malmö, Sweden (Figure 4.19). Commercial roadside strip landscapes are equally disorienting and a source of considerable stress when it is impossible for an individual to find an address because none are posted on the buildings, and buildings themselves are monotonous and indistinguishable from one another.[48]

**Bridging (B9)**—The thoroughfares of suburbia are often un-negotiable. Many traffic-clogged arteries have four lanes in each direction, together with a center median. Their crosswalks are barely navigable, in the best of conditions, even more daunting when cars are turning from intersections and constantly pulling in and out randomly from parking lots seemingly everywhere. Crossing excessively wide roadways is often like running the gauntlet in a firearms shooting gallery. For children, the physically impaired, and the aged, it is a no-go proposition, unfortunately. It is a formidable challenge to walk or ride a bike across these roadways, even at non-peak traffic periods. The non-bike and non-walk friendly boulevards of Los Angeles, Phoenix, Salt Lake City, Atlanta, and Houston come readily to mind. The strip in Las Vegas, with its notoriously busy cross streets, were the cause of so many traffic fatalities over the years that many of its most congested intersections now feature mandatory crossover pedestrian bridges. The pedestrian bridges are anchored at the street level by staircases and elevators, together with a network of access ramps connecting to the street level. Traffic calming measures may be unfeasible, especially in cases involving a highly traveled state or provincial highway. In these situations, construct unobtrusive yet universally accessible pedestrian overpass

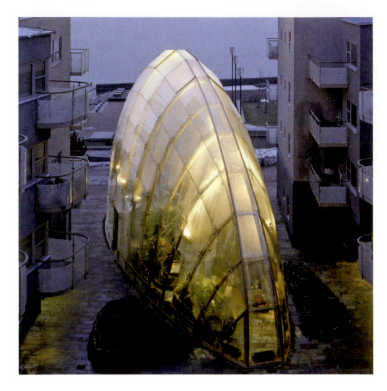

**FIGURE 4.19**  Glass Bubble, Malmö, Sweden. Photo courtesy of Ake Eson Lindman/Gora art&landscape

bridges (Figure 4.20). Pedestrian bridges should contain, ideally, three distinct, functionally distinguishable paths: a walking path, jogging path, and a bike lane. Where land allows, provide a sloping access ramp from street level on one or both sides. Where this is not possible, provide an elevator or pedestrian lift device to allow pedestrians and cyclists full, universal access. Provide effective lighting to encourage their use at night. Tunnels beneath roadways are often more expensive alternatives, but may be more feasible in some situations.[49]

**Multigenerationality (B10)**—In 2010 the number of people living under one roof in the U.S. reached its highest level in fifty years. Families are coping with job losses, unemployment, and fore-closure. According to a recent Pew Research Center Report, during the first full year of the Great Recession (2009), the number of Americans living in multigenerational households rose by 2.6 million, or more than 5 percent. When households contract in number, it is an indicator of more who are opting to move in with parents, other relatives, and unrelated others. This trend has been occurring since 1980 and is also driven by immigration, and a host of other socio-cultural and demographic determinants. Forty-nine million Americans—16.1 percent of the total population—currently live in households with multiple generations under the same roof.[50] Households with extended family structures were on the decline in the sixty-year-plus period after World War II, and this trend was largely due to the era of massive suburban expansion. Families in central cities moved out to new subdivision tract houses in places such as Levittown New York and elsewhere. Immigrants are accounting for a growing portion of the current trend in the U.S., and this pattern echoes the pre-World War I waves of European immigrants and others who came to America. They lived under

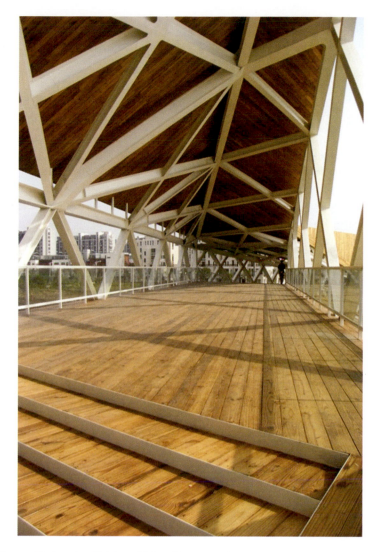

**FIGURE 4.20**   Qingpu Pedestrian Bridge, China. Source unknown

one roof with relatives until they could stand up on their own financially, move out, and eventually attain autonomy. The current rise in multigenerational households poses challenges with regards to suburban transfusion. Autos are more expensive to own and operate than ever before, as a percentage of annual income. Gasoline prices are going nowhere but up. Many destination points are out of reach via walking and cycling, due to unmitigated sprawl compared to ever before in history. The unemployed or underemployed become stranded, as if stuck on an island. In response, endeavor to establish housing and public health initiatives that encourage households to locate closer to the physical centers of their transfused suburban precincts. This can yield job opportunities, socialization options, and reduce the stress and anxiety otherwise caused by physical inactivity caused by being stranded in suburbia, especially among the aged.

**Echo Housing (B11)**—By no means new, this is especially prevalent in places with limited land for development, such as in Japan. Yet it is a relatively new proposition within conflated sprawl machines in the U.S. and in other rapidly suburbanizing parts of the globe. In the U.S., the lot sizes of the typical post-World War II middle-class suburban tract house provided ample space for a distinct and autonomous rear yard. The backyard was sized to allow children to play ball, with space for the swing set and the detached one or two-car garage. In time, the American backyard became an iconic and highly valued component of sprawl machines. They consume a tremendous amount of open space, in the aggregate, and in a resource-starved world they now afford an equally compelling and intriguing opportunity to achieve a higher degree of density in a given neighborhood without altering its fundamental visual character. Echo housing typically consists of the construction of a second dwelling behind the main front/streetside dwelling with the front dwelling typically facing the street or vehicular access point, or is situated between two neighboring dwellings (Figure 4.21). Ample land is currently available in most suburbs for this type of intervention. It will be essential to live closer in proximity to where one shops, works, and goes to school. Infill strategies such as this directly promote walking and biking—and in turn promote greater physical activity and healthier lifestyles. In addition it can relieve the pressures of multigenerational households on a single suburban site as the echo dwelling enables family members who may currently be sharing the same crowded dwelling to once again experience independance and autonomy without necessitating an additional land purchase. At present, antiquated, sprawl-inducing zoning laws in suburbia remain the major obstacle to this type of infill transfusion strategy. Sensitively sited and designed echo dwellings in

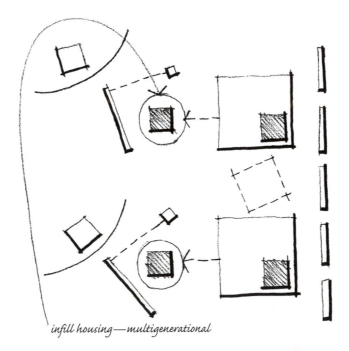

*infill housing—multigenerational*

**FIGURE 4.21**  Create Echo Housing

mid-block, side yard, and in rear yard configurations allow creative freedom for the architect, such as the Swiss architect Werner Schmidt's proposed *amphibious* infill housing (Figure 4.22).[51]

**Heliotropic Tectonics (B12)**—Horticultural species are heliotropic, gradually tilting back toward their sun source as a means to optimize solar energy absorption. Conventional sun-tracking solar panels often require the use of costly motors and electronic control systems. Recent advances in this technology have yielded the manufacture of heliotropic solar panels that far more cheaply capture solar energy with significantly less technical apparatus required. Lower cost-lower tech systems are needed in developing countries and in urban communities everywhere that lack the financial wherewithal to continue to support antiquated and overburdened conventional energy grids. A student team from MIT has recently developed an innovative prototype called *Heliotrope*. This system imitates the way plants track the sun across the sky, by using the temperature differentials between shaded and sunlit areas to modify the properties of the material supporting solar photovoltaic cells. This biomimetic system is completely passive, requiring no power source or electronics to control panel movement. Moreover, the system's panels are significantly cheaper to operate and maintain than existing sun-tracking systems and are constructible from materials readily available in developing parts of the world.[52] The demand will decrease for electricity to be transferred to individual buildings connected to a conventional power grid. This will liberate transfused suburban communities from onerous utility bills and the inefficiencies of conventional energy grid system brownouts and total breakdowns that routinely and widely occur due to system overload, extreme weather events, and the like. The cost savings incurred by the community will be substantial and this can help to promote further reinvestment in the transformation of dying suburbs everywhere.

**Historic Preservation (B13)**—In suburbia the preservation of historic buildings remains a controversial and delicate proposition. In most suburbs, the property owner has the ultimate say to elect to demolish without obtaining any prior approval or consent form any public oversight entity. While strong neighborhood and citywide preservation review boards exist in most cities, such

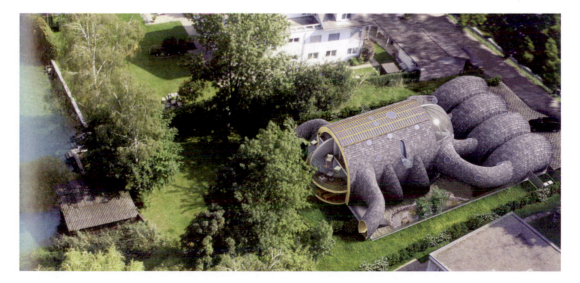

**FIGURE 4.22** Amphibious House (Proposal), Basel, Switzerland. Photo courtesy of Atelier Werner Schmidt

organizations do not exist within most sprawl machines. This is troublesome. As inner suburban communities age, their inventory of buildings is increasingly subject to designation as historic landmarks. The reappraisal of post-World War II architecture, i.e. churches, shopping centers, schools, housing types (such as the one-level ranch house), fast food restaurants, and so on is underway in America's suburbs. The Spirit of the Age was captured in the best buildings that were built in the post-World War II period in suburbia in a time of seemingly unlimited possibilities when anything seemed possible. Sadly, mid-century modernism, suburban and otherwise, is under particularly intense siege today in many places. Mid-20th-century modernist landmarks are being lost everyday due to demolition. Tens of thousands of meritorious buildings are threatened. The recent loss of Wayland High School designed by the Architects Collaborative (1960) and built in a Boston suburb, personifies this sad trend. Praised at its opening as an outstanding example of progressive school design in *The New York Times, Architectural Record, Time, Life* magazine, and in *The Nation's Schools*, it immediately became an important ingredient of its community's physical fabric and its collective cultural memory.[53] Not every building was a landmark at the time of its construction, of course. A prime example of this was the nondescript suburban American ranch house built in the post-World War II period. In Chicago, Atlanta, and elsewhere in the U.S., however, grassroots preservation efforts are now underway to designate in these aging suburbs noteworthy examples of their rich inventory of unique architecture as historic buildings, and as landmarked districts. The preservation of cultural landmarks and districts in suburbia needs to be of utmost priority as a core ingredient that defines a genuinely healthy community, and needs to be fused within a community's overall transfusion strategy.

**Vertical Intervention (B14)**—Landmark and potential landmark-status buildings in suburbs are a source of controversy where land values might be low at present but are predicted to increase in future years. Free market advocates (such as developers) remain highly skeptical of mandatory, and in their view overly restrictive, historic preservation requirements pertaining to private property. It is counterproductive to encourage preservation while disallowing the private property owner from altering the exterior size, color, or appearance of one's property. This is a source of heated debate where local preservation statutes forbid vertical additions from being added to the tops of buildings. The debate centers on whether or not this type of an addition will increase or decrease a building's market value by adding occupiable floor area. Will vertical expansion detract significantly from its history, façade, or the interior qualities of the building's envelope? Beijing is facing this dilemma across its historic traditionally planned and built *hutong* neighborhoods. New York City, with its infamously aggressive developers and entrenched preservationists, is a perennial hotbed of vertical expansion controversy. There, a number of recent municipally unapproved roof expansions side-stepped the legal review process, with myriad unapproved additions and penthouses having appeared throughout the city.[54] Lawsuits erupted on both sides. Developers have in some cases been forced to tear them down. In one case, a relatively obscure penthouse in TriBeCa narrowly avoided this fate although a similar addition in Chelsea wasn't so fortunate. In 2010 a building in the Dumbo neighborhood was forcibly stripped of six illegally added stories that were built in 2006 because the owners had never obtained a formal zoning variance for added residential space to their commercially-zoned property. This practice in New York City is known as *tenement topping*. In suburbia, increased densification pressures within transfusion catalyst sites will increasingly result in pressures to build upwardly versus horizontally, i.e. resuscitated dead malls vertically expanded with multi-family housing on their roofs. Inventory all occupied as well as abandoned buildings and suburban landscapes currently threatened with demolition that might be reborn vis-à-vis judicious vertical expansion, such as in the case of the Dutch firm RAU and its 2006 vertical expansion

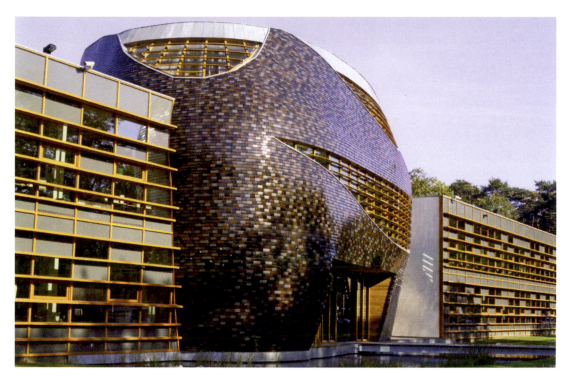

**FIGURE 4.23** Reclaimed WWF Agricultural Laboratory, The Netherlands, RAU. Photo courtesy of Kusters fotografie/RAU

and carbon neutral retrofit of an abandoned 1950s industrial complex in The Netherlands (Figure 4.23).[55]

**McMansion Epidemic (B15)**—The twenty-year American craze for ever larger homes built on sites formerly occupied by "teardown dwellings"—*McMansionitis*—has garnered much media attention internationally. A McMansion is a supersized new home typically seen as ostentatious, over-scaled, or an otherwise poor fit for its immediate neighborhood. The term was coined in the 1980s and is derived from the generic, inauthentic qualities of the fast food served at McDonald's. The debate centers on whether 4,000 square foot-plus houses are acceptable as infill construction in inner suburban neighborhoods surrounded by older "ensemble" housing that may be no more than one third the size of their new supersized neighbors. In older suburbs, supersized McMansions stand out for their lack of a coherent architectural style as much as for footprints significantly out of scale. Their envelopes typically push out far to the edges of their sites, overwhelming the context. They proliferated in many inner-ring American subdivisions built in the 1980–2005 period, particularly in the American Southeast and Southwest.[56] Marketed as *executive homes* yet of a quality not dissimilar from conventional spec homes, hundreds of thousands were built on greenfield sites where the land was cheapest. There, they tended to not draw strong opposition from existing neighbors. By 2010, fortunately, the American McMansion was itself history.[57] Resale values were in sharp decline due to the national and global economic doldrums and increasingly due to stronger NIMBY opposition. Also, builders turned their attention to smaller, more affordable residential types built on smaller lots because, by 2010, many places in the U.S. had passed laws to limit their construction, including in Austin, Texas, DeKalb County, Georgia, and Marin County, California. Austin in 2007 initiated a moratorium against their rampant proliferation in the city's older, established neighborhoods. The debate in these locales is centered on issues of architectural compatibility, infrastructural burdens, and the unintended consequences of forcing out longtime residents who cannot afford rising tax rates.[58] The challenge is to develop ecologically sensitive alternatives such as infill eco-housing that promote healthier, far less auto-dependent lifestyles. Calvin Chiu's wetlands reclamation submission to *Dwell* magazine's Reburbia competition in 2009 is instructive in this regards (Figure 4.24).[59]

**Ungate Communities (B16)**—A glaring expression of the depleted public realm in the U.S. is the *gated community*. In an Asphalt Nation the denial of the public's access to these "exclusive" residential enclaves symbolizes an inward-focused reality. It shuns broad-based social discourse, racial and ethnic diversity, denies spontaneity, and shuts off exposure to the idiosyncratic qualities of everyday life. The inhabitants of these places seek introversion, autonomy, and disengagement. Gated communities exploded in popularity in the late 20th century and, by 1995, 4 million Americans lived in them. In Bear Creek, in Seattle, four people stand guard, not unlike military sentries, guarding a military compound.[60] They acquired popularity as their inhabitants perceived them as safe havens from a nation that experienced rising rates of violent crime. They maintain particularly strong drawing power for transient professionals and their families, luring high-end corporate executives. In the U.K. more than 100,000 persons reside in Britain's 1,000-plus gated communities, walled off from the outside world. Bream Close, in northeast London, is situated on a peninsula on the River Lea, surrounded by water except for its entrance road—a road monitored with electronic gates and CCTV cameras. When Maida Vale, a neighborhood in an upscale part of West London, erected gates in 2007, it was in response to the rising number of crimes committed by local youth gangs, crimes that included the dumping of stolen cars, property theft, and numerous incidents of trespassing. This attracted considerable media attention and became a source of controversy locally. To critics, it symbolized a troubling, negative trend because it further discouraged those who opt to live in sprawl communities from otherwise living and working closer to the urban center.[61]

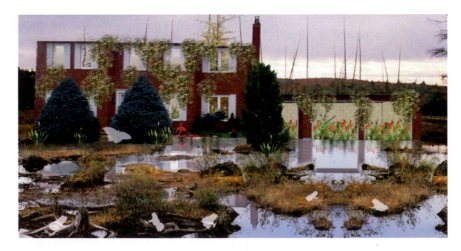

**FIGURE 4.24** Frog's Dream, Reburbia Competition (Proposal), Calvin Chiu. Illustration courtesy of Calvin Chiu

Seek to develop transfusion strategies that re-establish the infrastructural support. *Un*gate such prominent components of sprawl machines. Reconnect them with the rhythms of everyday civic life. Endeavor to do so in a manner that is safe and which promotes healthier lifestyles for everyone.

**Fluid Facades (B17)**—The sprawling, decentralized landscapes of suburbia render highly diffuse settlement patterns, isolating rather than drawing people together. Excessive horizontalism is counterintuitive to fluid, diverse, human-scaled communities. Jan Gehl, in *Cities for People*, argues for the nurturing of genuinely inviting streetscapes because they stimulate, reaffirm, and underscore the social bonds so critical in everyday life. Streets with mixed functions provide a broad range of activities. They are safer places, especially when housing is in close proximity to commercial and civic places of importance. A neighborhood's civic places for social interaction feeds off synergies generated by active, interactive storefronts, sidewalks, side paths, and streetscapes. Even if a street itself is deserted one can still *sense* its connectivity with adjoining buildings: perhaps viewing the lights on at dusk inside the surrounding buildings. This is especially meaningful during the winter months. In a city such as Copenhagen, where the buildings in the urban center are no more than five or six levels in height, visual connections between the street and upper levels of the buildings are also sustained. Above this height, such connections are lost (Figure 4.25). Gehl writes:

> Ground floor building design has a disproportionately large impact on the life and appeal of city space. Ground floors are what we see when we walk past buildings. . .people inside can follow what is going on outside, and vice versa. If populated. . .[or] even at night. . .furniture,

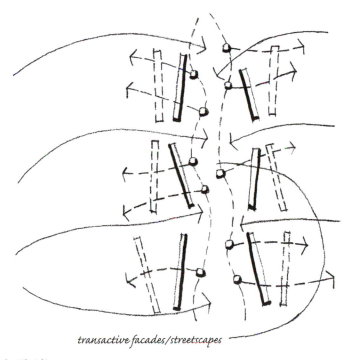

*transactive facades/streetscapes*

**FIGURE 4.25** Façade Fluidity

flowers, parked bicycles and forgotten toys are comforting witnesses of life and [our] proximity to other people. Light streaming from the windows of shops, offices and dwellings helps increase the feeling of safety in the street.[62]

By contrast, streets with metal shutters and/or blank walls concealing all interior functions within may be interpreted as symbols of an unsafe, even hostile environment.

**Light Manufacturing Interwoven (B18)**—Richard Florida is fond of describing cities as big idea labs, and views the existence of a prosperous creative class as a prerequisite condition in the eradication of blight and economic decline. In reference to New York's struggling garment industry, Tom Vanderbilt writes:

> Yes, cities are filled with the modern-day equivalent of the *luftmenschen* [literally, people who "live on air"], persons who breathe WiFi. But in many sectors of the 'creative industry,' there comes a point in time when something physical must be made, and when, because of financial or time constraints, it makes sense to have it produced locally. . .Having manufacturing close to the locus of creation isn't simply a matter of convenience; the process of production can inform and shape the creative process itself. So before another "industrial" loft is converted to a fantasia of Bosch appliances and Brazilian teak floors, before another productive building becomes a midrange hotel for tourists, take a closer look.[63]

Cities that function most successfully are those with the highest *velocity* of ideas, and the most efficient and direct links between people in terms of getting things done, getting things made. This requires the existence of strong interrelationships between designers, manufacturers, marketers, and so on. Traditional urban centers such as New York City are evolving into what sociologist Saskia Sassen calls a "postindustrial production site." It is a place built by and for the dissemination of ideas.[64] The same modus operandi is possible in transfused suburban landscapes. The points of contact, however, need to become sufficiently denser in order to support the types of human transactions necessary to spawn new economic life in these places. Endeavor to save and restore significant buildings in suburbia that can be transformed into platforms for the creative "making" of ideas and things by providing support for light manufacturing operations—right in the heart of the neighborhood where people live, worship, play, work and socialize. Support the production of products produced within the immediate community because it is counterproductive and self destructive to do otherwise.

**Electrocharging Stations (B19)**—Electrocharging stations supply recharges for alternative personal vehicles (APVs) and related plug-ins, and hybrids. At present, all-electropowered APVs are rechargeable on domestic wall outlets; in the future their battery cells will be rapidly replenished via high-speed commercial rechargers and indirect, inductive, recharging technologies. In the first half of the 20th century, internal combustion engines faced the similar hurdle of too few fossil fuel stations for the refueling of vehicles. In places with few gas stations and especially in expanding suburban and in rural precincts, motorists experiencing fossil fuel range anxiety often had to wait in long lines to refuel. This same thing is occurring with APVs in the 21st century until an adequate recharging network is in place. The Silicon Valley-based developer of the *Smartlet*, an individually controlled recharge station with locations in public and in private parking areas, introduced the first solar powered electric vehicle recharge station in the United States in 2009 in Chicago. It is a joint venture of Carbon Day Automotive and Coulomb Technologies. Chicago, a city with relatively few sunny days (fewer than 100 per year) proved successful for this corporate start-up despite its climatological limitations.[65] The town of Elk Horn, Iowa, as of the end of 2010 operated the only electro-charging station on Interstate 80 between Chicago and Denver. Prior, one would have had to "borrow" an electro-charge from a stranger or friend's house or private business along the route. Recharge stations currently cost $7,000 each, with an average recharge time of less than three hours. Electrocharging stations are in operation across the state of California, including 130 listings in the San Francisco bay area alone as of the end of 2011. In time the appearance of more stations in closer proximity to one another will diminish the range anxiety currently surrounding APVs.[66] *POD Point* in the U.K. currently publishes online the location and availability of recharge stations. There, APV recharge stations are proving successful, not unlike the system launched in Madrid, Spain in 2010.[67] Intercity transport will soon be far more practical because the two major impediments will have been overcome—a sufficient number of recharging stations, and a reduction in recharge time. Endeavor to establish APV recharge stations in and between suburban including zones, including or resuscitated dead mall sites.

**Indigenous Public Health Traditions (B20)**—The post-World War II suburban mall ruined thousands of traditional main street business districts, and in the process eviscerated many long-standing health promoting traditions. People were able to walk to downtown, but not to the mall.[68] Pay close attention to pre-mall precedents, however, when transfusing classic 1950s-era suburban malls to once-again vibrant centers. Peruse the narratives on the deadmalls.com website for insight in this regard. Conduct the due diligence to learn of its historical place in the community's social and architectural heritage. Research whether any specific local public health rituals were associated with it when it was in its prime. Developers of shopping malls in the late 20th century seldom bothered to take the time to learn of any such local traditions. Does a correlation exist between the rise and fall of a given mall and local health and wellness indicators? This information can guide in the restoration of once-popular events that promoted physical activity outdoors in the public realm. The annual Walk for Hunger in north suburban Chicago for many years drew people from all ages and backgrounds together for a common cause that simultaneously promoted both the activity of walking in suburbia, and global nutritional health. Old Orchard Shopping Center was a major sponsor. The Strawberry Festival in suburban Long Grove, Illinois, draws thousands of visitors every July from across all of Chicago's metro area to celebrate the strawberry's surprisingly diverse culinary expressions. People walk throughout the town's historic core, rediscovering the joys of being a pedestrian amid Chicago's encroaching sprawl machines. Identify and celebrate unique traditions, with a particular focus on the role of food, music and art as in the local culture manifest in sponsored civic events outdoors involving walking and cycling. The recent adaptation of a former vacant K-Mart store into the Lebanon-Lalede County Library, in Ohio, was enhanced by the inclusion of the products produced by local artisans, the site's reconnection to long-dormant pedestrian and cycling linkages with the surrounding neighborhoods, and through the use of architectural references inspired by local vernacular traditions.[69]

## C. Mall Transfusion

**Demise of the Megachain (C1)**—For thirty years, American consumers went on an all-out shopping spree. Their frenzy fueled the rise of the megachains and supersized retail outlets to the point where by 2010 consumer spending accounted for 71 percent of the total U.S. Gross Domestic Product (GDP), and thousands of traditional Main Streets died, or were reduced to near-death. Up until the Great Recession of 2008, American megachains raced to construct thousands of big box retail outlets, seemingly everywhere. The largest three magachains—Wal-Mart, Target, and K-Mart—were usurped by yet another group of mega-merchants, known as *category killers* and their (aptly named) *power centers*. In the US, category killer power centers include Bass Pro Shops and Cosco. These non-places are usually built on formal Greenfield agricultural sites. Somewhat smaller in scale but no less destructive companies of this new type include Staples, Zellers, Sam's Club, Kohl's, Big Lots, Family Dollar, Barnes & Noble, Whole Foods Market, Best Buy, Linens N'Things, PetSmart, the Home Depot, and Lowe's. A power center big box is a freestanding, low budget, one-level warehouse container that ranges in size from 20,000 to 280,000 square feet, and it is built expressly for retail use.[70] As of 2011, there were 2,913 Wal-Mart Supercenters in the United States, with the largest big boxes covering 260,000 square feet on two levels. As previously mentioned (see Chapter 3), Wal-Mart currently employs more than 1.5 million persons across the globe. Its critics argue that Wal-Mart in particular will no longer be capable of maintaining its "warehouse on wheels" now that fossil oil reserves have peaked. Gasoline prices will inhibit the ability of people to drive to these places.[71] The public may look back nostalgically on this era ending, but will just have to find consumer happiness elsewhere, perhaps differently from the extraordinarily compulsive mass consumerism of recent decades, as illustrated in the now-dead former Kroger's big box grocery outlet in Lafayette, Louisiana, photographed in 2011 (Figure 4.26). Why attempt to keep U.S. retail megachains and their global counterparts on life support in the form of government bailouts and the like? They should be allowed to die off as a species. Unfortunately, Wal-Mart continues to out-size itself by building ever larger power centers and then turning around overnight and abandoning the older carcass left behind: in 2011 it carried an inventory of more than 250 vacant big box carcasses due to its self-predatory practices—complete with no-compete clauses built in to

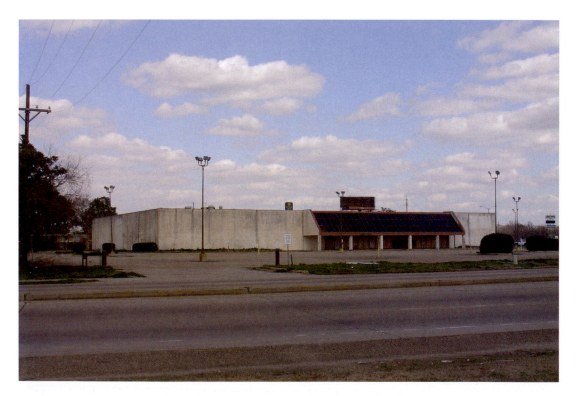

**FIGURE 4.26**  Dead mall, Lafayette, Louisiana

disallow any other retailer from claiming its abandoned carcasses. Meanwhile, local officials appear helpless to do anything to stem this suburban tragedy.[72]

**Small Box/Big Box Dialectics (C2)**—As James Howard Kunstler has pointed out, in the coming years suburbia will have to be rebuilt from the bottom up and it will occur within an entirely new, grassroots-based economic system. It will be rebuilt by resurrecting the locally based interdependencies that the post-World War II national chain megastore movement nearly completely destroyed. It will be a massive undertaking.[73] The locally owned bike shop, bakery, shoe store, and so on will experience a renaissance in a transfused suburban milieu. These small businesses will repopulate suburban dead zones in the wake of the decline and fall of the megachains and their behemoth outlet stores. New small businesses will be housed in them, in recycled modular ISOs, and in abandoned office and residential buildings, i.e. McMansions. They will be housed in clusters beneath the roof-shells of abandoned Wal-Mart superstores. It will be necessary, first, to overhaul conventional zoning ordinances thereby allowing for new land use overlay districts with tax and related incentives provided to those who elect to pioneer the redevelopment of the many thousands of carcasses left behind by the fallen megachains. Instead of hundreds or thousands of outlets, new start-ups will have a small number of outlets all in close geographic proximity to one anther. Opportunities will open up for architects to innovate in response to their new clients' rapidly evolving need for a rapid response architecture. Its public health affordances will be many if these establishments do not remain over dependent on the conventional automobile, and if located close enough in proximity to one's home whereby one can easily assess without always having to drive there. The coming wave of anti-big boxes should therefore be conceptualized as infill-destination points for a wide range of goods and services able to be accessed within close walking and cycling distance and close to public transport systems, i.e. light rail, electric buses.

**Deconstruction Strategies (C3)**—The power center box itself, with its low budget, minimal articulation, is woefully bereft of the *delight* component in the Vitruvian conceptualization of a true work of architecture as embodying *commodity, firmness, and delight*. Deconstructive strategies return dead malls and big box outlets to far more salutogenic and ecologically sensible land uses. Add by subtracting. A bizarre aspect of big box consumerism is that one has to actually *purchase* the privilege to shop there in the form of a "membership" card in order to gain access to a Sam's Club, Cosco, and most other U.S.-based big box retailers although they are nothing more than conduits for products shipped to the box then put on a high warehouse rack then sold for the lowest price to the largest number of people. The vast expanses of pavement surrounding big boxes are unaesthetic, geared to get the most consumers in and out of the box as fast as possible. The selective removal of portions of a big box—and its adjoining sea of pavement—affords many possibilities to re-connect these non-places to their immediate community in a far healthier manner from a public health perspective. Create courtyards, oases, opportunities to take a break from shopping by strolling past a garden, create play areas for kids or a daycare center (Ikea currently provides this service to its customers), outdoor pocket parks, places to sit and rest or eat where one can buy more than an overcooked hotdog shipped from thousands of miles away and served on a stale bun (Figure 4.27). Reconfigure the container and its immediate exterior environs, drawing inspiration from collective civic memory, genuine placemaking precepts, and local architectural tradition. *Addition-by-subtraction* is applicable to interior and exterior spaces, as well as formerly residualized in-between horizontal voids. With the help of EXED, a charter school developer, an Episcopalian congregation purchased an abandoned mall down the street from the group's offices near down town Los Angeles and transformed it into an elementary school. The Camino Nuevo Chapter Academy (2001), designed by Daly/Genik Architects, has become a catalyst within a once-neglected neighborhood, and effectively serves multiple functions through its transfusion from a dead strip mall by means of various deconstructive strategies (Figure 4.28).[74]

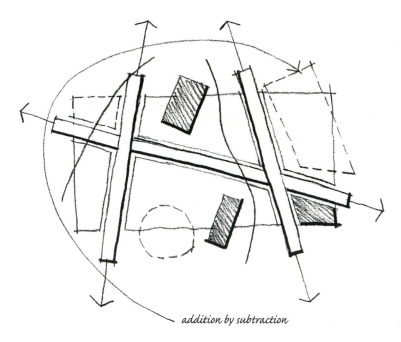

*addition by subtraction*

**FIGURE 4.27**  Deconstruct Dead Malls

**Transparency (C4)**—In big box megastores, storefront windows, if there are any, exist only on the front facade. In most, natural light is transmitted solely through the front doors at the entrance. These monolithic warehouses are stark, featureless, dominated by dreary, gray concrete masonry or tilt up prefabricated slab walls. Their scale is impressive if nothing else. This sole light source into the box causes excessive glare for those near to the portal. Light is transmitted through a miniscule aperture, and they don't want you to look out to the world beyond, anyway. With few or no skylights or clerestories, it gets worse: an army of oversized omnipresent mercury vapor and fluorescent light fixtures stare down at you from the upper reaches of the box, hanging conspicuously from the undersides of the exposed steel grid ceiling. This open grid reveals all in a bare one's aesthetic as if to proclaim, "We saved money on finishing out our building so we could pass the most savings on to you, Dear Shopper." Meanwhile, Mr. and Ms. Unsuspecting Shopper below circulate in a zombie-like funk up and down supersized aisles with a supersized cart filled with supersized foreign-made goods. The products themselves—ketchup, mayonnaise, juices, frozen foods, clothing, consumer electronics— are nearly always sold in large packaged quantities. How can an anti-salutogenetic marketing strategy such as this result in anything but an ever more obese clientele? Cleverly, a big box is designed and built with great subliminal care so as to not draw undue attention onto itself. One need not know anything about the world outside the big box while shopping in one. Any such attention presumably distracts from the main agenda—to immerse the shopper in the "Wal-Mart Experience." It does not have to always be this way. In stark contrast to the generic power center's blind box aesthetic, the Crate and Barrel national home furnishings and housewares chain in the U.S. employs abundant natural light in its retail outlets. Clerestories, spatial variability, laminated wood beams, and carpet proffer a far more transparent, open, immersive shopping experience. In transfused big boxes, endeavor to inject the natural environment. Reintroduce new elements and spatial experiences in a completely new aesthetic and functional configuration (Figure 4.29).

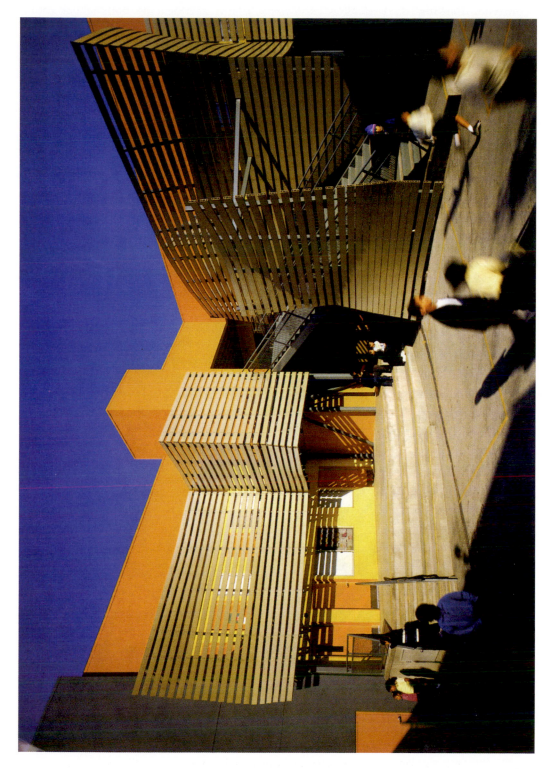

**FIGURE 4.28** Camino Nuevo Academy, Los Angeles, Daly Genik Architects. Photo courtesy of Daly Genik Architects

**Deconstruct Parking (C5)**—Endless expanses of asphalt pavement do nothing but choke sprawl machines. They are anathema to salutogenic public health precepts or to health promoting environmental design strategies. Open, agricultural land and forests give way to paved expanses that look and feel like deserts. They're hot, shadeless—horizontalism at its severest. This "aesthetic" dominates strip centers and shopping malls everywhere and undermines our daily lives and the health of our environmental ecosystems. Why has it become so hard to step back and critically reassess? Mark Crispin Miller, in his analysis of television, the second technological servant that came into mass acceptance in the 20th century (with the automobile being the first), sees the medium of TV as now so integral to our ambient culture that we can no longer isolate ourselves from it to acquire any reasonable perspective of our place within mass media landscapes.[75] There remains simply no safe vantage point from which one can survey its near-complete domination of popular culture. And the same is rapidly occurring with our growing addiction to our computer screens and handheld smart devices. This analogy is apropos. Seas of parking surfaces cut us off from nature. The automobile and the horizontal surfaces and parking decks invented for its storage and retrieval are both deeply ingrained in our collective conciousness. Our psyches have been rewired. As Jane Holtz Kay observes, this makes it virtually impossible for us to understand that in both cases the servant has become the master.[76] To mitigate the potentially adverse psychological public health consequences of drowning by chronic exposure to overpavement, endeavor to deconstruct large expanses of horizontal pavement vis-à-vis landscape urbanism strategies of selective removal, dissection, slicing, and layering within reclaimed natural ecosystems. Zoning laws of the past required parking capacity levels to be calculated based on peak use periods. This must change. Once, it was assumed everyone would come and go by private auto. This must also change.[77] In addition, the featureless, treeless pavement surrounding strip centers and shopping malls contributes to the urban heat island effect. Trees and pervious ground cover are mitigation tools thereby countering the pavement's severity while expressing a far more appealing aesthetic, not unlike *Dwell* magazine 2009 Reburbia

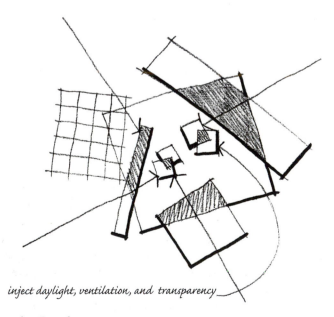

*inject daylight, ventilation, and transparency*

**FIGURE 4.29**   Buildings that Breathe

competition submittal for a dead mall's conversion into a suburban farming co-op, by Forrest Fulton (Figure 4.30a–b).[78]

**Terracing (C6)**—Terracing represents perhaps the best current example of the convergent blurring of the lines between landscape urbanism and architecture. It allows for the retention of existing green horizontal open space and affords new opportunities for innovative urban typologies and topographies. This is achievable by creating buildings that simultaneously function as ecological landscapes. Modulated stepping accommodates level changes which reflect topographic conditions, but can go far beyond the mere stepping of simulated naturalistic hillside configurations comprising gardens, water elements, and architectural amenities. The Fukuoka Prefectural International Hall (2000), in Fukuoka Japan, designed by Emilio Ambasz & Associates, remains a tour-de-force in the deployment of compositional terracing infused with a park-like landscape (Figure 4.31). The city was in need of a new government office building and the only available site was a large two-block parcel that also happened to be the last remaining horizontal green surface in the city center. Ambaz was awarded the commission for his proposal to reconcile otherwise contradictory aims: to retain (replace) the existing park on the site while simultaneously providing the city center with a new multi-use landmark building. Beneath the structure's fourteen one-level trays—terraces—lie more than 1 million square feet of office and commercial space, containing an exhibition hall, museum, 2000-seat proscenium theater, conference facilities, 600,000 square feet of government and private sector offices, and a large underground parking deck and retail mall. Its northern façade presents an elegant arrival portal that reconnects the city's busiest commercial artery with green civic space. Its

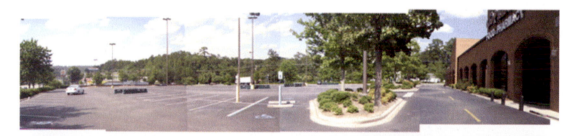

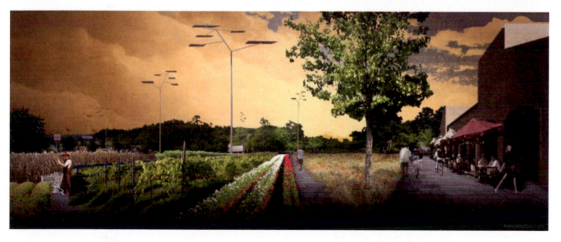

**FIGURE 4.30a–b** Big Box Agriculture, Reburbia Competition (Proposal), Forrest Fulton. Illustrations courtesy of Forrest Fulton

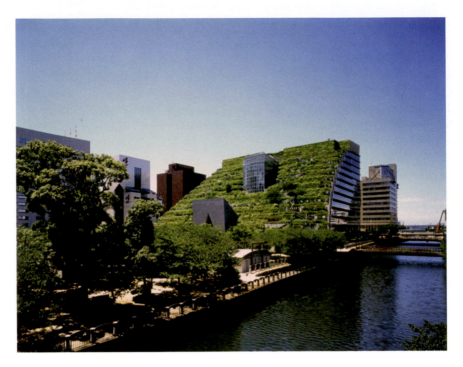

**FIGURE 4.31** Fukuoka Prefectural International Hall, Japan. Photo courtesy of Emilio Ambasz & Associates

southern side extends the existing park through its terraced gardens, ascending the full height of the building, culminating in a magnificent belvedere. This space affords magnificent views of the harbor and surrounding hillsides. This redevelopment of an otherwise underutilized urban zone has received numerous awards, including the 2000 *Business Week/Architectural Record* Award, the 2001 DuPont Benedictus Award, and First Prize in the 2001 Japan Institute of Architects Certificate of Environmental Architecture.[79]

**Spacesharing (C7)**—Sixty miles from Bangkok, Thailand, an open-air market operates directly on the tracks of a heavy rail commuter train line. Each time a train approaches this station-cum-market hundreds of merchants and their customers hurriedly scatter, hastily removing everything from the railway's right of way. Day in and day out, with each approaching train, this spectacle is repeated *ad infinitum*. As an urban ritual it may sound extreme but in point of fact, single-function commercial operations are a thing of the past in dense places where every square foot must count. Interest is rapidly growing in the ability to time-share space—*space share*. It is not a new concept. In the U.S., many local civic organizations have used a similar concept for generations. The Veterans of Foreign Wars (VFW) and the American Legion Posts across America constructed a network of hundreds of local lodges in the 20th century. These facilities were time-shared insofar as on weekends they were used for social events including pancake breakfasts for fundraising, i.e. the local Boy Scouts troop, and by various religious congregations. These places were built at or near the center of the town within easy walking or biking distance from nearby neighborhoods. Time-sharing allows multiple businesses to share the same space at different times to offset high rents and the high initial site development investment costs associated with building ownership.[80] An e-retailer, for instance, may only need the space three days per week for its use as a *nomadic warehouse* or part-time storefront operation. On the other days of the week a second e-retailer could do the same; and a third retailer, and so on, with specific day–only (or even hourly) uses scheduled in–between on a 24/7 basis. School facilities from pre-schools to universities should be reconsidered for their time-sharing amenity on weekends, evenings, holiday periods, and during the summer months. Gone are the days of one site, one function architecture in suburbia.

**Edge Sites as Coral Reefs (C8)**—Coral reef buildings represent one facet of an ecological architecture whereby a building is sited in sufficiently close proximity to other buildings as a means to spark *covariant synergies*, thereby contributing to greater transfusional vibrancy, economic viability, and livability. In the post-World War II American suburb, archaic zoning laws required buildings to be distanced far from one another by seas of horizontal surfaces that needlessly precluded their potential to meaningfully co-vary with one another and with the amenity of sidewalks, cycling paths, and related human (non–auto) scaled activity. Anti-pedestrian spaces now become walking and cycling paths, and buildings become interwoven and interdependent. This, as opposed to the deadening suburban condition whereby nonrenewable building and infrastructural resources are consumed without giving anything back. Reconsider the density and substance of edge sites. Recast them as vibrant, interconnected *coral reefs* full of life and as points of destination. The Winter Park Village is a 525,000 square foot mixed use "lifestyle center" located on the site of a failed regional shopping center in Florida in an affluent older suburb of Orlando. It now features a blend of retail, offices, and fifty-two loft apartments. This grayfield site was redeveloped on 40 acres and its transfusion featured numerous edge site interventions interspersed with open green spaces. In a second phase, additional housing is planned on the edge sites together with additional landscaped open space. Other recent examples of transfused edge sites at once-dead shopping malls include the Voorhees Town Center, in New Jersey, the Biltmore Village, in Asheville, North Carolina, and at Belmar, in Lakewood, Colorado. In each case, these redeveloped edges function as major contributors to the dead mall's makeover, as the majority of these examples were once dreary seas of horizontal pavement.[81]

**Soft Surfaces (C9)**—Sprawl machines produce hard, dreary, harsh surfaces. In the U.S., *asphalt-to-nature land trusting* is a concept that offers the possibility of turning hard pavement into soft, open green space. This will require the reversal of decades of mindless suburbanization, however, and a full court press on the part of the general public. San Francisco's streets and rights of way currently consume over 25 percent of the city's total land area and this is more space than exists in all of the city's parks combined. The city's recent "Pavement-to-Parks" initiative is ameliorating this condition by reclaiming dead pavement parcels for total makeovers into public plazas and park spaces. The Showplace Triangle (2009) on 8th Street between 16th and Irwin Streets in the Potrero Hill neighborhood, designed by ReBar Group, was transformed with nearly entirely recycled materials, including debris boxes redeployed as planters. It has proven to be a success with the community.[82] Additional similar projects are now currently underway in other parts of San Francisco. Seas of asphalt in urban and suburban communities are vestiges of a land use zoning system having gone off the rails. The deconstruction of massive expanses of pavement into soft surfaces and coral reefs reclaims these parcels and helps return these places to a more natural state. Endeavor to reduce the amount of off-street parking and correspondingly increase on-street parking on these sites. This makes it possible to create new open green space in formerly unbroken expanses of pavement. Reclaim this type of underused pavement with a focus on placemaking on the sites of dead shopping malls and commercial strip centers. Where space is limited, create layered matrices of hard and soft surface textures and material palettes. Overflow parking on-site is reconfigurable using permeable pavers and level changes, encouraging multifunctionality, i.e. the local farmers' market, art festivals, and for music and other health promoting

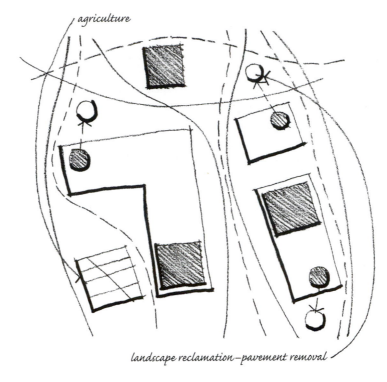

*agriculture*

*landscape reclamation—pavement removal*

**FIGURE 4.32** Reclaim Dead Pavement

community events year-round. During non-peak use periods these soft surfaced places can accommodate temporary overflow parking (Figure 4.32).

**Fast Food Restaurants (C10)**—There are currently more than 160,000 fast food restaurants in America, and these places generate sales of $65 billion annually. McDonald's alone operates 14,027 outlets in the U.S. and 32,737 outlets worldwide.[83] American fast food corporate chains have continued to aggressively expand their networks of franchisees since the 1960s. The effects of corporate overexpansion, the Great Recession, evolving consumer tastes, and unprecedented competition within the industry have recently dovetailed. In most U.S. metropolitan areas the inventory of fast food outlets is significantly overbuilt. Roadside, strip, and mall-based fast food outlets are being shuttered due to cannibalization of sales resulting from hyper-competitiveness wherever dozens of close-by fast food restaurants are concentrated cheek by jowl. Over time, the Wendy's was built next to the Sonic next to the Arby's next to the McDonald's next to the Burger King next to the Arby's across the street from the Hardee's that is next door to the Taco Bell that is right across the street from the KFC and next door to the Subway located across from the Popeye's, and so on. Not surprisingly, the most lucrative corporate expansion opportunities in fast food currently exist in developing countries. It is a corporate culture that remained remarkably impervious to its core markets growing clamor over the poor nutritional quality of its food offerings. Cheaper food is not necessarily better food. A factor in the industry's current supply-quality-demand problems in its core markets is its slow response to rising obesity and chronic disease rates. Why not take a vacant Hardee's, Wendy's, or KFC and transform it into an aerobics facility, Pilates center, or light-boxing emporium? Adapt them into childcare centers with their exterior environs adapted into play space. Remove the seas of asphalt and replace these hard surfaces with soft, pervious surfaces, i.e. green grass, trees, seating, and community gardens (Figure 4.33).

**Site Sharing (C11)**—Many post-World War II era suburban shopping malls, subdivisions, office complexes, medical centers, and allied building types were constructed in one fell swoop because the financing was available to do so. The developer owned the land as well as all the buildings. No longer may this be the case in an age of governmental deficits, cutbacks, far stricter bank lending practices, unemployment, layoffs, foreclosure, shifting demographics, diminished natural resources, and consumer retrenchment. Instead of once-greenfield sites where the developer owned and controlled everything insight, the challenge now centers on reclamation as a process of incremental redevelopment and of doing more with less whereby the landowner(s) and the building owner(s) may co-operatively share a transfused site. New, creative, entrepreneurial site leasing/occupancy strategies are called for. This will provide new life to abandoned buildings, vacant parcels, parking lots, and fallen salutogenetic in-between spaces scattered throughout the suburban landscape. It can work this way: a landowner relinquishes the idea of owning all the land plus all its "improvements'" thereby debunking most traditional conceptions of "property"—in a disassociation of the concept of land ownership from the concept of building ownership. With land valuations predicted to be in constant flux in the coming years, property ownership in a traditional sense may be a far less desirable proposition, and more risk-laden than in the past. Site sharing can consist of owning the site improvements (but not the land beneath), i.e. portable modules stationed on leased sites. Buildings can migrate

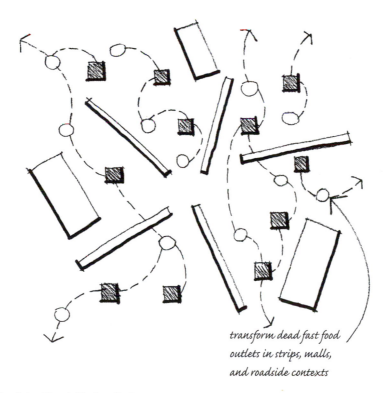

transform dead fast food
outlets in strips, malls,
and roadside contexts

**FIGURE 4.33**   Reclaim Dead/Dying Strips

elsewhere as needs change, i.e. healthcare facilities, because this concept recasts traditional landlord-renter agreements. Explore lease-to-own agreements. On site reclamation and the interplay between land sharing, residualized landscapes, and transportable buildings, Robert Kronenburg writes:

> A lot of buildings and sites are now unused. . .Think about all those millions of acres of road-sides, empty inner city building lots, ex-industrial land, and roofs. If these were accessible, serviceable and open for use, then long-lasting but moveable architecture would become viable.[84]

Most current zoning laws are obsolete in this regard. *Site sharing* stimulates private sector reinvestment in a downtrodden suburb. It starts with a dead mall, a locally owned neighborhood bakery, dentist's office, a Subway fast food outlet, a reclaimed factory, a complex of sixteen modular apartments that can be located or reconfigured, a reconfigurable mom and pop fresh food corner grocery—housed in a single mixed-use structure or in configurations of freestanding portable or fixed buildings.

**Landmarks and Anomalies (C12)**—As previously discussed, dead malls are often fondly recollected for that favorite toy store, shopping season, sitting on Santa's lap as a child, or merely for hanging out with old friends in the food court as a teenager. The long-demolished Capitol Court mall (a big box center was later built on its site) on the northwest side of Milwaukee, Wisconsin, was such a place, with Hagensick's toy store and the Kookie Cookie House. The latter was a freestanding wood frame house that looked like a North Pole toy factory. Shop windows featured miniature displays and they were changed on a frequent basis. Some days visitors had to wait in long lines to be a part of this spectacle: an "assembly" process that culminated with toy Tonka trucks leaving the "factory" on a small conveyor "road" and transporting cookies to the center of the mall's open air court.[85] A dead mall may warrant serious reconsideration as a civic landmark. Unheralded oddities may also be of merit and worth preserving, as in the case of New Orleans's Gentilly district, where a small frame house sits amid a busy intersection. Enormous billboards are perched on its roof and have been there since the early 1950s (see Chapter 5). While intrinsically unaesthetic (perhaps in some strange way not dissimilar from how the Eiffel Tower was first perceived when it appeared on the Paris skyline) it nonetheless has remained an accidental neighborhood landmark for over sixty years. Neighborhood anomalies need not be of an unselfconscious nature to be considered of landmark stature. In India, the firm Vāstu Shilpā Architects continually explores in its buildings the inner profundities of curvilinearity, including in its housing, incorporating domes, thin concrete shells, skylights, evocative massing, and imagery such as at Sangath, the architect's design studio/residence, completed in 2005 (Figure 4.34).[86] Endeavor to produce buildings and landscape of coherence, those which hold the power to generate positive recollective memories and in the case of historically significant buildings, salutogenically preserve and enhance them by restoring and/or adapting them in a way that promotes the public's health.

**Vertical Gardens (C13)**—Agricultural land of any type is becoming a scarce commodity in densely populated locales globally. The consequences of farming land loss include the aforementioned urban heat island effect, and its implications for food production. A vertical garden's ornamental and agrarian properties can exceed those of a green roof. Vegetated walls can aesthetically enrich otherwise harsh, featureless facades, adding color, texture, aromas, provide seasonal variability, and add biodiversity while yielding significant insulating and evaporative cooling properties to the immediate micro-setting (Figure 4.35). Soft, permeable vertical planted surfaces are referred to as biowalls, living walls, or *greenwalls*. The horizontal roof garden is the nearest precursor to the vertical greenwall although the cultivation of vegetated vertical surfaces is by no means new, as wall

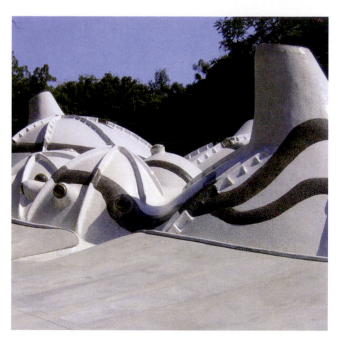

**FIGURE 4.34** Design Studio/Residence, Sangath, India. Photo courtesy of Vāstu Shilpā Architects/Consultants

vines and assorted plantings were integral to architectural facades and in spa and bathing complexes of ancient Rome. In their current incarnation, greenwalls are integral to theory and practice associated with sustainable environments and have recently been re-popularized by the French botanist Patrick Blanc in his Caxia Forum near Atocha Station, in Madrid. A primary school in Itabashi, Japan, is screened by a living wall comprised of melon plants. It is of aesthetic value and helped to meet LEED certification requirements. A greenwall requires a sophisticated irrigation system, however, as the wall may be subjected to direct sun exposure, winds, and of course the forces of gravity. Carefully select species that can thrive in such potentially challenging conditions. A rooftop rainwater collection system (rain cistern) can irrigate a greenwall. Plants purify slightly polluted water (graywater) by absorbing dissolved nutrients, such as the system used by the Brazilian firm Triptyque Architecture, in its housing complex (2007) for a suburban infill site in São Paulo, Brazil (Figure 4.36).[87] Popular species for temperate climates include Actinidia, Aristlochia, Campsis, Celastrus, Clematis, Cotoneaster, Hedera, Humulus, Lupulus, Lonicera, Pyracantha, Selaginella, and Wisteria.[88] An interior biofiltration wall was installed at the University of Guelph in its Humber Building, in 2005. Greenwalls can yield salutogenetic human health benefits by reducing symptoms of physical discomfort experienced within buildings.[89] Recent projects include the proposed Pyramid Farm, by Eric Ellingsen and Dickson Despommier, a skyscraper Urban Farm, by Jung Min Nam, the enormous insect-like Dragonfly Tower, by Vincent Callebaut, and the modular Harvest Green high-rise proposal by Romses Architects.[90]

**Roofscaping (C14)**—Dead malls can be ugly. But when viewed from above their expansive flat roofs can be even more unattractive. Roofs may be structured to withstand the weight of minimal landscaping as long as the specific drainage requirements for water runoff/retention can be met. Make possible their reclamation or portions thereof for this type of new use. It can be achieved by

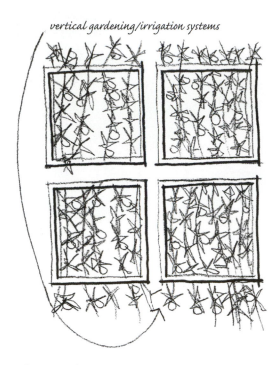

**FIGURE 4.35** Foster Vertical Horticulture

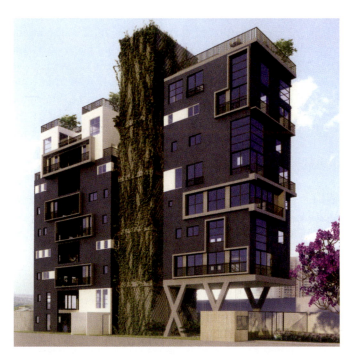

**FIGURE 4.36** Vertical Garden, Suburban Infill Housing (Proposal), São Paulo, Brazil. Illustration courtesy of Triptyque Architecture

selectively peeling away the roof plane, or by slicing away strips, replacing these segments with new, vegetated roof segments. An A/B A/B rhythm can be created with some roof segments landscaped and with intervening roof segments painted a light color to deflect solar gain, or to provide for instal-lation of photovoltaic modules. *Green roofs* are also referred to as ecoroofs, oikosteges, vegetated roofs, and living roofs. A green roof is therefore one that is partially or completely covered with vegetation, installed atop a waterproofed membrane. These installations can feature a root barrier, and sophisti-cated irrigation systems. They are becoming popular in metro areas globally because they provide an oasis of nature within otherwise harsh, non-landscaped surroundings, they allow for therapeutic benefits accruable through human interactions with nature, they afford fresh air, sunlight, can be a source of fresh food, and because they can be installed directly above (or adjacent to) one's dwelling or workplace. The City of Chicago has been at the forefront of this movement with respect to its city-owned buildings. Urban and suburban roofscaping counters the urban heat island effect by reducing ambient air temperatures. Installations are generally of two types: intensive roofscapes, able to support a broad array of plant species and requiring significant maintenance, often installed in small, concentrated areas; and extensive roofscapes, covered in a light layer of vegetation and signifi-cantly lighter overall, often covering a much larger area than an intensive installation. SITE Architects' prescient (yet unbuilt) Terrarium Showroom for BEST Products (1978) featured an entirely organic intensive roofscape (Figure 4.37).[91]

## D.  Suburban Agrarianism

**Suburban Farmers' Markets (D1)**—The movement to distribute fresh, locally grown produce has caught on in suburbia, where there are now many examples of successful farmers' markets. Many operate only one day per week, such as on Saturday mornings. The French Market in New Orleans's Vieux Carré is among the oldest farmers' markets in North America and is a precursor to many recent suburban farmers' markets of the past decade. It is open every day of the week. These places draw diverse individuals together and provide a healthier food alternative to "store bought" produce, and their presence often contributes to a more socially vibrant streetscape because people stop to interact casually who may not otherwise do so if always driving in their private cars to and from the local corporate-owned supermarket. Farmers' markets will continue to proliferate in suburbia due to consumer preferences, the unavailability of affordable store-bought fresh produce, and the rising cost of fossil fuel. It will simply be cost prohibitive for an 18-wheeler to transport grapes and carrots many hundreds of miles to a corporate-run supermarket. In New Orleans East, a 6,000 member Vietnamese community has since 1975 been engaged in suburban micro-farming with its produce sold in the local community and in New Orleans's nearby French Market. Many of these community farm-workers had previously been fishermen in Vietnam; others at one time worked in factories, hotels, and restaurants throughout the metro area. These plots are farmed communally along the fertile banks of a drainage canal. The community has developed a successful, locally owned agricultural enterprise. The Viet Village currently consists of 20 acres in the heart of the residential community on the city's outskirts, plus five 1-acre commercial plots, a poultry and livestock area for free-range chickens and goats, areas for recycling of organic wastes, and three market pavilions where growers sell their produce and meats. On this suburban farm tract these entreprenuers grow many varieties of vegetables and fruits. The Viet Village Suburban Farm project received a 2008 Excellence Award from the American Society of Landscape Architects (ASLA).[92] Suburban farming is central to the deconstruction of sprawl machines. It also adds life and interest to otherwise banal, lifeless places; successful examples can raise adjoining land values and foster the redevelopment of adjacent land.

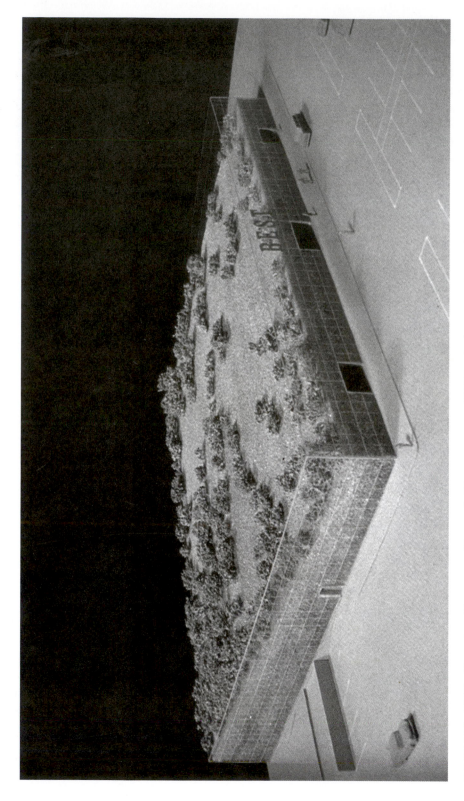

**FIGURE 4.37** SITE—Terrarium Showroom (Proposal). Photo courtesy of SITE—Architecture, Art & Design

Daniel Phillips's futurist submittal to the 2009 Reburbia competition envisions wind-powered vertical farming masts that hover high above traffic-clogged freeways of the future (Figure 4.38).[93]

**Microfarming (D2)**—In industrialized, developed countries, corporate-owned agribusiness produces milk, chickens, eggs, and pork on what are known as confined animal feeding operations (CAFOs). These places consume excessive water, generate many tons of waste, and confine their animals indoors nearly continuously. Being indoors means that if one animal gets sick, they all get sick. To alleviate this, corporate megafarms pump their animals full of antibiotics. Excessive antibiotics then flow into the groundwater supply and come in contact with bacteria—forming superbugs. Humans eat the unhealthful growth hormones fed to these animals. Conventional grocery stores sell as many CAFO products as possible because they hold their color and appearance longer. These food monopolies and their powerful, well-paid political lobbyists are doing their best to force mom and pop/privately-owned farmers out of business. For instance, Monsanto now controls most of the whole seed inventories in the world, since it successfully lobbied Congress to allow it rights to patent seed. Meanwhile, between 1997 and 2007, 52,000 family-owned agricultural enterprises in the U.S. alone went out of business. Farming is rapidly becoming a lost redevelopment tool in rural areas, but it can be an essential one in cities and suburbs in economic decline (Figure 4.39). Freedom Organix is a small diversified 20-acre farm located 70 miles from Chicago, a city of more than 8 million yet

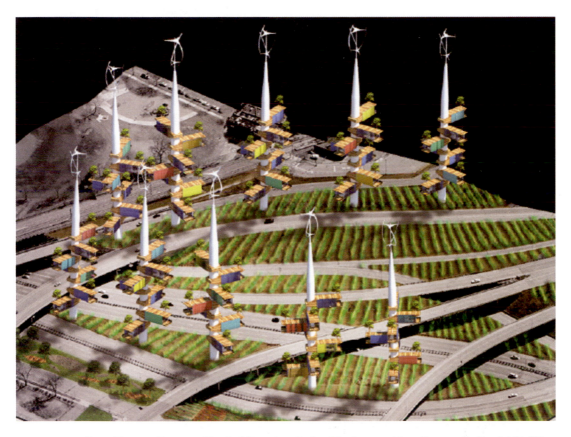

**FIGURE 4.38**   Inter Estates: Freeway Vertical Farming, Reburbia Competition (Proposal), Daniel Phillips. Illustration courtesy of Daniel Phillips

one only able to feasibly support very small-scale micro-urban and suburban farming at this time. Independent growers sell their fresh produce and vegetables in Chicago's neighborhood farmers' markets.[94] With 80,000 vacant lots in Chicago, the large City Farm Chicago was constructed on the grayfield site on the former (now demolished) Cabrini Green public housing complex. This 6-acre farm includes the Mobile Food Collective, a series of nomadic carts that facilitate the selling of fresh produce while providing space for seminars and training. Its produce is sold to local restaurants and to local residents.[95] In places with viable economies it still remains cost prohibitive to convert former industrial properties to open green space for agricultural use, although dead malls offer *microfarming* opportunities in this regard.

**Agrarian Stoa (D3)**—The tools and implements used in microfarming are many, diverse, and complex. They range from small hand-held tools to large irrigation and crop management equipment. These implements require an efficient, safe, and accessible storage structure. In the case of suburban infill microfarm plots, it is important to attempt to locate the microfarming plot near to a local farmers' market structure or complex. The ancient *stoa* is a timeless, practical, and adaptable architectural element for this purpose. Its narrow, linear configuration allows for one to three sides to be open-air with its rear wall remaining enclosed. The open front side of the stoa allows for the display of produce in the various stalls, with the rear zone along the stoa's rear wall providing space for centralized, lockable storage units for equipment used in the adjoining farming plot(s). In periods of inclement weather, the front-open side of the stoa can easily be shielded from the elements vis-à-

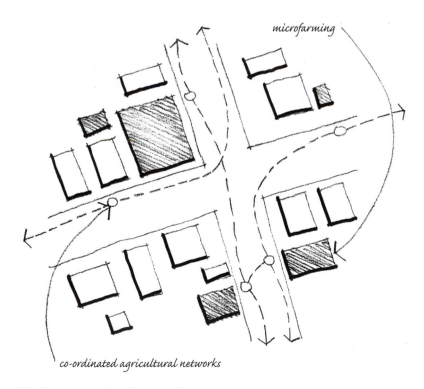

**FIGURE 4.39**  Suburban Agricultural Networks

vis a roll-down cloth protective membrane; this is precisely how it was done in ancient Greek towns such as Pergamon. Tools can be checked out on a daily or hourly basis and gardeners may bring their own tools and related equipment from home (Figure 4.40). Tools may be checked out only once per week, while sitting idle at other times. Co-ops are being established in many places for the sharing of farming equipment, much like a public library for hard copy book sharing. Tools therefore remain in active use, not unlike keeping a good book in circulation as it passes from reader to reader. Major issues in suburban organic microfarming include irrigation, land use efficiencies, and land co-ownership. In Detroit, there are currently more than 30,000 acres of vacant and abandoned grayfields and brownfields. Individual plots, community gardens, and a few larger sized farms are feasible, although larger acreage can be associated with increased human health and environmental risks, potential conflicts with adjoining non-farming land uses, and the impacts of NIMBY-ism. As the size of parcels increases attention will need to be devoted to design and site placement of an agrarian stoa in relation to the environmental, smell, and noise impacts of light and heavy machinery, trucks, chemical pesticides, herbicides, noise, and air quality, all of which may bear deleterious environmental side effects in suburbia. Conduct due diligence to test for the possibility of toxic soils in and near agrarian stoa as well as adjacent farming parcels that may require remediation.[96]

**Infill Agrarianism (D4)**—A community or private-plot fresh food garden created on residual infill sites can transform forlorn or underused land in suburbia into a valuable amenity, a source of food for a family. The typical U.S. suburban tract house built in the post-World War II period was sited squarely in the middle of its land plot, often resulting in residual side parcels and a large yard directly behind the house: on one side, the driveway leading to the garage, on the other, a

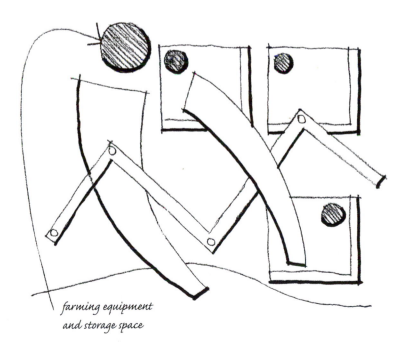

farming equipment
and storage space

**FIGURE 4.40**  Suburban Farming: Implements/Amenities

narrow swath of lawn. The British long ago mastered the art of infill gardening, a tradition dating back centuries. In Surrey, residents in 2007 were forced to unite to launch a "Hands off our back gardens" campaign as a means to protect their beloved yet endangered back gardens. The fight was on against local government ordinances that sought to reclassify back gardens as brownfield sites. Such land is given a greater priority for development, enabling new homes to be developed on formerly community-operated and semi-private "squatter" garden plots.[97] In places coping with the aftermath of disaster, such as in post-Katrina New Orleans, the demolition of thousands of densely packed 19th- and early 20th-century residential structures has resulted in many blocks pockmarked with weed infested parcels where dwellings once stood. In a city with 125,000 fewer residents due to the 2005 disaster, local officials saw it as an opportunity to establish infill gardens in these dead zones and in-between residuals.[98] More and more, suburbanites are growing their own produce in the underused parcels around their homes and businesses. In Los Angeles, a group of residents transformed a cinder block wall into a vertical garden of strawberries, tomatoes, herbs, and vegetables. The public health benefits of organic infill suburban farming include physical exercise and the knowledge that one's food is free of the harmful pesticides and related chemical additives so common in store-bought food products. In terms of architectural reclamation, as discussed earlier, abandoned industrial buildings can be peeled away and their interior footprints can be reappropriated for use as infill farming either by removing their concrete slabs, roofs, and by bringing in topsoil and drainage improvements.[99]

**Suburban Composting (D5)**—Compost is decomposed plant matter recycled as a fertilizer and soil supplement. It is a key aspect of organic farming and dates from the ancient Akkadian Empire in Mesopotamian Valley, based on information recorded on clay tablets produced 1,000 years before Moses was born. There is evidence of composting among the Ancient Greeks, and in the early Roman Empire from the time of Pliny the Elder (AD 23–79). References to composting are contained in 10th- and 12th-century Arab writings, in medieval church texts, and in Renaissance literature. Writers such as William Shakespeare, Sir Francis Bacon, and Sir Walter Raleigh all mentioned the use of compost. The first industrialized process for the transformation of urban organic materials into compost was in Weis, Austria, in 1921.[100] The process requires the sorting of waste in a container outdoors for a year or more. It entails a multi-step, closely monitored protocol with measured inputs of water, air, and carbon–nitrogen rich materials for gardening, landscaping, horticulture, and agricultural uses. The most common microorganisms found in active composts are bacteria, actinomycetes, fungi, protozoa, and rotifers.[101] The compost unit itself is beneficial for soil, including as a conditioner and a natural pesticide.[102] In landscape ecosystems, composting aids in erosion control. Most U.S. cities will eventually require food and yard waste to be sorted for composting. In 2009, San Francisco became the first U.S. city to mandate that all residents and businesses separate their recycling and compost material from their normal trash. This measure is anticipated to help increase landfill diversion rates by up to 75 percent.[103] The public health benefits of composting include land and stream reclamation, wetland construction and conservation, and its amenity as a topsoil layer in grayfield and brownfield site reclamation. This land is reconditioned for recreational uses with the aim of health promotion, i.e. walking, jogging, and cycling activities. Similarly, the earth beneath suburban parking lots can be reclaimed, restored, and hence transformed through the use of on-site composts together with the transport of compost-enriched soil from nearby processing centers.

**Cisterning (D6)**—Suburbia relies almost solely on publicly financed potable water sources and systems. The age of cheap freshwater available in seemingly endless supply is over, simply because current infrastructure is on the verge of collapse in many places. In the American Southwest, water consumption levels are now being severely curtailed routinely, with new laws that render the ability to maintain a bright and healthy "green" lawn highly impractical if not outright illegal. Cisterns are a viable and cost effective alternative. They are aboveground containers to capture and store rainwater and are distinguished from wells by their waterproofed inner linings. Modern cisterns range in capacity from a few to many thousands of cubic feet in capacity, and in effect function as miniature-covered reservoirs. Their use dates from the earliest Neolithic settlements in the Middle East, and are a common practice in areas where water is scarce due to sparse rainfall or due, as mentioned, to local overconsumption. Rainwater cisterning supports irrigation, cooking, and hygiene. A removable lid serves to protect the water source from bacteria, algae, and insects. In Brazil, cisterns are made of bright blue molded plastic with matching lids. In the U.S., cisterns are currently used in greenhouses, but still only infrequently in residential contexts.[104] Bermuda and the U.S. Virgin Islands now require rainwater-harvesting systems as a part of all new construction. Japan, Germany, and Spain offer direct financial incentives and/or tax credits for their installation and use. They also are of benefit as a water source for firefighting in areas with scare water resources. Cisterns must be kept clean, periodically disinfected with chlorine, and thoroughly rinsed at specific intervals. It is recommended that public policy and suburban transfusion strategies promote cisterning as an environmentally ecological and cost-effective practice. It can complement existing civic municipal and private ownership property infrastructures, while costing comparatively little to set up and operate. Incorporate rain drains with cisterns on rooftops, in backyards, parks, in neighborhood co-op microfarming, and in commercial and civic buildings (Figure 4.41). Public health benefits include the physical activity required to operate and maintain the units, and their provision of fresh water for multiple daily needs.

**Horticultural Education (D7)**—Microfarming requires specialized skill sets that very few suburban residents currently possess. But the time is right to educate suburbanites on the financial and health promotional benefits accruable to people who love fresh food and vegetables, who harbor heightened concerns over overall food safety and quality, or who share the growing disdain for modern food production and its far-flung food distribution systems. Microfarming can be a catalyst for the economic revitalization of a declining neighborhood, and this is leading many residents to learn more about gardening and agricultural techniques. As they ponder the potential and feasibility of transforming their currently inedible yards and lawns, more individuals and groups are seeking education on how to do so. Progressive community colleges and universities across the U.S. are launching certificate-training programs to teach people to farm in American cities and suburbs. Many non-profit neighborhood organizations are also stepping up to help fill this void in education and training. These include the Atlanta Urban Gardening Program, and Growing Power, in Chicago. The U.S. organization Beginning Farmers launched a resources web site on theory and technique.[105] In Boston, the Massachusetts Avenue Project's urban agriculture training programs feature practical, philosophical, and experiential opportunities to learn about successful strategies as well as pitfalls to avoid. Participants receive training in urban fish farming—*aquaponics*—livestocking, vegetable crops, composting, and attend seminars with experts on topics including how to start an Urban Youth Farm (UYF) for the benefit of providing useful activities for troubled adolescents and teens, as a source of life general enrichment, and community job creation. A single 1½ acre microfarm plot can currently yield $25,000–35,000 in gross income annually, if its owner-operator is properly trained and equipped on how to make it a success. Such an organization's goal is typically to rebuild the healthier local community vis-á-vis urban farming fuelled by entrepreneurship.[106] Health promotion through an active lifestyle is fused with new employment opportunities, personal self-empowerment, and the return of previously overlooked, dying, or dead spaces to viable new uses.

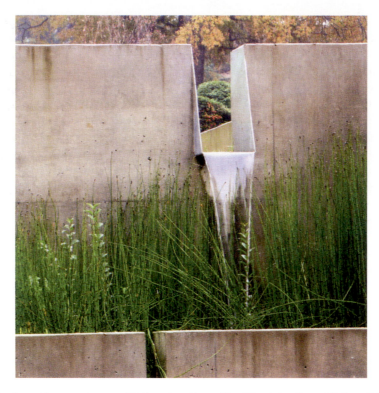

**FIGURE 4.41** Student Center, Averett University, Danville, Virginia, Pete O'Shea/Siteworks Studio. Photo courtesy of Siteworks Studio

## E. Implementation

**Transfusion Zone Diagnostics (E1)**—The importance of due diligence in selecting a neighborhood transfusion zone cannot be overestimated. It must possess a requisite core, baseline infrastructure to enable the transfused zone to grow and flourish through serialized improvement across time. Prerequisite infrastructural grid components include electricity, natural gas, water, sewerage, telecommunications, links to public transit, roads, adjacency to water, climatic factors, educational resources such as schools and universities, and careful historical documentation of prior land uses. Prior land uses may have otherwise unforeseen, even politically notorious consequences, such as the profundities of a former industrial site that is now a brownfield or grayfield site. Such sites often require costly remediation and can become a source of politically combustible situations.[107] The systematic analysis of the transfusion zone's economic redevelopment potential is of critical importance from the outset as well as at every subsequent step. The *transfer of development rights* (TDR) is a governmental mechanism (in the U.S) that assigns or reassigns an entity the authority to redevelop a zone to a private or quasi-private land use. The intent is to stimulate reinvestment, not unlike the goal of a TIF (tax increment financing district). The track record of TIFs and their policy derivatives in suburbia in recent years has been spotty at best. Rezoning will in all likelihood be of absolute necessity because conventional zoning laws in the U.S. are archaic with respect to most transfusion theories and methods.[108] Use Google Earth, GIS, and archival databases available in local libraries and museums, media outlets, combined with boot-on-the-ground grassroots recognizance to gather and analyze site information and then to be able to systematically document these data in a series of diagnostic base maps, videographics, and photographs. Mapping and documentation of the following are essential: the origins and history of the zone, all relevant geographical attributes, its cultural amenities and fabric, its educational institutions, its healthcare infrastructure, landmarks, and anomalies, residual buildings and land uses, LULUs and TOADs, public transport linkages, historic buildings and civic space, the effects of past natural and/or human-caused disasters, and current land use (zoning) patterns. Start with broad-stroked geographies and then move in successive waves of inquiry and investigation to more closely scrutinize *tissue samples* at the level of individual precincts, blocks, and individual buildings and their associated open spaces (Figure 4.42).

**LEED and Sprawl Mitigation (E2)**—Established by the United States Green Buildings Council (USGBC) in 2000, LEED (Leadership in Energy and Environmental Design) is today the preeminent accepted standard for certifying green buildings in the U.S. and around the world. It is currently used in more than 100 countries. To date (2011), LEED has certified over 4 billion square feet of built buildings. The system recently has instituted provisions and benchmarks intended to improve community health in the outdoor realm and the indoor health of building inhabitants. One requirement of LEED is the control of environmental tobacco smoke (ETS) through the ban on indoor smoking. In 2009, LEED adopted *social equity* metrics, measured by, among other factors, human health promotion criteria. LEED also functions as a vehicle for the development of metrics to gauge additional health-related benefits similar to those that measure a building's carbon footprint, overall water efficiency, and water

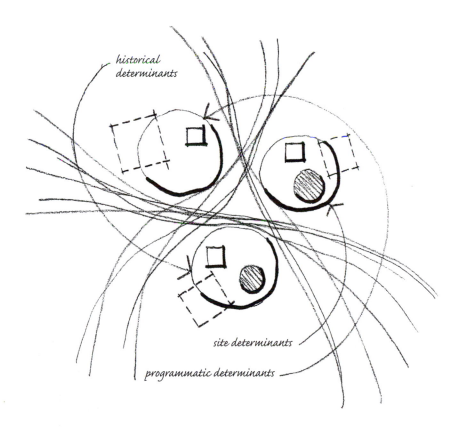

**FIGURE 4.42**  Transfusion Zone Diagnostics

fixture efficacy. An allied set of metrics, LEED-ND (Neighborhood Development), now focuses on linkages to health promotion within a LEED building's surroundings, i.e. improvements in outdoor air quality, the minimization of ozone depletion and heat island effects, and measures to reduce obesity within the community through the provision of sidewalks, cycling lanes, and associated amenities.[109] The LEED protocols and the massive machine it has spawned in Washington, D.C. have faced a backlash of heightened scrutiny, however. In recent studies, some LEED certified buildings at the Silver and higher level have been found to consume far more energy than initially touted, and are even unhealthy for their occupants. Meanwhile, every day, more government bodies, municipalities, educational institutions, and businesses are mandating their buildings to be LEED certified at the Silver level or higher (certification rating levels are currently Silver, Gold, and Platinum).[110] A recent report by a U.S. not-for-profit group concluded that highly energy efficient buildings actually increase occupants' exposure to toxigens, because air exchange rates between the indoors and outdoors are insufficient. Outdoor air is generally cleaner than indoor air, and these practices over-concentrate airborne particulates including gases and other chemicals, resulting in more intensive human exposure rates. Unfortunately, very few among the tens of thousands of chemicals that exist within buildings are tested for toxicity, and few members of the USGBC possess any formal medical, epidemiologic, or toxicological training.[111]

**Geomap Resourcing (E3)**—Every new building or renovation project in architecture is preceded by some sort of site-context analysis. A site survey is commissioned. This yields essential information about the site's physical attributes such as its physical boundaries, topological features, the presence and type of any ground vegetation and trees, the indication of adjacent roads and structures, pavement and barriers. Physical infrastructural systems are documented: above-grade and below-grade utilities, grid connectivity, and soil tests. This is intended to extract any and all data that might have a bearing on the design response. What exists determines what is possible. Additional analyses often include traffic patterns, land use classifications, access points to the site, location of local schools, parks, healthcare facilities, shopping districts, churches, libraries, local historical landmarks and neighborhoods, and civic places of significance. Digital mapping protocols examine the historical evolution of the site and its immediate neighborhood environs. The genesis of the design responses lies embedded in this database and in its representational accuracy. Digitalization has opened up new horizons. Google Earth's mapping digital software, fused with geographic information systems (GIS), now makes it possible to obtain a heretofore-unprecedented level of data about a building, its site, neighborhood, and city, anywhere. An equally extraordinary advantage of this database is that anyone, anywhere, can now access the same data and this capability is being applied by social scientists in the examination of human settlement patterns and class-based social hierarchies, especially in developing places, as a method to identify disparities in land ownership between rich and poor (Figure 4.43). Places that were previously undocumented now are accessible online. It is of critical importance for this mapping database to become more fully integrated on a global basis in the planning and design of communities everywhere and for it to remain accessible in the public domain.[112] Prior to the Internet, site data had to be painstakingly assembled on a case-by-case basis. Now, architects and urban designers are making use of online databases in analytical mapping worldwide. Sprawl machines globally are now being mapped and scrutinized. The challenge will be to further harness these technologies to expand global awareness of the unhealthful consequences of unmitigated sprawl.

**Stakeholder Engagement (E4)**—Not since the 1960s has a generation of activist architects, urban designers, and landscape architects been this motivated to reengage their client constituencies and the general public. Back then, the awakening was led by calls for massive social and political

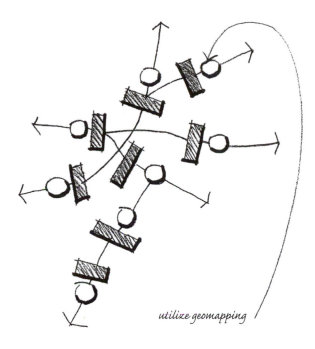

*utilize geomapping*

**FIGURE 4.43**  Geomap Resourcing

change in how institutions and governments operated and in the ways that cities were planned and built. It was then a call for the more equitable treatment of the underrepresented and marginalized segments of society. Governmental bureaucracies were challenged to their foundations, activism was the norm, and self-serving political and top 1% corporate interests were not to be trusted or tolerated in their then-current form. Planners and designers sought ways to more meaningfully engage their clients in ways that rejected the narrowness of the heroic masters of the 20th-century architecture such as Le Corbusier. Young, brash planners and designers developed tools for establishing common ground with their clients through interactive community design workshops, charrettes, and design reviews. Often, this occurred on the home turf of the client organization, that is, out in the neighborhoods. *Community design centers* (CDCs) were set up many inner cities in the U.S. These entities were established at the time with the primary goal to work with the disempowered and socially disenfranchised segments of society. C. Richard Hatch's excellent book, *The Scope of Social Architecture* (1984), documented the rise and later fall of dozens of CDCs.[113] In retrospect, two things stand out. First, theoretical discourse in grassroots social engagement was in time dismissed as quaint, naïve, and overly visionary. Second, as a result, many grassroots community engagement techniques, with the notable exception of the design charrette, a technique later to be championed by the New Urbanists, would eventually fall by the wayside due to benign neglect. Meanwhile, suburban mass consumer culture fell under attack and was critiqued in popular music, in film, and in literature in particular. Ironically, suburbia, and its attendant lifestyle of conspicuous consumption were seldom scrutinized in the popular culture. Exceptions included the Monkees' 1968 top-40 hit song "Pleasant Valley Sunday" and its scathing critique of suburbia and more recently, Arcade Fire's album "The Suburbs" (2010). Revive the CDC—only this time with an expanded focus on suburbia that is aligned with the occupy movement. This is not to imply that the social, political, economic, or built environment needs of inner cities are of any less urgency. Sprawl machines warrant the establishment of suburban CDCs (Figure 4.44).

**Gaming and Simulation (E5)**—Genuinely participatory tools—such as the design *charrette*—engage stakeholders in the design of their immediate neighborhood. Were rarely used in planning and constructing post-World War II suburbia. The typical American suburb was conceived *a priori* on the drawing board, with its streets, cul-de-sacs, homes, parks, shopping strips and malls, and civic institutions all neatly laid out in bubble diagram form, and that was that. Sometimes potential home-buyers were given the choice of their house style, choosing from a set of limited options from a catalog, or they could select the color of the exterior face brick of the front facade, the number of bedrooms, or if a one- or two-car garage, detached or attached. Larger planning-scale issues were seldom if ever presented to buyers for their input. The aforementioned participatory design move-ment of the 1960s was focused nearly singularly on inner urban core neighborhoods with compara-tively scant attention given to the then-burgeoning suburbs. It was not unlike a society having worn one gigantic set of horse blinders. For suburban transfusions, a gaming simulation prototype was developed in 2010 by Eva Behringer and Heather Bachman in the School of Architecture at Clemson University. Called "Dead Mall", it simulates how various transfusion scenarios can play out in simu-lated time prior to their implementation in real time (Figures 4.45–4.48). It is intended for use by grassroots neighborhood groups as a means to express what they want (or don't want) to happen with their local dead mall, for instance.[114] Participants are able to pre-select among six different redevelop-ment scenarios, which are then weighted, via a set of decision cards. The consequences of these deci-sions are played out in the format of a board game. The process consists of the decision cards, issue/

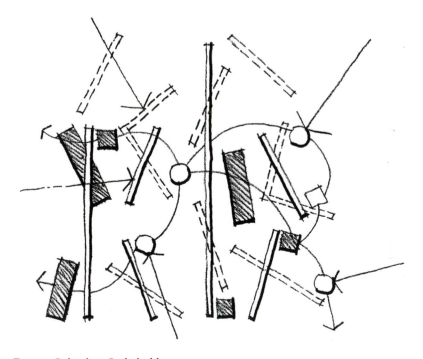

**FIGURE 4.44** Engage Suburban Stakeholders

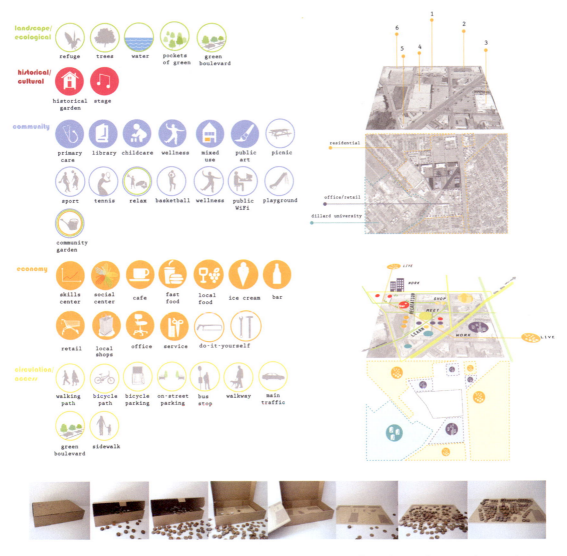

**FIGURE 4.45**   Dead Mall Game (Simulation). Illustration courtesy of Heather Bachman and Eva Behringer

priority cards, and a site plan playing surface whereby playing chips are distributed and redistributed iteratively across the transfusion precinct through a series of playing rounds whereby various stakeholder role players are required to negotiate with one another in a series of rounds. This allows players to experience what it is like to be in the shoes of other local decision makers in the transfusion, such as a banker who switches roles with that of a homemaker, or an auto mechanic who switches roles with the manager of the local outlet of a national drugstore chain. Each round is timed, therefore requiring precise negotiations, and decisions. The consequences (policy decisions) are displayed on the board game's playing surface itself and on an adjoining whiteboard. Color-coded chips are used for this purpose. When all role players agree upon a single collective strategy, it is played out across multiple rounds (implementation rounds 1–4) which may represent, say, four phases

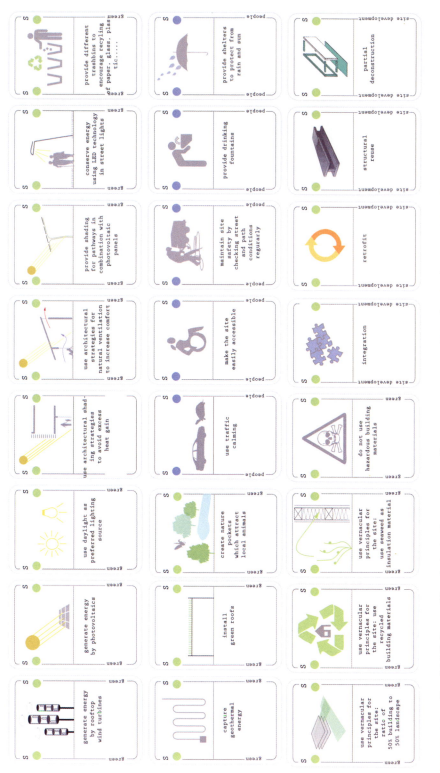

**FIGURE 4.46** Dead Mall Game (Simulation), Components. Illustration courtesy of Heather Bachman and Eva Behringer

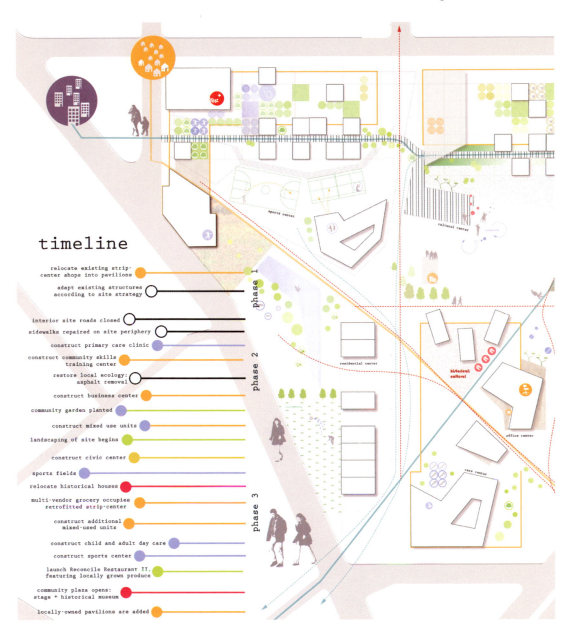

**FIGURE 4.47** Dead Mall Game (Simulation), Phases. Illustration courtesy of Heather Bachman and Eva Behringer

across the coming ten years. "Dead Mall" seeks to foster at the local level realistic redevelopment expectations as to what is and is not likely to occur premised on the assumption that change is to occur incrementally across many years, with many players involved, and not in one fell swoop, as might have been standard protocol in the past.

**Foster Innovation (E6)**—Design competitions and the mass media are but two mediums to critically examine the phenomena of sprawl machines. International design competitions function as

# design proposal

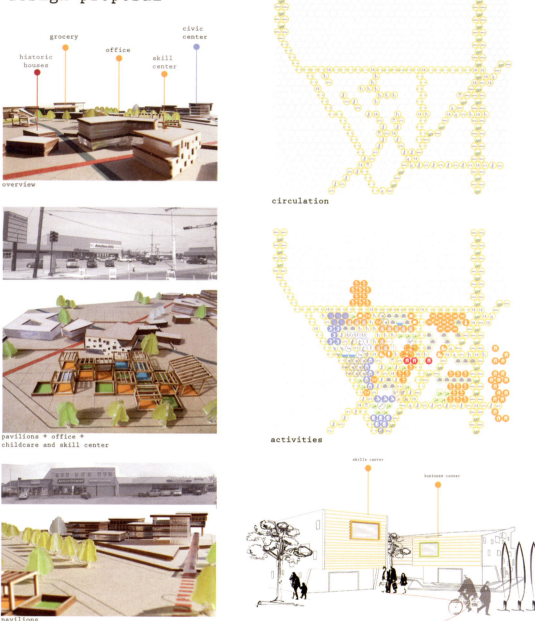

**FIGURE 4.48** Dead Mall Game (Simulation), Outcome Scenarios. Illustration courtesy of Heather Bachman and Eva Behringer

vehicles for innovation because they are able to question and extend beyond mainstream discourses. In 2009, *Dwell* magazine sponsored its Reburbia design competition for the re-envisioning of suburbia in the 21st century. Entrants were charged with conjuring future-oriented proposals within an open-ended site and project scope framework. The winners of the competition were featured on the websites Inhabit.com, Dwell.com, and Re-burbia.com, and in *Dwell*'s December 2009/January 2010 hard copy issue. Various proposals submitted addressed McMansions, big box stores and their power centers, strip malls, and parking lot reclamations, with proposals ranging from community agriculture and algae-based biofuels to transplanted tract developments to fantastical zeppelin-based on-demand public transport systems. The competition drew more than 400 entries from more than a dozen countries, and a set of twenty finalists was pared down to four wining entries:

- Grand Prize—Frog's Dream: McMansions Turned into Biofilter Water Treatment Plants (Calvin Chiu);
- Second Place—Entrepreneurbia: Rezoning Suburbia for Self-Sustaining Life (Urban Nature/F-S Design/Silverloin Design);
- Third Place—Big Box Agriculture: A Productive Suburb (Forrest Fulton);
- People's Choice Award—Urban Sprawl Repair Kit (Galina Tachieva).

Endeavor to advocate for (and even directly sponsor yourself) planning and design competitions focused on suburban transfusion vis-à-vis carbon reduction precepts. It is important to involve government at all levels—federal, state, and local—as well as the private sector, namely developers and venture capitalists. Instrumental leadership is called for at this time (Figure 4.49). The Moore Square design competition held in Raleigh, North Carolina, in 2009 drew more than 100 submittals (many with an anti-sprawl theme) for the resuscitation of a key block in the heart of that city. The intent of the competition's sponsor, New Raleigh, was to counter the Raleigh metro area's sprawling horizontalism.[115]

**Incremental Transfusion (E7)**—The era of grand redevelopment scheming is over. Money has run out in many places for grandiosity. Time is also running out. One recent grandiose effort in the

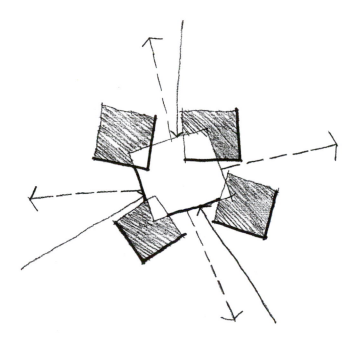

**FIGURE 4.49**   Foster Innovation—Design Competitions

U.S. was the 67-acre, $8.5 billion City Center in Las Vegas, a behemoth, one-fell-swoop redevelopment consisting of 6,000 newly built hotel rooms, forty-two restaurants, lounges, and bars, private residences, and a super-upscale retail mall. Funded and built just prior to the 2008 Great Recession, it was touted as the largest privately funded construction project ever in North America and an attempt to rebrand Las Vegas once and for all as a cosmopolitan destination city. It showcased the work of superstar designers including Daniel Libeskind. During its planning, its developers, the MGM Mirage, traveled to Shanghai and Dubai to capture the essence of international trends in high-end global urban redevelopment.[116] It now struggles amid the worst economic downturn in Las Vegas's history. Such one-fell-swoop strategies are antithetical (as defined here) to the aims of suburban transfusion, which must aim instead to implement more realistically grounded improvements in an entirely different approach—*incrementalism* (Figure 4.50). In Detroit, a city that experienced an historic decline in its population between 2000 and 2010, incremental, organic redevelopment, not "big bang projects," will be the only way the city will survive in the 21st century with one neighborhood at a time reborn, block-by-block. It is about the passion, the caring, commitment, and perseverance of local stakeholders. All it takes is a few pioneers. It started, on one block, in Detroit, in 2006, with one restaurant, then a woodworking shop, then additional businesses, all with support provided by a locally based not-for-profit, the Hudson Foundation. It has been all about grassroots

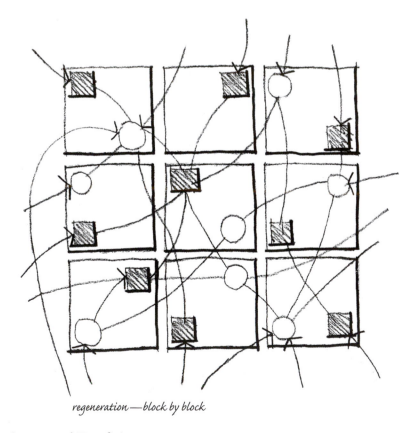

*regeneration—block by block*

**FIGURE 4.50**   Incremental Transfusion

progress, word of mouth, and it has captured the attention of national organizations such as CEOs for Cities, which held its Urban Leaders Summit in Detroit in 2010. Real estate experts, for their part, tend to always focus on physical assets in land valuation, while routinely failing to recognize the value of human capital assets, and yet this is by far the most critical building block in successful redevelopment. In a city and surrounding suburban area known for its rampant post-industrial decay, this initiative sends a far more resounding message: "Look at what we have left to work with!"[117]

## Fast Forward

As mentioned at the outset of this chapter, the theories and strategies presented here are merely a springboard, setting the parameters for further rethinking, expansion, and refinement by others elsewhere as more case studies are completed on the transformation of sprawl machines into denser, more livable, healthier, ecohumanist communities. In the following chapter this compendium of seventy-five design considerations infuses a case study for a battered yet globally significant city that urgently needs transfusion following the destruction wrought by Hurricane Katrina in 2005—New Orleans. The setting is an inner ring suburban district currently in the midst of massive recovery after having experienced a major catastrophe.

## Notes

1　Tachieva, Galina (2010) *Sprawl Repair Manual*. Washington, D.C.: Island Press, p. 7.

2　Shenson, Douglas, Benson, William, and Harris, Andree C. (2008) 'Expanding the delivery of clinical preventive services through community collaboration: The SPARC model,' *Preventing Chronic Disease*, 5:1. Online. Available at www.cdc.gov/pcd/issues/2008/html (accessed 8 April 2011).

3　Larson, N.I., Story, M.T., and Nelson, M.C. (2009) 'Neighborhood environments: Disparities in access to healthy foods in the U.S.' *American Journal of Preventive Medicine,* 36(1): 74–81. Also see National Association of County & City Health Officials (2010) *Building Healthy Communities: Lessons Learned from CDC's Steps Program*. Washington, D.C.: NACCHO.

4　Newberg, Sam (2011) 'The rush to build walkable grocery stores,' *Urban Land*, 22 March. Online. Available at www.urbanland.uli.org/Articles/2011/Mar/NewbergGrocery.html (accessed 21 April 2011).

5　Strauss, Richard (1999) 'Childhood obesity,' *Current Problems in Pediatrics*, 29(1): 5–29. Also see Freedman, Daniel, Khan, L.K., Dietz, W.H., Srinivasan, S.R., and Berenson, G.S. (2001) 'Relationship of childhood obesity to coronary heart disease risk factors in adulthood: The Bogalusa Heart Study,' *Pediatrics*, 108(3): 712–718.

6　Centers for Disease Control and Prevention (2002) 'Barriers to children walking and biking to school—United States, 1999,' *Morbidity and Mortality Weekly Report*, 51(32): 701–704.

7　Howle, Julie (2009) 'New Wal-Mart shopping center to go on U.S. 123 site in Easley, SC,' *The TIW Blog*, 3 August. Online. Available at www.word.truthintheword.org/south_carolina/new-wal-mart-shoppin-center.html (accessed 19 March 2011).

8　Lerner, Jonathan (2010) 'Turning failed commercial properties into parks,' *Miller-McCune*, 28 December. Online. Available at www.miller-mccune.com/business-economics/turning-failed-commercial-properties-into-parks-26410/.html (accessed 24 February 2011).

9　Duran, Sergi Costa and Eguaras, Marina R. (2010) *1000 Ideas by 100 Architects*. Boston: Rockport, p. 12.

10　Dewey, Fred (1997) 'Cyberurbanism as a way of life,' in *Architecture of Fear*. Princeton, NJ: Princeton University Press. Reprinted in Graham, Stephen, ed. (2004) *The Cybercities Reader*. London: Routledge. Also see El Nasser, Haya (2011) 'Will "intelligent cities" put an end to suburban sprawl?' *USA Today*, 30 January. Online. Available at www.usatoday.com.html (accessed 2 February 2011).

11　Summer, Stuart (2011) 'Making cities smarter with technology,' *computing.co.uk*, 22 February. Online. Available at www.computing.co.uk.html (accessed 25 February 2011). Also see Arieff, Allison (2011) 'Trailer parks as models for affordable housing,' *The Atlantic Cities—Places Matters*, 21 September. Online. Available at www.theatlanticcities.com/design/2011/09/trailer-park-new-model.html (accessed

1 October 2011).

12 Farr, Douglas (2008) *Sustainable Urbanism*. New York: John Wiley, p. 52.

13 Hayden, Dolores (2004) *A Field Guide to Sprawl*. New York: W.W. Norton & Company, p. 106.

14 Anon. (2010) 'Grant could redevelop suburban Dixie Square Mall,' *ABC7News*, 23 September. Online. Available at abclocal.go.com/wls/story?section=news/local&id=7686112.html (accessed 11 April 2011).

15 Noble, G. (1992) *Siting Landfills and Other Lulus*. Basle: Technomic Publishing.

16 Hayden, *A Field Guide to Sprawl* pp. 108–109.

17 The New Orleans land trust concept, as proposed, would require the homeowner to purchase one's home but lease the land beneath it for $25.00 per year with a renewable ninety-nine-year lease. The Lower Ninth Ward essentially has devolved from a quasi-urban neighborhood, with a walkable infrastructure, to one where, at present, there are no full service grocery stores, only one gas station, and only one school.

18 Sullivan, Zoe (2011) 'Own a home, but not the land,' *Miller-McCune*, 18 February. Online. Available at www.miler-mccune.com/business-economics/own-ahome-but-not-the-land.html (accessed 24 February 2011).

19 Lerner, 'Turning failed commercial properties into parks,' p. 4.

20 Farr, *Sustainable Urbanism*, p. 176.

21 Kellert, Stephen (2005) *Building for Life*. Washington, D.C.: Island Press.

22 Wasser, Walter (2003) 'Designing with water: Promenades and water features,' *Topos*, 14(3): 24–38.

23 Sutton, Samuel B., ed. (1971) *Civilizing American Cities: A Selection of Frederick Law Olmsted's Writings on City Landscapes*. Cambridge, MA: MIT Press.

24 Kellert, Stephen R., Heerwagen, Judith H., and Mador, Martin L. (2008) *Biophilic Design*. New York: John Wiley & Sons, pp. 54–56.

25 Ibid., p. 56.

26 Anon. (2011) 'Cities use brownfields to go solar,' *Sustainable Cities Collective*, 13 April. Online. Available at www.sustainablecitiescollective.com/dirt/23753/cities-use-brownfields-go-solar.html (accessed 16 April 2011).

27 Kalita, S. Mitra (2011) 'Bruised feelings and skinned knees litter suburban sidewalk politics,' *Wall Street Journal*, 8 March. Online. Available at www.online.wsj.com/article/SB100014240527487043291045761386 21423895138.html (accessed 10 March 2011).

28 Gehl, Jan (2010), *Streets for People*. Washington, D.C.: Island Press, p. 44.

29 Ibid., p. 155.

30 Blue, Elly (2011) 'How bicycling will save the economy (if we let it),' *Grist*, 28 February. Online. Available at www.grist.org/biking/2011-02-28.html (accessed 29 April 2011).

31 Wiggins, Ovetta (2011) 'D.C. expands network of cycling lanes, bike-sharing program,' *Washington Post*. Online. Available at www.washingtonpost.com/wp-dyn/content/article/2010/12/24.html (accessed 29 April 2011).

32 Gehl, *Streets for People*, p. 7.

33 Tachieva, *Sprawl Repair Manual*, pp. 40–41.

34 Russ, Caesar (2009) *The Crown Fountain: Millennium Park, Chicago*. New York: Realviews.

35 Pfeiffer, Bruce B. (2009) *Frank Lloyd Wright Complete Works, Volume 3: 1943–1959*. Berlin: Taschen.

36 Burney, David, Farley, Thomas, Sadik-Khan, Janette, and Burden, Amanda (2010) *Active Design Guidelines: Promoting Physical Activity and Health in Design*. New York City Department of Design and Construction/ Department of Health and Mental Hygiene.

37 Lukez, Paul (2007) *Suburban Transformations*. New York: Princeton Architectural Press, pp. 99–100.

38 Anon. (2009) 'Sylvan Slough Natural Area,' *Conservation Design Forum*. Online. Available at www.info@cdfinc.com.html (accessed 14 April 2011).

39 Benedict, Mark and McMahon, Ed (2006) *Green Infrastructure: Linking Landscape and Communities*. Washington, D.C.: Island Press, pp. 258–259.

40 *SITE: Architecture as Art* (1980). New York: St. Martin's Press, pp. 84–87.

41 Verderber, Stephen and Fine, David J. (2000) *Healthcare Architecture in an Era of Radical Transformation*. New Haven: Yale University Press.

42 Jones, Stephanie (2011) "Cargotecture: 13 massive container architecture projects," *WebUrbanist*, 18 February. Online. Available at www.weburbanist.com/2011/02/18/cargotecture-13-massive-containers-as-building-bocks/html. (Accessed 12 March 2011).

43 Kronenberg, Robert, Scoates, Christopher, Urback, Hincy, and Betsky, Aaron, eds. (2003) *LOT/EK: Mobile Dwelling Unit*. Santa Barbara, CA: D.A.P/University Art Museum.

44  Sawyers, Paul (2008) *Intermodal Shipping Container Small Steel Buildings*. 2nd Edition. London: Create Space. Also see Duran and Eguaras, *1000 Ideas by 100 Architects*, p 171.

45  Gehl, *Streets for People*, p. 181.

46  Christensen, Julia (2008) *Big Box Reuse*. Cambridge, MA: MIT Press, p. 5.

47  U.S. Department of Health and Human Services (1996) *Physical Activity and Health: A Report of the Surgeon General*. Atlanta and Washington, D.C.: Centers for Disease Control and Prevention/National Center for Chronic Disease Prevention.

48  Duran and Eguaras, *1000 Ideas by 100 Architects*, p. 188.

49  Gehl, *Streets for People*, pp. 131–132.

50  St. George, Donna (2010) 'More generations live under one roof,' *The Times-Picayune*, 18 March, p. A11.

51  Duran and Eguaras, *1000 Ideas by 100 Architects*, p. 241.

52  Anon. (2010) 'Biomimicry of heliotropic plants—more efficient solar panels.' Online. Available at www.bobaid.com/bionics/biomimicry-of-heliotropic-plants-more-efficient-solar-panels/html (accessed 30 March 2011).

53  Cipriani, Christine (2011) 'Days numbered for midcentury-modern school by the Architects Collaborative,' *Architectural Record*, 25 February. Online, Available at www.archrecord.construction.com/news/2011/02/110225wayland_high.html (accessed 1 March 2011).

54  Smith, Stephen (2010) 'Development as preservation,' *Market Urbanism*, 26 November. Online. Available at www.marketurbanism.com.html (accessed 21 January 2011).

55  Duran and Eguaras, *1000 Ideas by 100 Architects*, p. 269.

56  Kunstler, James Howard (2005) *The Long Emergency*. New York: Grove Press, pp. 56–70.

57  Fletcher, June (2009) 'McMansions out of favor, for now,' *The Wall Street Journal*, 29 June. Online. Available at www.online.wsj.com/article/SB124630276617469437.html (accessed 11 April 2011).

58  Solomon, Christopher (2009) 'The swelling McMansion backlash,' *MSN Real Estate*, 14 May. Online. Available at realestate.msn.com/article.aspx?cp-documentid=13107733.html (accessed 11 April 2011).

59  Chiu, Calvin (2009) 'Frog's dream: McMansions turned into biofilter water treatment plants.' Online. Available at www.re-burbia.com.html (accessed 7 July 2010).

60  Kay, Jane Holtz (1997) *Asphalt Nation: How the Automobile Took Over America and How We Can Take it Back*. Berkeley: University of California Press, p. 31.

61  Rubin, Gareth (2009) 'Gated communities: Life behind bars? Yes, please,' *The Sunday Times*, 29 November. Online. Available at www.property.timesonline.co.uk/to/life_and_style/html (accessed 29 April 2011).

62  Gehl, *Streets for People*, pp. 99–100.

63  Vanderbilt, Tom (2011) 'Long live the industrial city,' *The Wilson Quarterly*, Spring. Online. Available at www.wilsonquarterly.com/article.cfm?AID=1809.html. (Accessed 14 April 2011).

64  Sassen, Saskia (2008) *Territory, Authority, Rights: From Medieval to Global Assemblages*. Princeton: Princeton University Press.

65  Kelly, Matt (2009) 'Nation's first solar powered electric vehicle charging station unveiled in. . .Chicago?' *Examiner.com/Los Angeles*, 6 April. Online. Available at www.examiner.com/alternative-transportation-in-Los-Angeles.html (accessed 2 April 2011).

66  Anon. (2010) 'Elk Horn, Iowa: An oasis for electric cars,' *Carbonday*, 9 September. Online. Available at www.carbobday.com/index.php?s=Charging+stations.html (accessed 2 April 2011).

67  Anon. (2010) 'Endesa and Telefónica launch first electric vehicle telephone booth recharging station.' Online. Available at www.endesa.es/Portal/en/press/press_releases/our_companies/enter.html (accessed 2 April 2011).

68  Hardwick, M. Jeffrey (2004) *Mall Maker*. Philadelphia: University of Pennsylvania Press.

69  Christensen, *Big Box Reuse*, pp. 145–149.

70  Ibid., p. 5.

71  Kunstler, *The Long Emergency*, pp. 256–257.

72  Christensen, *Big Box Reuse*, pp. 5–6.

73  Kunstler, *The Long Emergency*, p. 257.

74  Kimm, Alice (2001) 'Camino Nuevo Academy: Los Angeles,' *Architectural Record*, February, pp. 134–137.

75  Miller, Mark Crispin (1988) *Boxed In: The Culture of TV*. Evanston, IL: Northwestern University Press.

76  Holtz Kay, *Asphalt Nation*, pp. 33–34.

77  Farr, *Sustainable Urbanism*, p. 165.

78  Fulton, Forrest (2009) 'Big Box Agriculture: A Productive Suburb.' Online. Available at www.re-burbia.com/2009/08/01/a-new-business-model-a-productive-suburb/html. (Accessed 7 July 2010).

79 Anon. (2001) Fukuoka Prefectural International Hall. Online. Available at www.emiloambazandassociates. com/portfolio/type.cfm?type=2.html (accessed 8 April 2011).

80 Lukez, *Suburban Transformations*, p. 98.

81 Field, Katherine (2009) 'Toast of the town,' *Chain Store Age*, June 2009, pp. 47–49. Also see Shaer, Matthew (2009) 'After the mall: Retrofitting suburbia,' *Christian Science Monitor*, 22 May. Online. Available at www.csmonitor.com/Money/2009/0522/after-the-mall-retrofitting-suburbia.html (accessed 7 July 2010).

82 Lee, Lydia (2009) 'Planting in the streets,' *The Architects Newspaper*. Online. Available at www.archpaper. com/news/articles.asp?id=3813.html (accessed 1 May 2011).

83 Anon. (2011) 'McDonald burger prices teach inflation,' *USA Today*. 15 April, p. A–16.

84 Kronenburg, Robert (2007) *Flexible: Architecture that Responds to Change*. London: Laurence King Publishing, p 100.

85 Nosacek, Gary (2010) 'Memories of Milwaukee's Capitol Court Shopping Center,' 11 October. Online. Available at www.watter.com/Default.aspx?tabid=348.html (accessed 22 April 2011).

86 Duran and Eguaras, *1000 Ideas by 100 Architects*, pp. 96–99.

87 Ibid., p. 195.

88 Blanc, Patrick, Lalot, Veronique, Bruhn, Gregory, and Nouvel, Jean (2008) *The Vertical Garden: From Nature to the City*. New York: W.W. Norton & Company.

89 Fjeld, Tove, Veiersted, Bo, Sandvik, Leiv, Riise, Geir, and Levy, Finn (1998) 'The effect of indoor foliage plants on health and discomfort symptoms among office workers,' *Indoor Built Environment*, 7(3): 204–209.

90 Despommier, Dickson (2010) *The Vertical Farm: Feeding the World in the 21st Century*. London: Thomas Dunne Books.

91 *SITE: Architecture as Art* (1980), pp. 90–93.

92 Hanson, David (2010) 'Vietnamese gardeners in New Orleans offer much food for thought,' *Grist*, May 2010. Online. Available at www.grist.org/article/fod-elderly-Vietnamese-gardeners-in-New-Orleans-/ html (accessed 6 July 2010).

93 Phillips, Daniel (2009) 'Inter estates: Reclaimed freeways turned farms.' Online. Available at www. re-burbia.com/finalists/html (accessed 7 July 2010).

94 Barnes, Michael (2011) 'Locally grown, organic food available in Chicago,' *Chicago Conservative Examiner*, 29 March. Online. Available at www.examiner.com/conservative-in-Chicago/locally-grown-organic-food.html (accessed 29 March 2011).

95 Anon. (2010) 'City Farm Chicago.' Online. Available at www.homerownevolution.com/2009/05/city-farm-chcago.html (accessed 6 July 2010).

96 Chaoui, Hala (2009) 'Why urban farming needs to be organic,' *Innovative Science: Agriculture and Food Edition*. Online. Available at www.files.inovatve-science.com/1_innov_science5.html (accessed 1 May 2011).

97 Fairbank, Lawson (2007) 'Hands off our back gardens,' 15 March. Online. Available at www.lawson fairbank.co.uk/backgarden-development-campaign.asp.html (accessed 12 March 2011).

98 Reid, Molly (2010) 'Urban farming begins to grow in New Orleans,' *The Times-Picayune*, 27 February. Online. Available at www.nola.com/homegarden/index.ssf/2010/02/urban_farming_begins/html (accessed 12 March 2011).

99 Corn, Jessie (2010) 'Gardening is a small way to fight urban sprawl,' *Gainesville Times*, 9 April. Online. Available at www.gainesvilletimes.com/archives.31881/html (accessed 1 May 2011).

100 Heckman, James (2006) 'A history of organic farming: Transitions from Sir Albert Howard's War in the Soil to USDA national organic program,' *Renewable Agricultural Food Systems*, 21: 143–150.

101 Epstein, Elliott (2011) *Industrial Composting: Environmental Engineering and Facilities Management*. 2nd Edition. Boca Raton: CRC Press.

102 Coyne, Kelly and Knutzen, Erik (2008) *The Urban Homestead: Your Guide to Self-Sufficient Living in the Heart of the City*. Port Townsend: Process Self Reliance Series.

103 Meinhold, Bridgette (2009) 'San Francisco signs mandatory recycling and composting laws,' *Inhabitat*. Online. Available at www.inhabit.com/san-francisco-mandates-recycling-composting/htm (accessed 11 March 2011).

104 Thomas, Justin (2005) 'Tacoma man installs sizeable rainwater cistern,' *Treehugger.com*, 24 May. Online. Available at www.treehugger.com/files/2005/05/seattle_man_ins.php.html (accessed 11 March 2011).

105 Kongs, Jennifer (2010) 'Urban agriculture and garden training,' *Mother Earth News*, 17 October. Online. Available at www.motherearthnews.com/grow-it/urban-agriculure-raining-zb0z10zkon.aspx.html

(accessed 30 March 2011). Also see (2011) 'Beginning farmers: An online resource for farmers, researchers, and policy makers.' Online. Available at www.beginningfarmers.org/urban-farming/html. (accessed 30 March 2011).

106 Anon. (2011) 'Massachusetts Avenue Project (MAP).' Online. Available at www.mass-ave.org/spring uatreg.htm (accessed 30 March 2011). Also see Anon. (2010) 'Mobile Food Collective.' Online. Available at www.archeworks.org/proj0910_moblefoodcollective.cfm.html (accessed 21 June 2010).

107 Lukez, *Suburban Transformations*, pp. 100–110.

108 Duany, Andres et al. (2000) *Suburban Nation: The Rise of Sprawl and the Decline of the American Dream*. New York: North Point Press, pp. 220–227.

109 *Active Design Guidelines: Promoting Physical Activity and Health in Design* (2010), pp. 110–113.

110 Hincha-Ownby, Melissa (2011) 'LEED woes continue,' *Mother Nature Network*, 10 January. Online. Available at www.mnn.com/money/green-workplace/blogs/leed-woes-continue/html (accessed 14 April 2011).

111 Anon. (2010) *LEED Certification: Where Energy Efficiency Collides with Human Health*. North Haven, Connecticut: EHHI.

112 Gupta, Pankaj Vir (2011) 'Urban journal: Mapping the city,' *Wall Street Journal*, 8 March. Online. Available at www.wsj.com/indiarealtime/2011/03/08/urban-journal-mapping-the-city.html (accessed 11 March 2011).

113 Hatch, C. Richard (1984) *The Scope of Social Architecture*. New York: Van Nostrand Reinhold.

114 This game was developed in the context of a design studio in the Graduate Program in Architecture + Health at Clemson University, in 2010.

115 Geary, Robert (2009) 'What's wrong with Moore Square?' *Citizen*. Online. Available at www.indyweek.com/citizen/archives/2009/04/21/html (accessed 1 May 2011).

116 Jones, Jay (2009) 'City Center—the beginning of a new Las Vegas,' *Los Angeles Times*, 29 November. Online. Available at www.travel.latimes.com/articles/la-trw-citycenter29-2009nov29.html (accessed 6 April 2011).

117 Gratz, Roberta Brandes (2010) 'Rebuilding Detroit the sane way—a block at a time,' *Citiwire.net*, 24 December. Online. Available at www.citiwire.net/post/2458/html (accessed 5 April 2011).

# 5

# CASE STUDY: NEW ORLEANS

The kids have a new take
A new take on faith
Pick up the pieces
Get carried away
I came home to a city half erased
I came home to face what we faced

This place needs me here to start
This place is the beat of my heart

Oh my heart
Oh my heart

Storm didn't kill me
The government changed
Hear the answer
Hear the song rearranged
Hear the trees, the ghosts and the buildings sing
With the wisdom to reconcile this thing
It's sweet and it's sad and it's true

Oh my heart
Oh my heart

Mother and father I stand beside you
The good of this world will see us through
This place needs me here to start
This place is the beat of my heart

Among American cities, New Orleans has endured more than its share of hard times. In its nearly 300 year existence, this settlement near the mouth of the Mississippi River has been a fulcrum in a delicate balancing act between the forces of nature, geography, and sheer determination of the human spirit. Plague, pestilence, wars, floods, hurricanes, and economic vicissitude left an indelible mark on its culture, economy, politics, and its people. The city's rich cultural traditions—its music, food, architecture, and civic traditions centered on the annual Mardi Gras celebration—set this place apart from anywhere else in America. From its inception, New Orleans has been controversial. In 1718, Bienville went against the advice of his own team of French engineers, who recommended against his choice for the initial settlement. They argued the land was unsuitable for permanent settlement due to its swampy marshland and the annual spring floods caused by the post-winter thaw of the mid-section of the North American continent. This "land" was in fact an alluvial plain created by the silt deposits accrued over 2,000 years by the Mississippi River's delta. Even the river itself had changed course numerous times over the past two millennia, forming natural banks alongside its various paths through the southernmost parts of the Louisiana Territory.[1] A single strip of "high ground" straddled the east and west banks of the Mississippi as it flowed through this region and it would eventually become home base to a metro area of 1.5 million inhabitants.

The questionable decision to locate the initial settlement where it is today has therefore been an issue since 1718. It poses a chronic dilemma to the city's survival. The term *dilemma* is defined as "a problem involving a difficult or unpleasant choice" which can bring unintended consequences. By the mid-1850s, New Orleans was the third largest city in the United States.[2] In the 18th and 19th centuries the city's inhabitants contended with waves of public health epidemics including yellow fever, typhoid, malaria, and dysentery due to the semi-tropical climate and the city's rising stature as an international port of call. Sailors and Merchants arriving from foreign locales brought with them various new diseases and the local population, it seemed, was continually fighting this influx. The city, from its inception, therefore has maintained a love–hate relationship with its prosperous port. The history of New Orleans's built environment has revolved around the interdependency between water, climate, drainage, and public health. Public health crises unfolded with regularity while by the first half of the 19th century New Orleans was the epicenter of the entire Mississippi Valley.[3]

Prior to the 1890s, drainage, and the sanitary disposal of sewerage in New Orleans were viewed as one and the same. Both caused severe problems, with disastrous consequences for public health. The city government was unable to cope with the city's subtropical climate and its peculiar geography. A lack of both scientific understanding and basic sanitation left the city vulnerable to successive waves of deadly epidemics. As the city's population increased, so did the number of deaths from disease. In 1818, 1847, and 1853, 2,200, 2,800, and 9,000 persons respectively succumbed to yellow fever. After the 1850s, improved epidemiological prevention, treatment, and public awareness helped with containment. Up until then, the period of July through October each year was dreaded more for "Yellow Jack" than for hurricanes, and the seasonal evacuation each year approached one-third of the total population of the city. In 1848, one cholera epidemic resulted in over 3,000 deaths. Mosquitoes were the evil foe, causing yellow fever and malaria. The great yellow fever epidemic that struck many southern U.S. cities in 1878 began in New Orleans. Not until 1895 would a modern underground drainage plan be adopted for implementation and this new, state-of-the-art system was not completed for nearly ten more years.[4] By 1900, New Orleans was recognized as a leading center in public health research on its troublesome tropical diseases.[5]

Engineering, commerce, and politics have always been uneasy bedfellows in New Orleans's historical development. Its history has largely been shaped by landmark engineering feats, each as an attempt to sidestep Mother Nature through constructed acts of water diversion and/or containment.

The greatest hydrologic feat consisted of the taming and virtual walling in of one of the largest and most powerful rivers in the world by the United States Army Corps of Engineers. It constructed a levee system that would eventually surround much of the city and its metro area. This enabled the drainage of additional marshy low ground. The continuous battle for the control of water profoundly shaped patterns of settlement in the city. The high ground was the first to be settled and is known as the *sliver by the river*. It runs the length of the river's banks on its east and west banks and varies from approximately a half mile to a mile "back" from the riverbanks.

The earliest section—the French Quarter, or *Vieux Carré*—was laid out by Bienville's chief surveyor, Pierre La Blonde de la Tour, and his assistant engineer, Adrien de Pauger. This site was situated at a 90-degree turn in the river, and it afforded maximum visual surveillance of potential invaders sailing up from the mouth of the river 60 miles to the south. Fourteen squares extended along the river with a depth of six squares back. A ditch encircled each square, and a large open canal surrounded the whole city. A nearly continuous protective wall provided the city's enclosure. The ditches around the squares flowed into two larger ditches and a canal that, in turn, emptied into a large swamp lying directly behind the original city. Nearly 200 years later this would become the entire suburban section of the city, stretching northward to Lake Pontchartrain. The area behind the rampart (city wall) was referred to as the "back o' town." It was essentially a semi-drained swamp. This sanitation system became chronically overwhelmed during rainstorms; streets were completely flooded and each square became a virtual island[6]

In 1819, architect Benjamin Latrobe described New Orleans in three words: "mud, mud, mud."[7] The earliest suburbs were developed downriver from the Vieux Carré. By the 1830s there were three main sections of the city along the river: the original *Vieux Carré*, the American Sector, and the Faubourg Marigny.[8] In 1878, a topological and drainage map of the city was published, showing precisely where the built-up areas began and ended. It foreshadowed precisely the parts of the city that would become submerged in the intense hurricanes of 1915 and 2005—still swamps yet to be developed in 1878.[9] This low-lying land has been scored and scoured through the centuries. It has been a constant battle to remove water and to keep it away from the growing urban center. These constructions, while designed to protect, have also at times turned against the populace, becoming at times serious hazards and a risk to human life. In the city's history, the aftermath of one disaster has been the prelude to the next.

Cotton was the principal export, and much of it was shipped to Liverpool and other British ports. The city never did develop as a major manufacturing center for the raw products it shipped, financed, or stored:

> Cotton was the sinews of business in antebellum New Orleans, the economic rhythms of the city revolving around the cotton seasons. Cotton was picked and baled from September through December. . .with most of the year's crop exported by May. In summer, the port was virtually deserted as the heat, humidity, and falling water levels [in the river] slowed dockworkers. . .and hindered river traffic. . .many merchants and their families left the city to avoid the heat, yellow fever, cholera, and hurricanes. However, between January and March, many plantation owners and their families would visit the city, partaking of the social whirl of Mardi Gras, shopping, and meeting with their cotton factors, who acted as agents, bankers, and financial advisors. . .businesses, for the most part, were small-scale master-apprentice operations [unlike] the factory system emerging in the industrializing Northeast.[10]

Retail trade expanded exponentially in the late 19th century, when many large department stores were established. These businesses traced their origins to the pre-Civil War (pre-1860) boom years.

As a seaport and major entry gateway to the U.S., New Orleans always had a transient population of seamen, immigrants, and tourists; its "hospitality" industry—restaurants, theatres, operas, bars, gambling houses, and red light establishments.[11] The city's population had reached 168,675 by 1860, the last pre–Civil War U.S. census. Eight percent (13,385) were slaves.[12]

As the city grew upriver, plantation boundaries came to determine development patterns. As one plantation was turned over to urbanization, its boundary lines became major streets.[13]

New Orleans's rich heritage has often been described as a cultural gumbo.[14] After the Louisiana Purchase of 1803, a mix of French, and later Spanish, Creole, and American cultures flourished. As businesses prospered, new commercial buildings were constructed. Building façades, fences, signposts, billboards, and street furniture were canvases for visual advertisements. These commercial buildings and their districts contributed significantly to neighborhood cohesiveness and identity as much as to civic discourse and to racial and ethnic diversity.[15] In New Orleans's central business district (CBD), as elsewhere, commercial buildings and their signage competed for attention, such as the Falstaff beer billboard perched atop a building at the intersection of Common and Rampart Streets, shown in 1946 (Figure 5.1). It was an immense building-sign and at night was emblazoned in floodlights. This tradition of large commercial billboards that sit on buildings in the CBD persists to this day.

As the pre-suburban city expanded, commercial buildings soon lined its main thoroughfares, not unlike cities elsewhere. As new neighborhoods were built in the early 20th century, further back, or away from, *the sliver by the river*, the newly built main arteries were made much wider to accommodate a rapid rise in private automobile ownership. This would be the case from the 1930s onward. Mom and pop corner grocery stores dotted the intersections of these neighborhoods. These places were modest in scale, in the middle-class and poorer neighborhoods. Their signage was directed towards passersby and persons waiting at streetcar stops and, later, bus stops. This was the case at the corner of Dryades (now Orthea Castle Haley Boulevard) and Philips Streets in the Central City neighborhood, shown in 1954. This mom and pop "Dollar Store" market was covered with commercial signage (Figure 5.2). From the late 1920s, long-established businesses in the CBD, such as bakeries, florists, banks, and clothing stores, continued to open branches in the newly developing parts of the city.

Artists provided commercial signage and these artifacts were installed across the neighborhoods of the city, new and old alike. A sign advertising JAX Beer was hand painted in April 1943 on the exterior wood siding of a neighborhood corner bar (now Marie's). Marie's is located in the Faubourg Marigny neighborhood (Figure 5.3). Numerous hand-painted signs such as this one were the norm and typically adorned bars, grocery stores, bakeries, butcher shops, laundries, and many other commercial building types throughout the city's 18th- and 19th-century neighborhoods.[16]

By the late 1940s and early 1950s, these commercial buildings began to line the city's main streets in the former swamps being developed further and further away from the Mississippi River—along major streets including Carrollton Avenue, Claiborne Avenue, Elysian Fields, Broad Street, parts of lower St. Charles Avenue, Tulane Avenue, and along Gentilly Boulevard. In New Orleans, as elsewhere across the U.S., commercial buildings were erected in shopping strip configurations along these main arteries. In 1952, the Community Food Store and Cabibi's Pharmacy were built in a single strip center on Carrollton Avenue (Figure 5.4). The Airline Shopping Center was built on Airline Highway in Metairie in 1956 (Figure 5.5) and the Gentilly Woods Shopping Center dates from the late 1940s (Figure 5.6). The commercial strip center in Gentilly featured an H.G. Hill Supermarket, F.W. Woolworth's, and a Katz and Bestoff's pharmacy outlet. These three shopping strip-centers were among the earliest built in New Orleans in the post–World War II period, and all three, architecturally, expressed a blended conflation of art deco with 1950s streamline moderne motifs and imagery. They quickly became prosperous

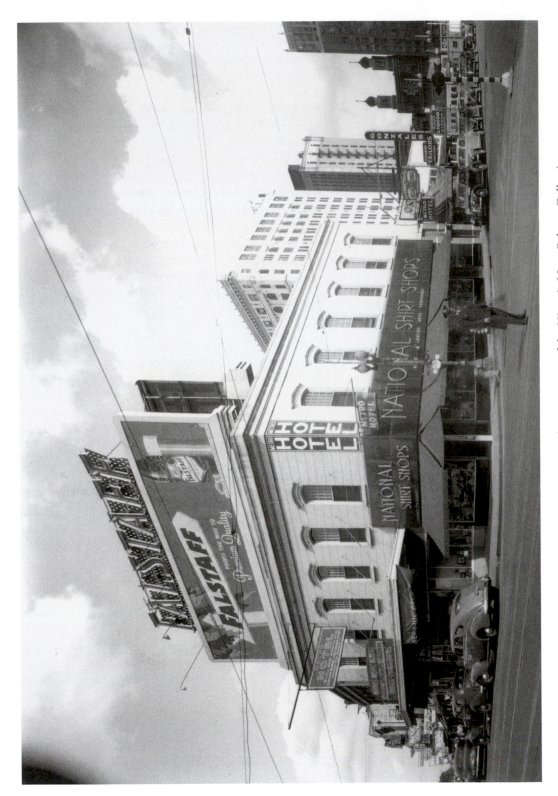

**FIGURE 5.1** Common and Rampart Streets, New Orleans, 1946. Photo courtesy of the Historic New Orleans Collection

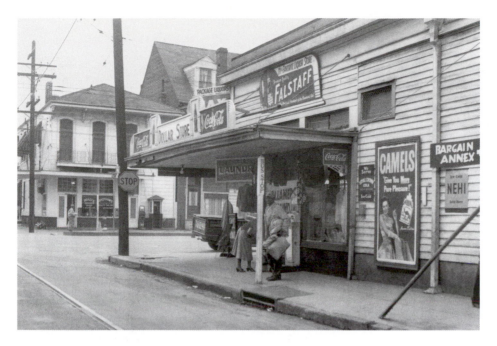

**FIGURE 5.2** Dollar Store Corner Market, Dryades Street (now Orthea Castle Haley Blvd.), New Orleans, 1954. Photo courtesy of the Historic New Orleans Collection

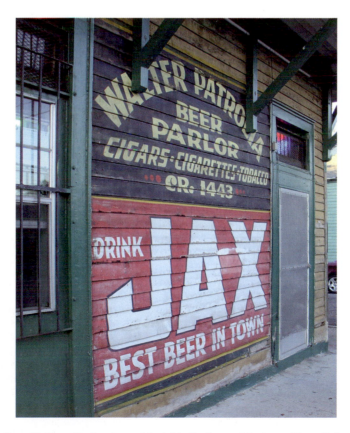

**FIGURE 5.3** Walter Patrolia Beer Parlor (now Marie's), Faubourg Marigny, New Orleans, 2011

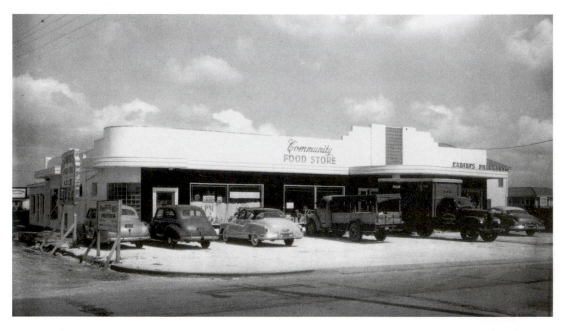

**FIGURE 5.4**   Community Food Store-Supermarket/Cabibi's Pharmacy, Carrollton Avenue, New Orleans, 1952. Photo courtesy of the Historic New Orleans Collection

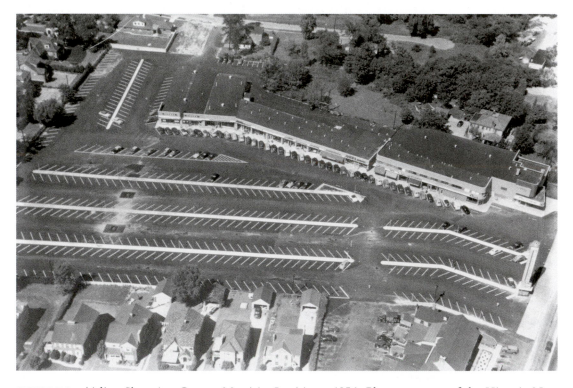

**FIGURE 5.5**   Airline Shopping Center, Metairie, Louisiana, 1956. Photo courtesy of the Historic New Orleans Collection

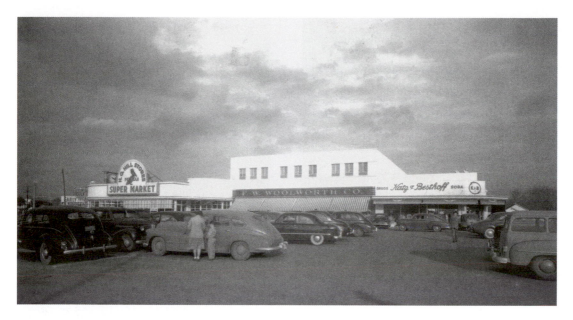

**FIGURE 5.6**  Gentilly Woods Shopping Center, New Orleans, 1949. Photo courtesy of the Historic New Orleans Collection

because they were built adjacent to the new neighborhoods to which people were moving, in a pattern of post-World War II suburban flight from the older urban core nearest to the Mississippi River.

## New Orleans as Urban Text

An urban analysis is presented below of New Orleans's morphological development across time and physical space. It represents an attempt to *read* the urban fabric as a narrative *text*, as a means to convey the urban expansion pattern which occurred in New Orleans throughout the 20th century. A series of iterative maps document key variables in this narrative within the overall city proper while also pinpointing the catalyst site for a case study to be discussed below. This catalyst site is indicated as an open white rectangle on the accompanying series of urban analysis maps. Pre- and post-World War II patterns of constancy and change are emphasized, as is the impact of Hurricane Katrina in 2005. All water and land elevation heights, which accompany this set of urban analysis maps, are reported in feet. The patterns of growth, change, and constancy are of particular relevance to any discussion of any city's suburbanization in the 20th century. In the case of New Orleans, these consist of the following four urban morphological dimensions:

### Pre-World War II Suburbanization

By 1940 the city's urban street grid was built-out in the neighborhoods nearest to the Mississippi River (Figure 5.7a–d). The Mid-City and Broadmoor neighborhood street grids were established and hundreds of single-family homes were built on low-lying sites at the bottom of the *urban bowl*—the lowest land below mean sea level. The city's water control network, consisting of six immense pumping out-flow stations, were also built near or at the bottom of this bowl, and were built at roughly equidistant intervals along the entire 4-mile length of Broad Street, a main thoroughfare that

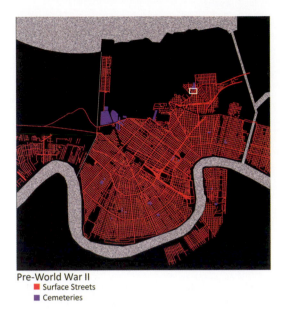

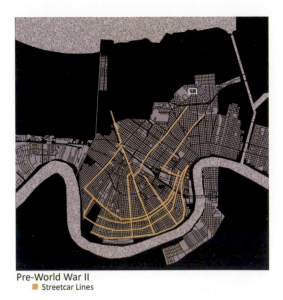

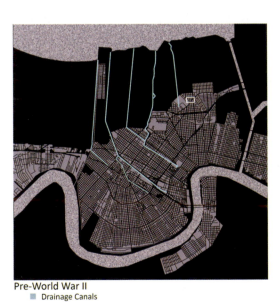

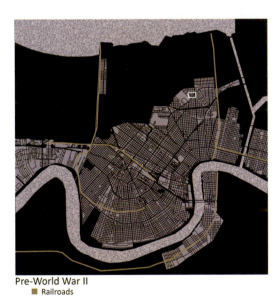

**FIGURE 5.7a–d** Pre-WWII Development, New Orleans (Orleans Parish). Drawings by S. Verderber/ Annette Himelick

transverses the city. Broad is a wide boulevard with a neutral ground functioning as its center median. This thoroughfare runs from east to west generally following the crescent shape of the Mississippi River. The lower section of *Gentilly*, nearest the river, was nearly fully developed by 1940. This land had been dredged in the 1920s and 1930s. Gentilly was the northern suburban edge of the city at the time with the areas depicted in black remaining undeveloped swamp. The majority of cemeteries in the city were built in sections within the "old city;" each cemetery was typically one square block in size, surrounded by residences and small businesses. The city's largest open drainage canal (New Basin Canal) linked the old city with Lake Pontchartrain to the north.[17] The city's streetcar lines prior to 1940 were concentrated nearest to the Mississippi River, and these also followed the crescent shape of the river.[18]

## Post-World War II Suburbanization

The street grid was extended across the city and to the north to touch the shoreline of Lake Pontchartrain (Figure 5.8a–d). It was further articulated by a network of major and secondary arteries constructed, linking the old city with new sections. Streetcar lines began to disappear and by 1963 only the St. Charles Avenue streetcar line remained. The interstate highway system, begun in 1956, had reached New Orleans by the late 1950s, with Interstate 10 (I-10) now traversing the city adjacent to the down-town and Vieux Carré , and later, a bypass was constructed: via Interstate artery (I-610). This second interstate highway crisscrossed the city from east to west, cutting across lower Gentilly and the middle of the nearly 5,000-acre City Park. The first vehicular bridge built across the Mississippi at the city center opened in the mid-1950s. This pattern of grids/grains that emerged in the post-World War II period expressed a layered quiltwork of overlapping street grids, bisecting and appearing to abruptly crash into one another at random intervals. Primary and secondary street grids and their interlocking grains become discernable. When the layered circulation patterns, comprised of green boulevards, streetcar lines, cemeteries, and drainage canals are diagrammed simultaneously, the close interrelation-ship between water, vegetation, and transportation becomes discernable. Large open spaces consist at the present time of the two large urban parks, Audubon and City Park (Figure 5.9a–d). Pontchartrain Park was built on the lakefront in the late 1950s. Land was set aside for few parks in the rapidly subur-banizing parts of the city during this period. This was attributable to a combination of the scarcity of land for new development, developer-based greed, and the city's expanding population.[19]

## Water, Green Space, and Suburbanization

By 1945 the last of the remaining swamps within the city proper had been drained and prepared for suburban development. The analytical mapping of the presence of water and water control devices relative to suburbanization tells a story onto itself. The system of federally built levees reveals a monumental struggle to contain and control the flow of water. As discussed earlier, this complex and very costly system to build and maintain has been the total responsibility of the United States Army Corps of Engineers (USACE). The main natural ecologies of open green space, notably City park (Figure 5.9a), swamps, and lake bottoms that later gave way to suburban expansion, are revealed through this analysis (Figure 5.9b). Gentilly, specifically, the case study site (see below), stands apart from these natural water ecologies (indicted once again here as a white rectangle on the accom-panying maps) because the initial area developed in the early 20th century sat on a strip of high ground and this narrow strip is what it's erstwhile trio of developers would dub the "Gentilly Ridge." The pre-suburbanized natural ecologies, when diagrammed in direct relation to the area's post-World War II development patterns, reveal the striking codependency between urban habitat and water. It is noteworthy that no sizeable parks were created in the swampland that would become suburban Gentilly (Figure 5.9c). The very lowest sections of the built city lie more than 10 feet below sea level. These suburban neighborhoods were developed nearest to the Lake Pontchartrain lakeshore. Areas depicted in black on the accompanying map are those at or above mean sea level (Figure 5.9d).

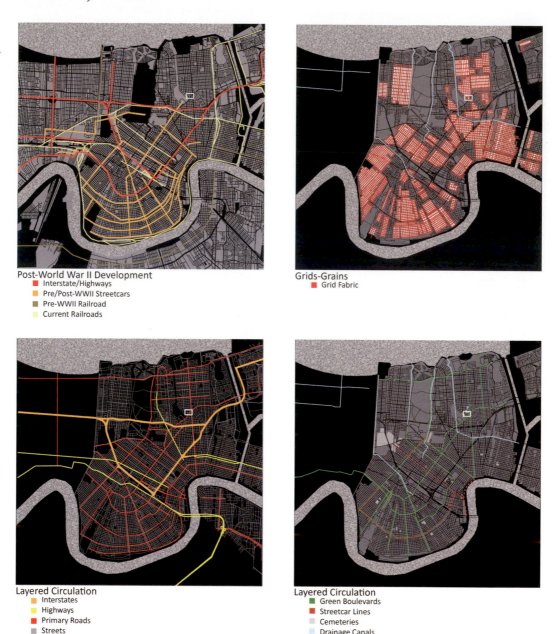

**FIGURE 5.8a–d**   Post-WWII Development, New Orleans (Orleans Parish). Drawings by S. Verderber/ Annette Himelick

## Suburbanization and Hurricane Katrina

An analysis of the flooded city in Katrina's aftermath in 2005 reveals that 80 percent of the city's total land area became submerged, with the lowest lying sections remaining submerged for up to three weeks (Figure 5.10a–b). The city's infrastructural systems sustained severe damage. Electric, sewerage, natural gas, and telecommunications systems were destroyed. Once again, areas represented in black

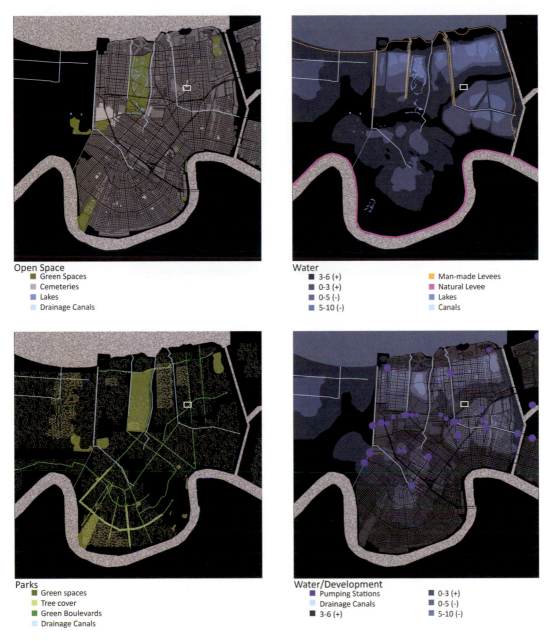

**FIGURE 5.9a–d** Natural Ecologies/Open Space, New Orleans (Orleans Parish). Drawings by S. Verderber/ Annette Himelick

did not flood; these consisted of the neighborhoods nearest the Mississippi River: the Esplanade/ Metairie Ridge, including the narrow strip of land known as Gentilly Ridge. Post-Katrina patterns of urban rebirth and renewal have been inconsistent across the city and these are illustrated in Figure 5.10b. Reconstruction activity has been most robust in the areas submerged for the shortest period of time or were not at all flooded, closest to the Mississippi. The least–rebuilt neighborhoods have been those farthest from the river including suburban Gentilly. Residents there have been

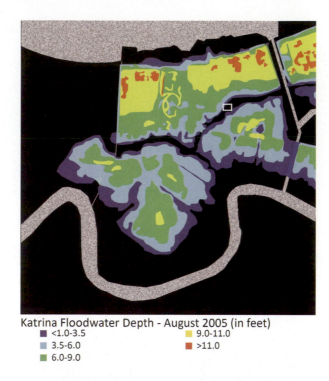

Katrina Floodwater Depth - August 2005 (in feet)
- <1.0-3.5
- 3.5-6.0
- 6.0-9.0
- 9.0-11.0
- >11.0

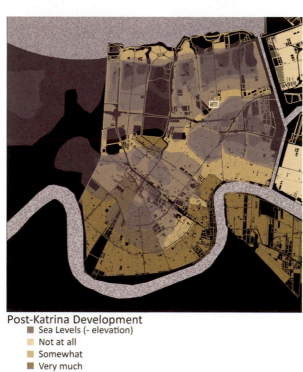

Post-Katrina Development
- Sea Levels (- elevation)
- Not at all
- Somewhat
- Very much

**FIGURE 5.10a–b**  Hurricane Katrina/Post-Katrina, New Orleans (Orleans Parish). Drawings by S. Verderber/Annette Himelick

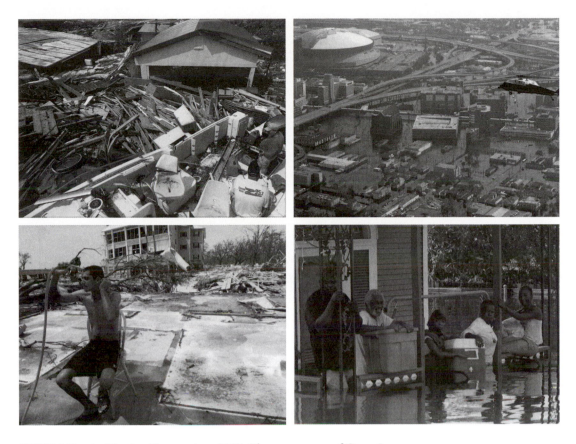

**FIGURE 5.11a–d** Katrina Devastation, 2005. Photo courtesy of Getty Images

challenged by insufficient rebuilding funds, lack of insurance, a lack of schools and businesses, and innutrition caused by a lack of places to buy healthy fresh food. Numerous schools never reopened and even landmark churches were demolished. However, grassroots neighborhood organizations across the city have demonstrated a remarkable resiliency, revealing the sheer determination of residents to recover and restore as much of their prior way of life as possible. While the fact remains that the hardest hit areas continue to suffer the most from infrastructural ruin and disinvestment, signs of progress are discernable as one drives, cycles, or walks through the neighborhoods deepest within the flood's strike zone. It remains these areas where property owners sustained the heaviest losses and where many homeowners and business owners may never be able to return (Figure 5.11a–d).

## Suburban Gentilly

Gentilly, the first 20th-century suburb built in the back-o'-town swamp, was drained just prior to World War I. Its origins date from a document called *The New Century New Orleans Master Plan*, which recorded that Mathurin Dreux, a militia officer who came to New Orleans with Bienville, acquired substantial property on the Bayou Savage Ridge in 1727 and established a very successful plantation that remained in the family for more than two generations.[20] The ridge's high ground had long provided access into New Orleans from the east. However, regular seasonal flooding limited its development until the early 1900s. The district's highest ground would later be the site of the city's first 20th Century suburban development, *Gentilly Terrace*. Development in the Gentilly area occurred after 1909 and then boomed after 1945.[21] Prior, save for scattered development along the Gentilly Ridge, and an earlier settlement built on the lakeshore, known as Milneburg, little growth occurred. Back in 1924 the New Orleans Levee Board had adopted a plan to drain the entire swath of "swampland" and in its place provide flood protection for the entire lakefront area. Over the next thirty-five years suburbia was built on top of swampland, obliterating this entire natural water ecology.

In 1909 a trio of local entrepreneurs had formed the Gentilly Terrace Company. Gentilly previously had been part of the extensive back-o'-town swamp. The aforementioned engineering innovations of the early 20th century had now made it possible to drain and stabilize large portions of this swamp that lay between the high ground situated along the Mississippi River, and Lake Pontchartrain directly north of the original city. Gentilly came to be known as the collection of neighborhoods situated between Mid-City to the south, the Industrial Canal to the east, Lake Pontchartrain to the north, and Bayou St. John to the west. The ridge of a former bayou was named Gentilly Boulevard, as this was to be the main, most prestigious street in this new residential section. By the early 1920s development had begun in earnest. Neighborhoods on both sides of the high ground along Gentilly Boulevard were built first. These enclaves consisted of middle-class residences in a variety of prevailing architectural styles. The most prevalent styles were the then in-vogue California bungalow, the California patio home, and updated variations of house styles prevalent in the older, established uptown section of the city. Historians continue to debate the origins of the name "Gentilly."[22] The developers, self-styled Men of Vision, seized the moment.

In 1909 the Gentilly Terrace Company published a full-color brochure outlining its vision for the new suburb. It was to be a suburban haven, a world away from the high population and density, decay, crime, and congestion of the old city. It was to be easily accessible via rail and streetcar. It was promoted as a *healthier lifestyle*—a spacious antidote to the dreaded public health epidemics that had plagued the city in prior decades. The developers clearly used public fear as a tactic to attract attention to their vision. The memory of the past still was vivid in the minds of those who had lost close family members and friends to the ravages of past cholera, dysentery, and yellow fever epidemics. The developers played upon public health fears in an attempt to sell lots to make money. It was a successful strategy. An appealing civic vision had been born for this newly christened suburban section of New Orleans that set it apart from the unsafe, crowded urban status quo. Major sections of the Gentilly Terrace Company's rather fascinating marketing brochure from 1909 are presented here:

## *GENTILLY TERRACE*

## *Where Homes Are Built on Hills*

## *A Piece of Our Past*

## *To Home Builders*

TO the man or woman who wants a home either for the home's sake or as a means of saving in a definite, regular way, Gentilly Terrace offers a most unusual opportunity. This home section of New Orleans possesses many advantages which are partly set forth in this book. The many homes already finished and those in course of construction and under contract are a safe warrant for the character of the neighborhood. This is the most important feature. The property being the most elevated ground in or about New Orleans insures perfect natural drainage at all seasons.

The terraces make for beauty, and the elevation of the property adds materially to the appearance. And so we could enumerate many more advantages in the beginning, but prefer to take them up one by one, discussing them in a truthful, straightforward manner, without a single ray of artificial coloring. The careful reading of every page in this book will, we hope, prove of material advantage to every home seeker to whom it may come.

## To Investors

NEW ORLEANS has passed the stage of experiment and resolved itself into a question of *where* to invest.

To the investor of either limited or unlimited means, Gentilly Terrace is very alluring because of its promise as a home neighborhood. Within the first sixty days of the opening of this tract there were six hundred lots actually sold. Some of these lots have been since resold at an advance of as high as one hundred percent over the purchase price. Some were purchased purely for investment, but the majority were acquired by intending home builders.

The terms are liberal. Ten percent of purchase cash and $5.00 per lot per month with interest at six percent per annum.

The prices of these lots with the above terms include the paving in front thereof, also the shillinger walks and concrete curbing, thus making the site ready for immediate building and solving forever the problem of additional cost to which the home builder is generally subject in other locations. We are making on our subdivision *fourteen miles* of paved streets and *thirty-five miles* of artificial stone sidewalks and concrete curbing.

## Available Building Sites

WITH the exception of low ground, nearly all residential property in New Orleans is today too congested for a comfortable home-site.

In evidence of this even the main avenue of the city now shows a crowded condition and one can count on the fingers of one hand the desirable unimproved locations on this avenue. Prices of desirable property, for the above reason, are too high to warrant the home builder or the investor in making a purchase. For this same reason, Gentilly Terrace offers a solution of the problem by making possible to both home-seeker and investor the most desirable lots at a mere fraction of cost as compared to what one would have to pay in less desirable neighborhoods.

Ten lots can be purchased in Gentilly Terrace for the price of what one lot would cost the same distance from the business center either on Canal St. or St. Charles Ave. This means pure air, beautiful lawns, health and the real joy of living as compared with "stuffy" rooms. It means that the worker has room to "breathe better" and consequently work better. It means "living" in the true sense.

## The Terrace Idea

COMPARATIVELY speaking as to soil, location and distance, Gentilly Terrace has many advantages and yet these fade in importance as compared to the great advantage of the Terrace, which is only possible in this particular part of New Orleans. If there is one community in the world where the terrace will be welcome, it is right here in New Orleans, because of the monotonous levels which prevail.

As a matter of fact, the very lowest lots in Gentilly Terrace are fifteen inches above the street grade. Thus every home will be built on a hill above the street, where some are as high as sixty inches above the street grade.

The advantages are too evident to even enumerate, although for the benefit of the unaccustomed to the terrace idea we suggest the following few:

By means of Terraces —

The home builder is saved at least $150.00 per lot for filling each lot to the city grade.

It makes possible the use of basements.

It saves a large portion of foundation costs.

It enhances the beauty of the lots.

It saves the cost of hedges or fences.

It minimizes noises from the street.

## Little California

IT has often been noted by strangers visiting New Orleans that while the climate and soil of our city is practically the same as that of Southern California, there is a lack of beautiful residential districts here, which are so common in the Golden West. With this one object in view the streets and avenues of Gentilly Terrace have been laid out on plans very similar to those which have proven so successful in Los Angeles. The map on the following page shows those arrangements. Cement sidewalks, paved parked streets, cement curbing, lawns, flowers, palms, and trees form the foundation for this great work. The bungalow style of architecture, which has proven of such universal success, has been practically adopted as the standard among Gentilly Terrace home builders.

(While we do not insist on this style of building we feel that it will prove the most desirable.)

To carry out the idea, a large central park has been set aside in this tract. This park will be laid out by an expert park builder and by the summer of 1910, will be a marvel of flowers, fountains, trees, and driveways.

## Elevation

THE average elevation of Gentilly Terrace lots is twenty-seven feet above the Cairo Datum Line, which means that it is the most elevated residential section in the City of New Orleans. This fact is best brought out by the Engineer's Rod shown on this page. To those seriously contemplating the building of a home in Gentilly Terrace there can be no greater point of interest than that of elevation.

When one considers the immense advantage of high ground in a low ground community, the advantages will be more evident. If we could move one hundred lots of average grade from their present location in Gentilly Terrace to St. Charles Avenue, the same distance as they now are from Canal Street, they would be worth a fabulous sum *because of their elevation*. But the map tells the story plainer than anything we can say in cold type.

## Distances

CONSIDERED from a strictly business point of view, real estate is generally valued by its actual distance from the business center of a community. In the case of Gentilly Terrace, however, this is not true since an investigation will show that the present price of the lots equi-distant in any other district from the business center of New Orleans.

A study of the map, and statistics on this page will show that by actual measurement Gentilly Terrace is closer to "town" than many locations which could not be purchased at many times the price per front foot in delightful location.

(This map and figures have been taken from official records and can be easily verified by any one so desiring.)

And here's another distance feature:

The streets leading to Gentilly Terrace are straight line, while the streets leading to uptown residence sections are crescent shaped, thus lengthening the actual distance to be traveled by twelve percent.

## Distance Statistics

Corner Canal and Baronne Streets to Gentilly Terrace, three miles.
Corner Canal and Baronne Streets to St. Charles and Peters Avenue, three miles.
Corner Canal and Baronne Streets to Audubon Park, four miles.
Corner Canal and Baronne Streets to West End, six miles.
Corner Canal and Baronne Streets to Carrollton Avenue and St. Charles, five miles.

## The Road to Gentilly

AS the crow flies it is just three miles from the corner of Canal and Baronne Sts. to Gentilly Terrace. The same distance to the corner of St. Charles and Peters Ave., as a horse travels, it is four miles. And this road to Gentilly is on of the most beautiful in the whole South. There are a hundred points of interest, and a constantly changing panorama of semi-tropical views that speak volumes. The road to Gentilly passes both the Quaint Creole Quarter, where may be seen the French and Spanish architecture of Ante Bellum days, and through streets lined with modern homes.

It touches on several beautiful parks, and leaps over historical Bayou St. John where the sluggish oyster lugger, and the modern steam launch vie for supremacy of beauty in the sunset. This hard, white, shelled roadway passes several wayside inns, where a quiet dinner, such as only New Orleans' chefs can produce, is always obtainable. Churches, convents and monasteries cast their shadow of silent mystery across the path.

Hundreds of automobiles travel this road every day and after sunset it closely resembles the Paséo of Mexico. It is lined on both sides with beautiful vistas.

The picture at the top of the proceeding page was taken from Gentilly Terrace and shows clearly the city in the distance and the road does not terminate at Gentilly Terrace.

## To Chef Menteur

CLOSELY adjacent to Gentilly Terrace is Chef Menteur, perhaps the most celebrated fishing and hunting ground in the South. In Spring and Summer one could leave home at five A.M., fish the Green Trout, Pompano, Spanish Mackerel, Sheep Head, and many others and have them fresh broiled on his breakfast table. In the Fall and Winter low land surrounding "The Chef" simply teems with game birds, Canvas back, Mallard, and Teal Ducks, Snipes, Pappabots, Plover, and other luscious morsels. The road from Gentilly to "The Chef" is in many ways as interesting as is the "Road to Gentilly" and includes some of the wildest natural views possible to imagine. This road is constantly being improved and promises to be the great Auto Boulevard of New Orleans within the next two years.

## Dairies and Poultry Farms

Many farms border the road to Gentilly Terrace on both sides for several miles, thus bringing the supply of Milk, Chickens, Eggs, Vegetables, and Berries to the very doors of Gentilly Terrace residents before they reach the city markets.

While on this point, we wish to state that the extreme eastern tier of lots in Gentilly Terrace, have been reserved for business houses and that no business will be conducted on the residence lots.

## Automobiling

THE Automobile and Driving Clubs of New Orleans have practically made the road to pass Gentilly Terrace to "The Chef" of their own. They are expending thousands of dollars in the improvements of these roads and the City Government is also assisting to this end.

The parkways, and road houses which dot the way make this the most beautiful drive adjacent to the city, and a constant stream of vehicles pass the property. This roadway is to be continually oiled which will eliminate dust and make it one of the most celebrated drives in the country.

The tendency of all large cities is to provide good driveways and in doing so the City of New Orleans not only does a great service to the public, but enhances the value of the property in Gentilly Terrace.

## Auto Transit Service

THE problem of transportation from home to business is one which weighs very heavily in the balance of decision in selecting a home site.

The street car line between Gentilly Terrace running along Franklin Ave., will land passengers at Canal St. in twenty minutes, but we have contracted for a far better service of transportation that this, one modeled on the same lines as have proven successful in the suburban districts of Brooklyn and Detroit. Five auto busses make regular trips from Gentilly Terrace to the corner of Canal and Baronne Sts. On a fifteen minutes regular schedule by day, and a half hour schedule by night. Each coach carries twenty passengers with comfort and is perfectly weather proof. The busses are furnished by the Gentilly Automobile Company.

## Our Closing Argument

GENTILLY TERRACE is being placed on the market by New Orleans men – by men who were born and reared in New Orleans and who know the requirements of a home in this climate. They are men of Financial and Moral responsibility whose interests are centered in the development of New Orleans as a city and Gentilly Terrace in particular. They have confidence in Gentilly Terrace sufficient to build their homes there and live in them.

The money that is paid for Gentilly Terrace property will be kept in New Orleans and used in the development of New Orleans. The organization of the Gentilly Terrace Company is under the laws of Louisiana and for Louisiana.

We thank you for the consideration given this book and we unqualifiedly endorse every statement set forth herein.

GENTILLY TERRACE COMPANY
M.A. Baccich, President
E.E. Lafaye, Vice President
R.E.E. De Montluzin, Sec'y-Treas.[23]

The brochure also featured dozens of beautifully hand-drawn color illustrations of a range of houses spanning from borderline stately to imminently livable, accompanied with floor plans (not shown here due to space limitations). A large panoramic rendering of the city, with Gentilly at its forefront, was prominently featured (also not shown). Four different types of street cross-sections were depicted. These illustrated the man-made dirt elevation of all of the home types. Houses were built on trucked in dirt 3–4 feet above the mean sea level of the street out in front. Local historians have pointed out that this brochure contained a number of distortions of fact. For one, it was asserted this new suburb was to be the highest, most flood-free "ground" in the area. This was never true nor is it true today (as Hurricane Katrina proved in 2005). Development in Gentilly was actually centered along a narrow "high" ridge in the heart of a large surrounding "swamp." Streets tapered downward from this ridge: it was a natural water ecology that remained extremely flood prone until (and even after) the area's extensive federally built levee system was constructed in the post-World War II decades. Second, bold claims were made in this marketing literature as to the establishment of high-quality and frequent public transport between Gentilly Terrace and the downtown CBD. This assertion would never be realized. Gentilly boomed along with the automobile after 1945 and was completely built-out by 1965. In 1995, Gentilly Terrace was placed on the United States' *National Register of Historic Places*.

## Enter the New Urbanists

In the months immediately after Hurricane Katrina, federal, state, and local planning efforts remained in utter disarray. There was very little coordination among the myriad agencies involved in reconstruction planning, and scant funds were made available for any organized planning efforts beyond the initiative sponsored by the Urban Land Institute (ULI) in the fall of 2005, Bring Back New Orleans. With various citywide and neighborhood-based grassroots planning efforts stalled out for lack of funding and/or political support, by April of 2006, a member of the New Orleans City Council invited the Miami firm of DPZ (Duany Plater-Zyberk & Company) to execute a design charrette for the Gentilly section of New Orleans. Funding was not available for the charrette, and therefore Andres Duany sent out a call for volunteers among the membership of the Congress for the New Urbanism (CNU). Duany received more than thirty offers from CNU members who wished to volunteer their services. This team, plus ten staff members from DPZ, carried out a design charrette on April 18–26 at the School and Church of St. Leo the Great, on Paris Avenue in the heart of Gentilly.

In their words, the five guiding provisos of DPZ's design charrette were as follows:

> *The Requirement of Participation.* Citizens have the right to take the lead in the planning of their own communities. They must also assume the responsibility to arrive at consensus. The planners who assist them must advise them frankly on the feasibility of their ideas and then serve as conduits of their proposals. Elected and appointed officials, for their part, owe them their best effort to enable their proposals and remove legal, bureaucratic or other obstacles. Public participation must be personal or by proxy. Since it is impossible to consult with everyone, the planners must take pains to find representation from a broad cross-section of incomes and ethnicities that constitute their neighborhoods. The process of any planning effort must be accessible by Internet and in print, so absentee citizens can follow as well. Discussions over important questions must be held in the open. Personal and political relationships are to be valued, but not when they affect the quality of the work to be done. Leadership through crisis must be maintained at the peak of probity.
>
> *The Requirement of Return.* Citizens must have the right to return to the houses and businesses they own. They deserve to receive accurate and timely information in order to decide if it is wise to do so. Once informed, they must be allowed to take calculated risks if they so desire. For a just repopulation of New Orleans, the neighborhood, city, and nation must concentrate on replenishing the supply of affordable housing. This is extremely difficult to accomplish. No proposal, be it legal, financial or technical, should be beyond consideration.

*The Requirement of Place.* Places require protection of the character of their architecture. All neighborhoods have their traditions, not just the famous ones. Existing conditions deserve sensitive analysis. Where the current zoning codes impede contextual rebuilding, new ones must be enacted. These codes must exclude neither modernist nor traditional architecture so long as the human scale and the primacy of the public realm is preserved. Neighborhoods have the right to rebuild better than before. Not every place should revert to August 28 (2005, the day before Katrina struck the city). Responding to the challenges of diminishing fuel supplies and global warming patterns, an urban future may involve an increase in economic diversity, mixed use, walkability, density, transit, green building, and sustainable landscaping.

*The Requirement of Expertise.* New Orleans is a superb city that requires, deserves, and can attract the best planning professionals in the world. History shows that after major disasters, cities enter intensely creative periods. No person or group should be excluded from contributing with his or her best efforts. Outside professionals must work together with local experts, who play a critical role in adjusting general principles and techniques to local circumstances.

*The Requirement of Urgency.* As people are suffering while waiting to get on with their lives, those in authority must take no longer than absolutely necessary to make decisions and process their work.[25]

The commercial heart of Gentilly lies at Gentilly Boulevard and Elysian Fields Avenue. This area was built-out in the period 1952–1960 and consists of an eclectic mix of strip shopping center buildings with pre-World War II one- and two-level modest wood frame structures. One of the strip center structures features a parking deck on its roof. The buildings are unremarkable, individually. Collectively, as an ensemble, they possess some merit because they document the rapid rise of suburban automobile culture in post-World War II New Orleans—a place for the most part built as a pre-automobile city (Figure 5.12). For this reason alone Gentilly merits serious attention on the part of historic preservationists. Nonetheless, hundreds of structures in the low-lying sections of Gentilly and across other low-lying neighborhoods sustained serious destruction from Katrina (Figure 5.13a–l), prompting the question, "How much is to be saved, and how much is to be replaced?"

The New Urbanists spent a week in earnest deliberations and fact gathering, documenting, and analyzing. They then put forth a set of recommendations. They zeroed in quickly on the 1952–1960 commercial shopping aggregation. They concluded that this strip center needed to be entirely replaced and reinvented in a nostalgic, neo-19th-century vision that had virtually nothing to do with its post-World War II vintage 1950s suburban strip aesthetic, nor with its current economic realities. It apparently meant nothing that the targeted area was post-World War II New Orleans *first* genuinely suburban commercial shopping precinct, and therefore it just might be worthwhile to try to save it or key parts thereof.

Most of the businesses in the neighborhood were looted in the aftermath of Katrina. Pre-Katrina tenants had included such bottom-feeders as Dollar Store, Right Aid, a Blockbuster DVD rental store, several low-end fast food restaurants, and local mom and pop-owned and operated businesses such as a soul food restaurant, hip hop clothing store, car detailing place, Laundromat, and three cash advance stores. Most of the storefronts remained empty at the time of the spring 2006 DPZ/CNU charrette and it was (prematurely) concluded that they would not be coming back. A major frontis-piece rendering presented in the team's final report (on page 66) depicted an unabashedly neo-19th-century town square on this site, featuring a church with steeple and a bell tower on one corner intersection, cute brick-paved streets and sidewalks, pitched roof buildings with stores on the street

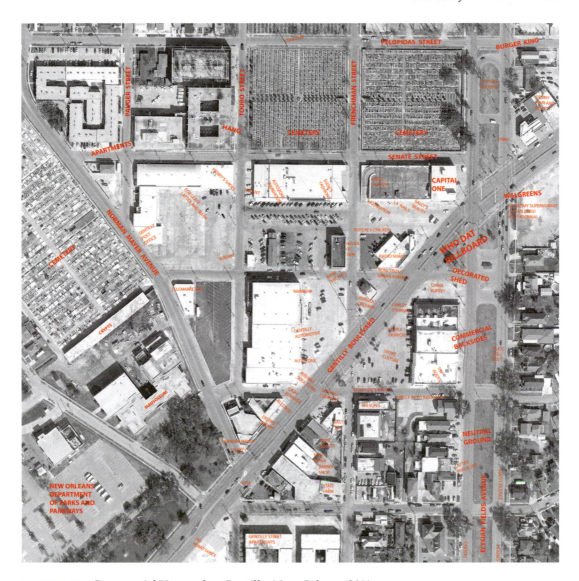

**FIGURE 5.12** Commercial Vernacular, Gentilly, New Orleans, 2011

level abutting the sidewalks and housing above, with balconies and buildings depicted in wood-frame cladding. All this was to be thoroughly traditional Vieux Carré-type, nostalgia-inspired buildings for a past that Gentilly never knew in the first place.

The New Urbanists decreed:

> This area should be repositioned as a *town center* instead of a strip shopping center, as it is today. . .The Gentilly Civic Improvement Association must hold to this design or one similar to it. Then, the reconstruction of the shopping center can take place regardless of the owner, in such as way that the center forms the town center of Gentilly and does not revert back to an interchangeable strip shopping center of no particular character.[26]

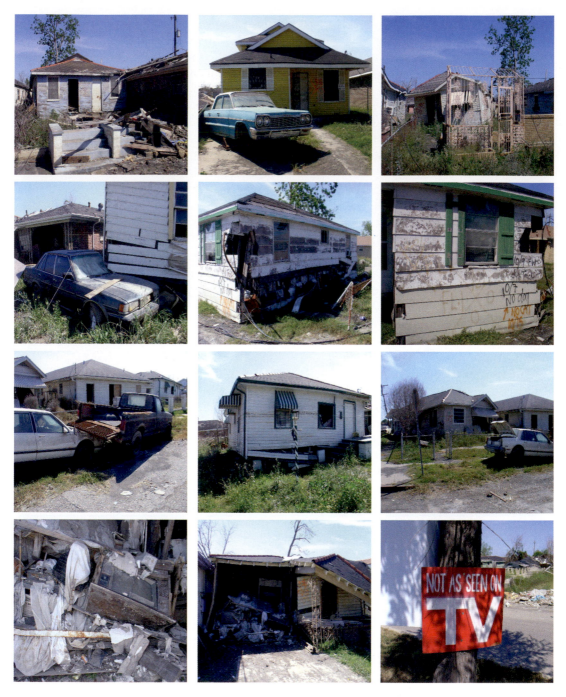

**FIGURE 5.13a–l**   Neighborhood Devastation, Post-Katrina, 2005. Photos courtesy of Alexander Verderber

The vintage shopping center aggregation was discarded, in favor of by-now generic caricatured imagery expressed in New Urbanist upscale enclaves such as Seaside, in Celebration, both in Florida, and elsewhere. Create a bucolic, romanticized town square by rerouting the existing street grid, and close any supposedly extraneous streets due to their "contaminating" effects. These moves would yield a roughly two-by-two city square block town square, with only oblique, if any, reference to what was there currently. The town square would be built in the same geographic location where parking lots presently stood together with the set of apparently "dismissible" commercial structures. The New Urbanists surmised it all had to go. This was further justified, in the DPZ/CNU team view, because currently the strip shopping structures along the major streets were underused, perceived to be poorly maintained, and aesthetically of poor quality. In actuality, these buildings did not suffer major damage from either wind or flood, although floodwaters did reach up to 5 feet in some buildings and in surrounding homes (but, fortunately, this land was part of the original Gentilly Ridge).

On the final evening of their week-long charrette, Duany and associates scheduled a forum to present their vision of a rebuilt Gentilly. This event occurred at St. Leo the Great Catholic Church. The event itself took on highly religious undertones for several reasons. First, it was a rainy evening and people had to brave the elements to attend. Despite this, the church was packed when the presentation began promptly at 7:00pm. As a hush came over the audience in the pews, Duany began to speak softly from the altar, in a carefully measured tone. It was as if he were the high priest speaking to the unwashed masses. After a half hour or so, due to the storm, the power went out in the church and throughout the neighborhood. This caused total silence for a few moments. Then, as if all at once, dozens of people in the audience opened up their laptops and together the screens created an eerie glow that bathed the faces in the audience, and Duany's face as well, on the altar. Duany, garbed in all white, pontificated from the darkened church altar that night. I was struck by the total self-confidence in his words and actions and in the drawings he attempted to display on a set of easels perched next to him on the altar. The charismatic Duany held the audience's rapt attention throughout. To me, the scene was totally surreal and bizarre. He basked in the glow of the moment: he on the altar, addressing his subjects. The meeting lasted over two hours.[27] The DPZ/CNU report proceeded to list twelve provisos, each stated as a need, each mandatory:

> 1. Create this town square as a green civic space; 2. Plant a double row of trees around it and leave its center open as a large lawn; 3. Design the square to accommodate future streetcar lines; 4. Reverse the current location of autos from the front to the rear of the buildings, and with public funds construct a parking deck; 5. Bring in out of state developers to develop a merchandizing plan; 6. Build gateway markers at major vehicular entry thresholds; 7. Seek gentrification in the form of attracting new upscale restaurants around the new town square; 8. Construct a multiplex cinema or a large department store to provide a strong commercial anchor (versus the mom and pop businesses that had been there for decades); 9. Preserve some existing historical buildings (but not any of the 1950s–1960s shopping center buildings); 10. Create a pedestrian link between nearby Dillard University and this new town square; 11. Realign several of the neighborhood side streets; and 12. Work to "encourage two main building types in the town center—apartments above shops, and live–work units."[28]

The DPZ/CNU team called for the adoption of its *Smart Code*, and its mandate for architectural standards that are code-compliant, and "attractive and compatible." Transects and streetscape designs were to overrule current zoning regulations. In other words, its form-based codes would henceforth govern all redevelopment in Gentilly. The charrette team's deliverables included a redefinition of the core neighborhoods that comprise Gentilly, and even its geographic boundaries. An assessment was conducted of existing demographic and socio-economic factors and limitations based on interviews with residents. Perceived prospects for the area's future were enumerated as well. A "recovery vision" was presented for rebuilding, as were strategic goals. Detailed maps were produced of prototypical block structures, neighborhood centers, major public amenities, and all pedestrian sheds that would be constructed and walkable within a ¼-mile radius of this new "town center". Public transport was addressed as were detailed narratives for existing and proposed new open spaces, schools, civic sites, and mixed-use commercial zones. Finally, an inventory was included on architectural typologies, their condition, and an architectural revitalization plan based on strategies for dwelling elevation combined with selective demolition. The implementation strategy identified urgent (1 year or less), intermediate (2–5 years), and long-term (up to 10 year) priorities, and a timetable. A Neighborhood Planning Center was proposed. Various public agencies and NGOs that might be housed in such a center were identified, including a field office of the U.S. Federal Emergency Management Agency (FEMA), an insurance claims center, a clearinghouse for information on rebuilding options, zoning information, demolition versus renovation options, and general legal assistance.

From the outset, the New Urbanists operated from highly flawed assumptions. First, New Orleans was not like anyplace else they had worked before (or since, with the possible exception of the DPZ/CNU charrette conducted in Port au Prince Haiti in late 2010). It is an insular city, a parochial place, one content to exist within its own world of political, business, and cultural traditions. Family, personal friendship ties, social class, and traditions supersede all else. Since the city's inception, a deep distrust of outsiders has permeated the air, and this was especially so in the weeks and months following Katrina. This was because it had been well documented in the local newspaper and in the international mass media that numerous outsiders had in fact, tragically perpetrated fraud with respect to locals' unfortunate circumstances. Gentilly residents were at the time of the charrette dealing with a widespread epidemic of contractor fraud. Hundreds of unscrupulous out-of-state "pretender" and shadow contractors and assorted charlatans routinely demanded upfront payment from unsuspecting homeowners and business owners. They required all insurance damage reimbursements and personal savings—referring to these pre-payments as "deposits" for building materials. Then they disappeared. The fleeced victim was left with virtually no money to rebuild. Besides this tragic spectacle, most locals were dealing with deep insurance company woes. Intransigent insurers were regularly denying legitimate property claim losses. Many locals simply became overwhelmed, and some despondent. The suicide rate was rising.

Second, and making matters worse, government agencies at all levels remained overwhelmed and unable to provide any tangible help. Federal, state, and local governments remained completely ineffective in the aftermath of the catastrophe. At this time, the State of Louisiana was in the process of formulating its infamously dysfunctional *Road Home* program, funded with federally provided funds.[29] This program channeled billions in federal Community Development Block Grant (known as CDBG funds) disaster funds to the state and local level for distribution. An individual homeowner could qualify and receive a grant for up to $150,000 to rebuild their home. As could have been predicted by any causal observer of Louisiana politics, the Road Home program was fraught with management ineptitude from the get-go. The chaos in people's daily lives was already enough cause for extreme stress and uncertainty among Gentilly residents. The DPZ/CNU team came off as too far out. This, despite the fact that it had only four weeks earlier conducted a similar week-long charrette in nearby St. Bernard Parish that was poorly received.

Third, perhaps most importantly, the New Urbanists' bucolic, romanticized small-town image of a neo-19th-century town center was completely off the mark, and ill-suited for Gentilly's working- and middle-class population. It was never an upscale place on the order of say, Uptown, or the Garden District. Historically, from 1909, its earliest developers envisioned a fundamentally *suburban* community and not a semi-autonomous small town.[30] It was a misguided notion from the outset, one that caused the locals to scratch their heads in disbelief when it was presented to them on that rainy night in April of 2006 on the altar of St. Leo the Great Catholic Church. It was a classic case of outsider "experts" coming in with an artificial, ungrounded vision—more accurately (and offensively, to some) a generic template. Undeniably, Duany's intent was for the local residents and business owners to grasp his every phrase and buzzword as part of a larger message meant to sound reassuring and compassionate. The result revealed a major disconnect between an ersatz romanticized urban utopianism thrust upon a flood-ravaged suburban area. Seldom if ever had the New Urbanists operated so far afield, so entirely ungrounded, and disassociated relative to the physical context and people they were working in/with.

To the DPZ/CNU team's credit, however, it was the first (in Gentilly) after the disaster, and worked on its own dime. The team paid its own expenses that entire week. The locals were appreciative of this act of professional *pro bono* work. The team's motives may not have been completely altruistic, for Duany et al. had hoped to inspire funding support from City Hall and the myriad government agencies responsible for distributing CDBG funds across the city. They knew attraction of any substantial federal CDBG funds would be absolutely essential if their vision were to be realized to any meaningful extent. Optimistically, they equally hoped that private investors would also be inspired to favorably step up to support their romanticized vision of a past that in fact never existed in Gentilly in the first place. Neither would occur. Out-of-state private investors, naturally, were scared to death to invest at all in a city with such poor flood protection, a track record of such significant population losses in recent years, and political corruption, long before Katrina.

Just four weeks earlier, the DPZ/CNU team had prevented its aforementioned grand-scaled proposal for the virtual reinvention of Chalmette, in St. Bernard Parish. Chalmette is a suburban bedroom community of 29,000 (67,000 persons prior to Katrina). All but a few buildings in the entire parish were completely destroyed by Katrina. Duany had judged Chalmette to be thoroughly ugly and publicly stated his view that it was one of the worst cases of uncontrolled, auto-centric sprawl that he had ever encountered anywhere. The DPZ team proposed a series of Venetian canals throughout, amid neighborhoods of new structures built on top of elevated dirt berms. I was also in the audience on the night of the first formal public presentation of that week's work (I video recorded these proceedings as well as the Gentilly presentation). The crowd that night was so emotional, completely absorbed in, and distracted by their own troubles that few could barely connect with anything Duany was saying. The audience viewed his proposals as "dreaming" and, without question, pie in the sky. One middle-aged crying woman sitting next to me whispered to her daughter, "But where will all of us live during the many years it will take to build all of this?"

The following week, Duany urged the St. Bernard Parish Council to quickly adopt his recommendations for an adapted version of the DPZ Smart Code that would supersede the six existing zoning ordnances that governed all land use. This version of the Smart Code was currently being developed for the city of Miami, and was inadvertently being paid for with a $1 million grant by that city for the work in Miami. The DPZ team presented its recommendations to more than 1,000 persons at the Parish Courthouse on the evening of 15 March 2006. Recommendations in Phase I of the plan called for a much-shrunken footprint for the parish, a total demolition (*cleanslating*, in planners' parlance) of over 1 square mile of flood-damaged structures, the implementation of the DPZ Smart Code, raised homes everywhere, a new town center with civic green, and a completely new network of surface water ecologies, i.e. retention ponds. As in the case of Gentilly, it was unabashed romanticism, complete neo-19th- century revivalism—although perhaps more so here due to its radical rejection of the entire present suburban condition. Duany told the Parish Council in a meeting soon thereafter, "You launch it, and if it gets funding, then you worry about it."[31] Nothing tangible ever came of either the Gentilly or the St. Bernard Parish charrettes, with the notable exception of the Katrina cottage prototype (from the St. Bernard charrette).[32] The New Urbanists had failed in their quest to conquer a ruined New Orleans.

## Suburban Transfusion

The DPZ/CNU design charrette in Gentilly and its prior charrette in St. Bernard Parish seemed so out of balance that I was inspired to react. I would focus on Gentilly as the site of an urban/suburban analysis and proposal for phased-in design interventions. A team of graduate students and I conducted research in New Orleans with work commencing in the Spring of 2010. The results of this field research comprise the remainder of this chapter. It is a reaction. It seeks to redress. In the past decade, many have harshly critiqued the formal and symbolic aspects of suburbia. Architect and academician Paul Lukez has critiqued contemporary suburban theorists, specifically the New Urbanists, for their fascile methods and arguments for how to re-establish civicness place-identification, and genuine authenticity in a suburb.[33,34]

To its critics sprawl is tantamount to inauthenticity—where everyplace looks like everyplace else. Genuine connections to a given place's past history and its evolution across time are negligible, even to be entirely dismissed.[35] This occurs, as Lukez cites, through a premeditated process of erasure and iterative re-imprinting (re-making on the same spot) that leaves a suburb culturally poorer than it was before. It is a common suburban condition that he contrasts with how the great cities of the world such as Venice, Rome, and Munich were able to rebuild themselves on their existing sites, but usually far better than before (if not always healthier from a public health standpoint). He paraphrases Aldo Rossi's assertion that time is of the essence in the re-making of meaningful cities.[36] His argument is premised on how the historical record shows how urban environments in history have been repeatedly erased and rebuilt in a manner fostering higher forms of cultural expression, the continued evolution of place identity, and uniqueness.[37] On this, Lukez writes:

> [American] suburbs developed from a set of policies and bureaucratic controls unparalleled in history. Post war housing construction was a process that resulted in massive demographic shifts in a relatively short time period. . .[raising the] question of whether an environment constructed in such haste can serve as an appropriate [mechanism for] collective memory representing the work of a civilization. . .the amount of space and services generated in the suburbs, per unit of infrastructure development, is highly inefficient when compared to more compact urban settlement patterns.[38]

Memorable architectural elements—landmarks—allow a society to gauge its bearings both in space and time. They enable people to orient themeselves relative to these markers as if part of a larger narrative, a type of inscription making. Sacred landmarks, such as churches, and rivers, streams, and mountains, facilitate in us strong cognitively-based place attachments, help us feel secure in our everyday lives, and help orient us to our individual place in a larger civic world. However, such landmarks, physical and/ or historic, are often absent in the suburbs because development has wiped away most traces of any such past or never sought to establish any such cultural legacy in the first place.[39]

Lukez recounts in some detail the history and growth of the New Urbanism movement in the U.S. He lists its contributions to current discourse yet faults its translation into practice as it relies too heavily on a romanticized vocabulary based in nostalgia and predictability, and is likely to sidestep or outright dismiss local idiosyncrasies and the unpredictable, funkier, grimier aspects of daily life. He concludes that New Urbanism is not the answer because it does not readily engage "vibrant and contemporary architectural language and relies more on historical precedents" and that further experimentation is needed to generate more effective strategies that take cognizance of a place's uniqueness, its own sense of precedent, and its authenticity. All this, within a paradigmatic framework that far better accommodates change across time.[40] Static re-creations of a past that no longer exists no longer hold relevance.[41]

The messiness of suburbia in its current condition can be the genesis of its reinvention. This messy past is reinterpretable through a process of selective yet comprehensive *suburban transfusion*. It involves re-building up/out from within. Selective, surgical transformation occurs, allowing the body of the sick patient to once again live and thrive. This process is not unlike an organ transplant or a blood transfusion and it is *absolutely not* about creating something entirely different than what existed there before. It builds upon the best of what is there now. The slate therefore need not be wiped clean, as so often happens in "redevelopment" initiatives.[42] Suburban transfusion is a both/and proposition and paradigm and is inspired by sources as diverse as Robert Venturi, Denise Scoot Brown, and Steven Izenour's seminal 1972 book *Learning from Las Vegas*[43] and Mario Gandelsonas's *The Urban Text*.[44]

An alternative suburban analysis of Gentilly yields a set of observational narratives. These morphologies are documentable and able to be layered and juxtaposed in varied configurations in a series of two-dimensional graphic collages inspired by Gandelsonas's urban texting methodology.[45] Twelve such analyses are depicted in Figures 5.14a–d, 5.15a–d, and 5.16a–d and these iterations seek to capture various salient narrative layers of New Orleans' and Gentilly's suburban morphology:

1.  *Land Use*—At the macro scale the Gentilly suburban milieu is a mix of residential single- and multi-family residences, commercial establishments, schools, related institutional land uses, a small number of industrial land uses, and the linear lakefront park that borders the levees along Lake Pontchartrain.
2.  *Roads*—Main thoroughfares are depicted, with the neutral ground in the center of Elysian Fields Avenue bisecting Gentilly, creating a north–south axis. Urban recreational spaces are to the east (Pontchartrain Park), north (Lakefront—University of New Orleans campus), and west (City Park) of the catalyst site.
3.  *Urban Fabric*—A pattern of collaged and colliding street grids exists in Gentilly. Primary grids are depicted in red, indicating their influence in shaping the suburban infrastructural grid as it criss-crosses the catalyst site. Secondary grids/grains take on a somewhat randomized pattern closer to the suburban periphery.
4.  *Circulation Nexus*—Walking distances of five, ten, fifteen, and twenty minutes are depicted in a series of concentric rings emanating from the catalyst site. Primary and secondary arteries are layered upon existing healthcare clinics in Gentilly.
5.  *Catalyst*—The primary existing structures that comprise the 1950s-era shopping center are depicted in red. Offset, colliding urban grids straddle and bump up against and sometimes harshly bisect the catalyst site. Vehicular arteries clearly dominate over the local secondary streets and these arteries cut abruptly through an otherwise orthogonal suburban street grid.
6.  *Pervious and Imperious Surfaces*—Now-obscured natural ecologies, current vehicular arteries, and large parking lots surround the aggregation of disconnected shopping strips that lie at the core. People underutilize its overpaved parcels, with autos filling no more than one fourth of the total parking capacity at any one time.

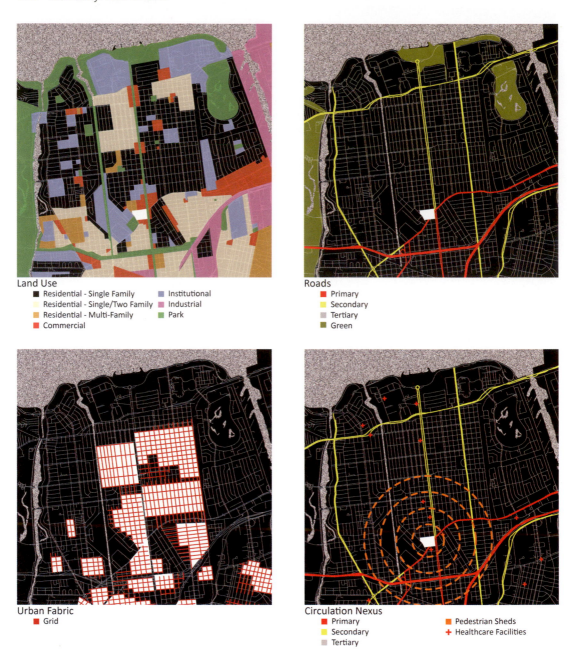

**Land Use**
- ■ Residential - Single Family
- ■ Residential - Single/Two Family
- ■ Residential - Multi-Family
- ■ Commercial
- ■ Institutional
- ■ Industrial
- ■ Park

**Roads**
- ■ Primary
- ■ Secondary
- ■ Tertiary
- ■ Green

**Urban Fabric**
- ■ Grid

**Circulation Nexus**
- ■ Primary
- ■ Secondary
- ■ Tertiary
- ■ Pedestrian Sheds
- + Healthcare Facilities

**FIGURE 5.14a–d** Urban Fabric 1. Drawings by S. Verderber/Annette Himelick

7. *Figure-Ground*—The 1950s–1960s shopping strip-center aggregation dominates the suburban figure-ground, as viewed against the broader suburban fabric. Five commercial structures dominate, these collectively define a "loose" commercial footprint. Residential dwellings and small commercial establishments comprise the surrounding fabric.

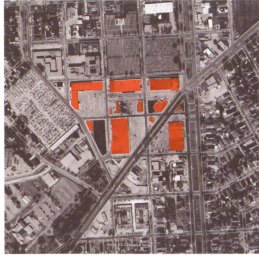

Catalyst

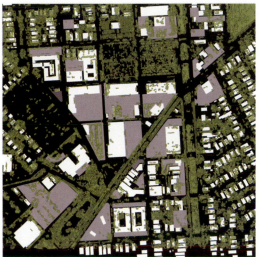

Pervious and Impervious Surface
- Trees
- Parking
- Roads

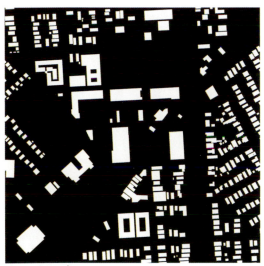

Figure-Ground

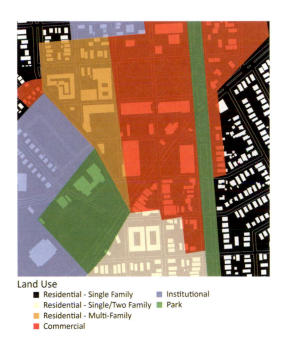

Land Use
- Residential - Single Family
- Residential - Single/Two Family
- Residential - Multi-Family
- Commercial
- Institutional
- Park

**FIGURE 5.15a–d**  Urban Fabric 2. Drawings by S. Verderber/Annette Himelick

8.  *Land Use (Collage)*—Land use is defined by the network of local primary, secondary, and tertiary street grids. The neutral ground of Elysian Fields Avenue is revealed as a primary green space, linear in configuration, and is used by neighborhood residents as recreational space throughout the year.

9.  *Sound-Circulation*—Vehicular traffic dominates the commercial precinct. The network of primary and secondary streets that bisects the shopping precinct generates considerable noise that bleeds

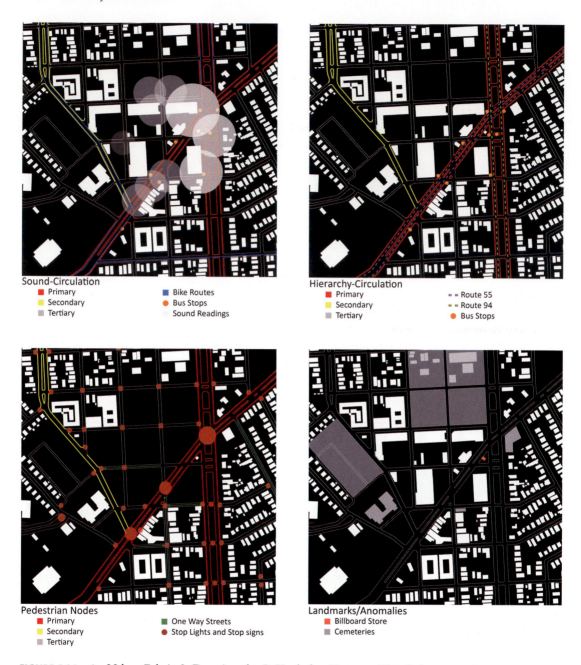

**Sound-Circulation**
- 🟥 Primary
- 🟨 Secondary
- ⬜ Tertiary
- 🟦 Bike Routes
- 🟠 Bus Stops
- ⬜ Sound Readings

**Hierarchy-Circulation**
- 🟥 Primary
- 🟨 Secondary
- ⬜ Tertiary
- ⬛ Route 55
- ⬛ Route 94
- 🟠 Bus Stops

**Pedestrian Nodes**
- 🟥 Primary
- 🟨 Secondary
- ⬜ Tertiary
- 🟩 One Way Streets
- 🔴 Stop Lights and Stop signs

**Landmarks/Anomalies**
- 🟥 Billboard Store
- ⬜ Cemeteries

**FIGURE 5.16a–d** Urban Fabric 3. Drawings by S. Verderber/Annette Himelick

into the surrounding residential zones. The noise epicenter is the intersection of Gentilly Boulevard and Elysian Fields Avenue.

10. *Hierarchy-Circulation*—Figure-ground patterns are collaged against primary, secondary, and tertiary thoroughfares. Public transport stops are located at street corners, and these nodes attract

significant pedestrian activity (and crime). Few amenities at present exist for pedestrians to make them feel safe while waiting at transit stops or when walking outdoors.

11. *Pedestrian Nodes*—Traffic control devices (traffic lights, stop signs) are ineffective, by and large. Auto and pedestrian traffic movement occurs randomly and is haphazard due to individuals' inability to predict the movements of drivers traversing the precinct. This causes severe personal safety problems.

12. *Landmarks/Anomalies*—Two cemeteries, predating suburbanization, function as foils to the precinct's present aggregation of commercial strips. The most iconic commercial vernacular structure in the district is diminutive, and sits on a triangular land parcel at the Gentilly precinct's epicenter. It shoulders a pair of immense billboards perched high above.

A closer examination of the immediate site environs, building upon the prior set of urban text analyses, reveals further insights into the everyday quality of life and its ramification for public health. Eight such fine-grain dimensions of everyday life in Gentilly include the following:

1. *Decay*—New Orleans is an old city, especially by American standards. Its ruins take on exceptional aesthetic properties onto themselves. To some, this visual decay is one of the city's major assets and its "tumbledown charm" remains a major attraction for tourists. It also gives the place a deep authenticity and sense of its history and of its once-proud position among major American cities. Its tens of thousands of decaying buildings take on properties of the natural environment, some with vegetation sprouting from their roofs and cornices, with cascading vines, as if drapes covering their facades. In many cases these buildings continue to be inhabited. The city's monuments to its heroes lean to and fro on their pedestals due to the soft, spongy soil beneath them. The city has perfected the art of deferred maintenance of its civic resources. This applies equally to infrastructural resources you can clearly see—as much as to those you can't. Nearly 50 percent of the fresh drinking water leaks from the city's belowground pipes each and every day of the year.[46] In many cases, individual property owners simply do not have the funds to renovate or rebuild, as is the case with the "Air Tire Car Wash" business (Figure 5.17a) and a tire repair shop close by (Figure 5.17b).

2. *Abandonment*—Six years after Hurricane Katrina more than 64,000 structures remained vacant across the city.[47] In the Gentilly section alone nearly 1,500 buildings remained vacant. Many had not been gutted since the flood in 2005. As they sat rotting in the hot, humid climate, residents who had returned to the neighborhood became increasingly exasperated. The inactivity associated with these abandoned homes and businesses angered residents to the point that they demanded action from the city. They wanted these structures either rehabilitated or demolished, and quickly. The level of blight caused by post-Katrina abandonment reached epidemic proportions in the hardest hit areas. The result was what planners like to refer to as the "jack o' lantern effect" where at night the lights of the returned families stood out in stark contrast amid a sea of surrounding vacant lots and abandoned structures. In 2010 the city launched yet another effort to fight neighborhood blight, including in the Gentilly section, and the results of this effort remain to be seen. Preservationists fear, and rightfully so, however, that this blind impulse to demolish now versus a more reflective resource conservation policy of urban homesteading or a similar initiative will result in the loss of thousands of historic buildings. Many of these places would have been rescued had there been an owner willing to take on this responsibility, such as the case with this single family dwelling on Elysian Fields Avenue (Figure 5.18).[48]

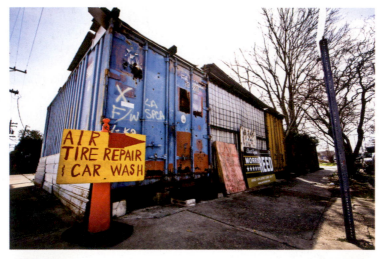

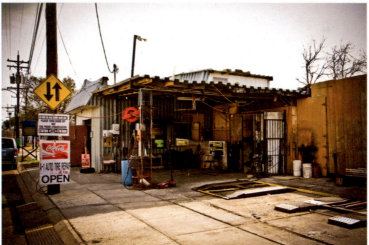

**FIGURE 5.17a–b** Decay. Photos courtesy of Derrick Simpson

3. *Signs*—The neighborhood is at present dominated by commercial establishments of modest scale. The buildings reflect a wide spectrum in terms of their age, appearance, and upkeep. Some have been in the neighborhood since the 1930s, others opened as more established businesses moved out of the area or went bankrupt. In the 1950s the Gentilly Plaza strip mall housed the first Maison Blanche department store outlet outside of the CBD, as well as numerous upscale clothing stores, specialty shops, and a full service grocery store, the landmark Economy Market. While businesses came and went, the commercial area fell into a precipitous decline in the 1970s and 1980s as more residents fled the neighborhood for newer suburban areas, leaving behind the poorer residents who had fewer options in terms of their mobility or purchasing power. These families and individuals had far less disposable income and therefore the range of stores in Gentilly Plaza and on adjacent streets continued to fall in quality. By 2005 the neighborhood had acquired a reputation as a place where one might not be safe at night.[49] This applied equally to the two graveyards in the immediate area. Similarly, the signs on the façades of the stores reflect

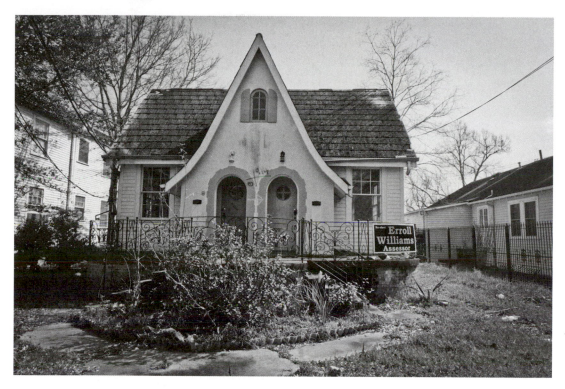

**FIGURE 5.18**   Abandonment. Photo courtesy of Derrick Simpson

this downward spiral insofar as many are handmade, while others appear to be about to fall to the ground. These ad hoc signs are interspersed with those of national chains who remain committed to this aging, dying shopping district (Figure 5.19a–t).

4.  *Parking Typology*—The Gentilly Plaza strip mall is dominated by large expanses of asphalt. There are very few trees or other types of vegetation. As one approaches the commercial district, parking lots become visible. The buildings appear to sit forelonely in a sea of paving. It is in many instances hard to distinguish where the street, sidewalks, and parking areas begin and end because they run into one another like poorly constructed sentences. The lack of differentiation between street, walking paths, and auto traffic has been the cause of untold accidents over the decades. It is unsafe to walk in the commercial district, particularly in the areas dominated by the strip malls. Cars are constantly coming and going in unpredictable patterns. Many drivers do not seek out sanctioned access drives as they enter and leave the area. Instead, in many cases, they make random use of any available path, be it over a curb, or in the direct path of pedestrians attempting to negotiate a labyrinth of randomized access points. The stores located along the older streets in the commercial district generally were built up to the sidewalk in a zero lot configuration. This tends to promote pedestrian safety as the sidewalks are buffered by the adjacent storefronts. One of the original 1950s strip mall structures features a roof parking deck (Figure 5.20a–b).

5.  *Gravesites*—Two graveyards in the immediate neighborhood predate the 1950s-era strip mall and associated suburban development in this part of Gentilly. These are the Mount Olivet Cemetery and Garden Mausoleum, located to the immediate west of the strip center (Figure 5.21a), and the

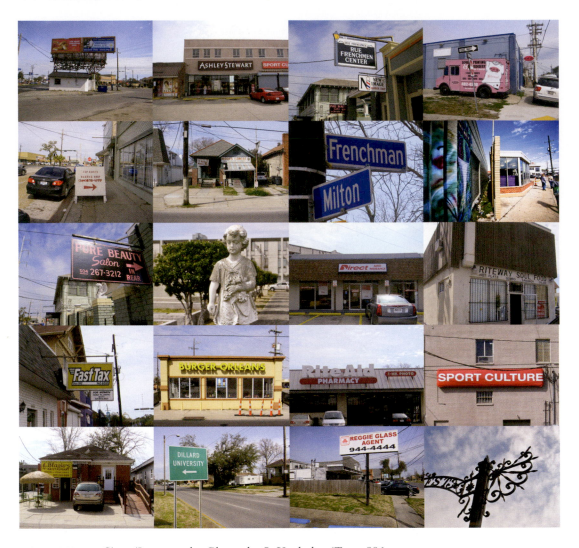

**FIGURE 5.19a–t** Signs/Iconography. Photos by S. Verderber/Team 896

Number 1 Hebrew Rest Cemetery, located to the north of the strip center (Figure 5.21b). Both feature above-ground gravesites. This is of necessity due to the high water table and the below sea level elevation of the two cemeteries. The bodies are therefore stationed above ground, and the tombs are subjected to a variety of maintenance challenges ranging from water intrusion, vandalism, wind damage, and the erosive effects of climate on the gravesites. It remains a strong local tradition for families of means to purchase, beginning generations ago, multiple sites in a contiguous parcel. As members die, the family is eventually reunited in its gravesite plot. The clusters of elevated gravesites and tombstones form a pattern of blocks and streets not unlike an urban grid. This attribute, combined with the elaborate tombstones and crypts built by middle- and upper-class families, has led to New Orleans cemeteries being widely referred to as "cities of the dead."[50] Because both cemeteries are considered unsafe at night, pedestrians, as a rule, avoid walking through them.

6. *Housing Typology*—The types of housing in the immediate area include a mix of one- and two-level cottages, shotgun houses, two-level flats, split-level bungalows, raised bungalows, and rental apartment buildings that generally fit into one of the aforementioned housing types (Figure 5.22a–t and Figure 5.23a–t). The neighborhood is dotted with 1950s-era suburban ranch houses that were built directly on slab. These slab houses sustained the most severe flooding, with floodwaters often completely above the roof and with most submerged up to their roof eaves. The remaining house types are raised up 3–4 feet in elevation above the street. Many dwellings are what are referred to as raised basement houses—implying that the living quarters are elevated one floor above an at-grade "basement level" that typically houses a garage and an adjacent laundry or storeroom. The condition of the dwellings varies widely based on the street, the income level of the occupants, the level of crime in the immediate area, and the degree of damage sustained by Katrina. In general, the dwellings located furthest from the Gentilly Ridge sustained the greatest flood damage. Hundreds of homes have been demolished in the years since the disaster, yielding vacant lots that contribute to the jack-o'-lantern effect in the immediate vicinity. Landscaping suffered greatly at Katrina's hands, also. The highly toxic floodwaters destroyed lawns, bushes, and trees throughout the area. The neighborhood sits barren compared to before Katrina.

7. *Residual Space*—The 1950s–1960s shopping strip center aggregation and nearby older commercial structures form a visual hodgepodge within a sea of residualized open land parcels (Figure 5.24a–k and Figure 5.25a–m). Enforcement of zoning regulations has been lax, with many zoning variances having been granted ad hoc. Few buildings genuinely address or "speak to" one another, i.e. many have front façades that directly face the backs of nearby buildings. Many spaces in between buildings are generally dysfunctional. The siting of the buildings often resulted in spatial voids too narrow for passageways with the darkest of these spaces becoming little more than receptacles for trash. There is, however, a notable absence of graffiti within the precinct. This is perhaps attributable to the high visibility of many of its wall surfaces, combined with their direct visibility to passersby on foot or in vehicles. These backsides are often loading docks and the service entrances to businesses but often they are merely blank windowless walls that inexplicably face public streetscapes. Collectively, an entire class of such orphaned façades and awkward figure-ground relationships functions to usurp the front façades of the businesses, and therefore undermine the entire precinct. This inexpiable condition, ironiclly, extends to the pair of nearby historic cemeteries, where the backsides of tombs there also often face the fronts of other nearby tombs.

8. *Landmarks/Anomalies*—Throughout New Orleans, ornate church steeples dominate the neighborhood skyline, and this is particularly so along the city's main boulevards and their neutral grounds. By contrast, in unexpected places, anomalous buildings and urban artifacts often provide another, totally different glimpse into the inner life of the city. These include the aforementioned massive billboards perched precariously on top of a small building at the intersection of Elysian Fields Avenue and Gentilly Boulevard (Figure 5.26a). The billboards are visible from afar not unlike a large church spire, and they dominate the district's skyline even as viewed from the downtown CBD. They remain, however, in the opinion of many locals, eyesores that have been there for fifty years, and yet because they have been there for decades they have become ingrained in local place-identity and in Gentilly's collective civic memory. Whether one views this accidental landmark as ugly or otherwise its presence remains unquestioned, by and large. Certain commercial vernacular types have acquired a near-mythical stature of their own in the Gentilly's collective civic psyche. One such architectural landmark is the Gentilly outlet of the locally famous McKenzie's

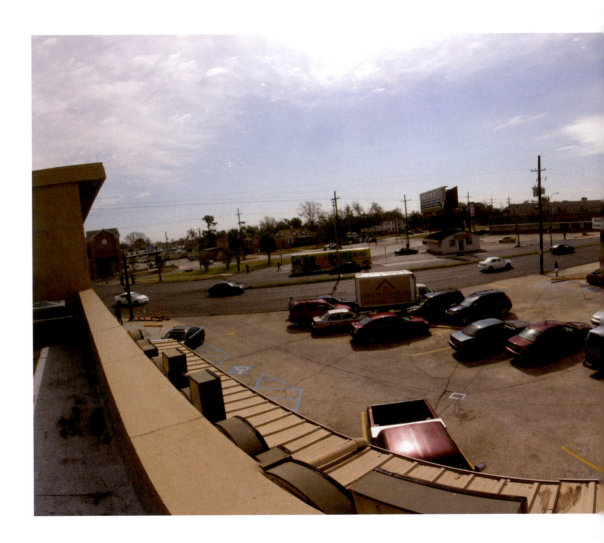

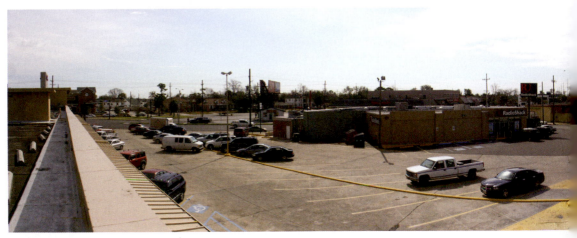

**FIGURE 5.20a–b** Seas of Parking. Photos by S. Verderber/Team 896

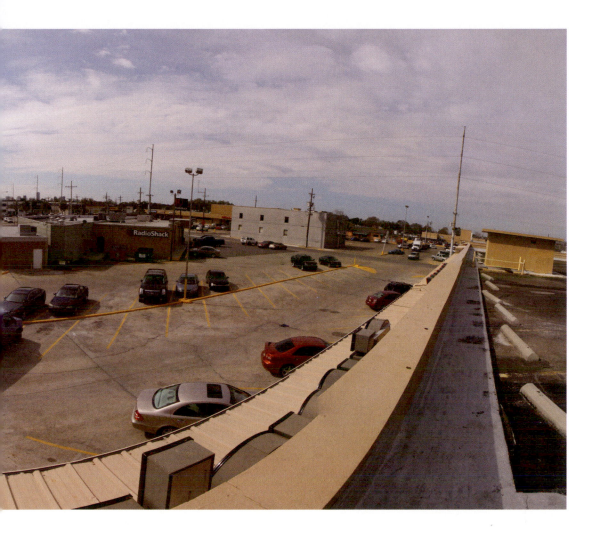

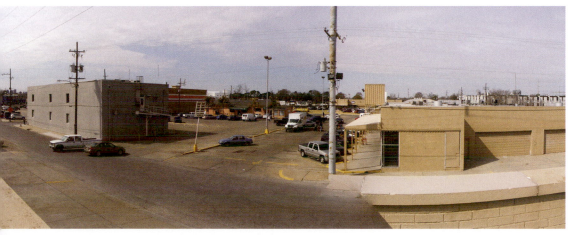

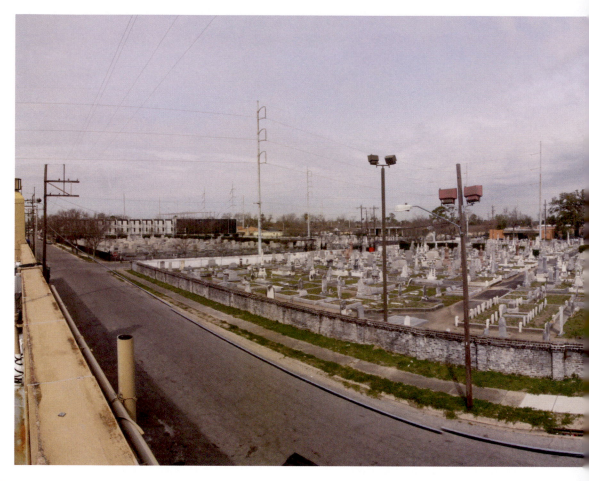

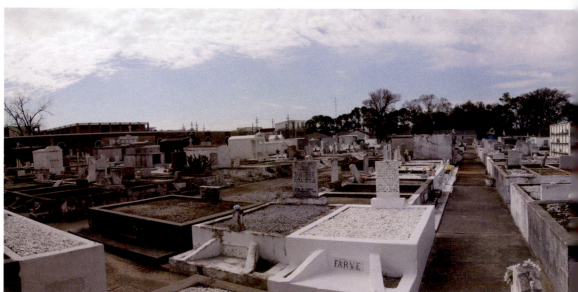

**FIGURE 5.21a–b**   Places of the Dead. Photos by S. Verderber/Team 896

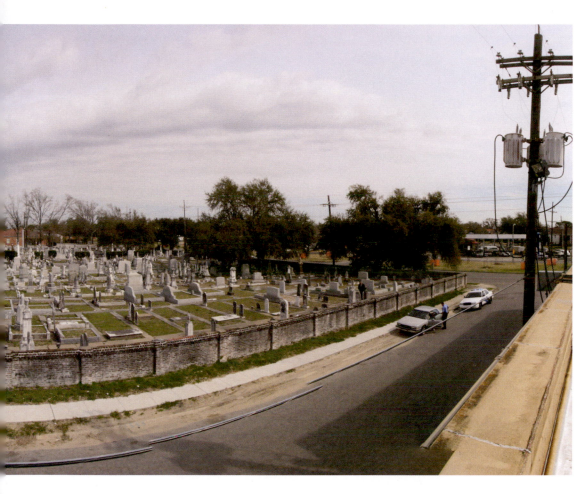

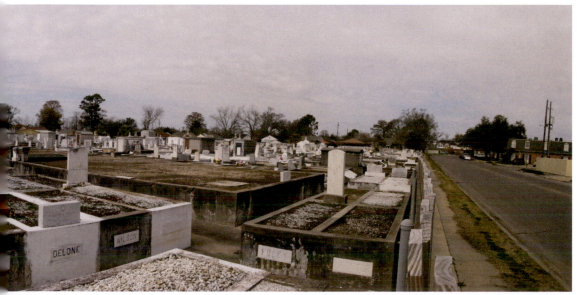

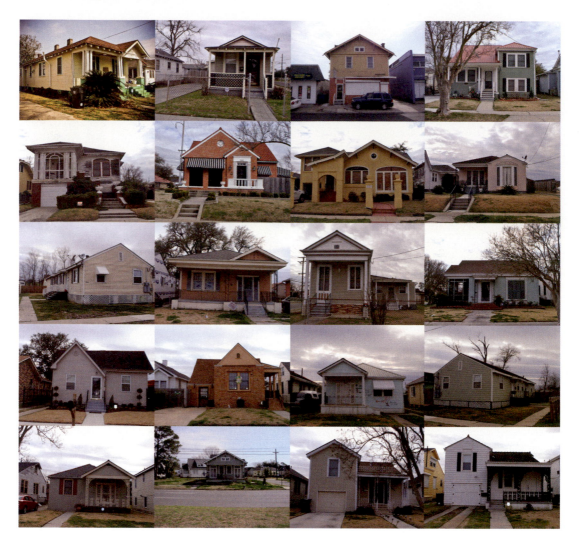

**FIGURE 5.22a–t**  Dwelling Typologies. Photos by S. Verderber/Team 896

bakery chain. Founded in the early 20th century, McKenzie's became famous for the colorful King Cakes it sells during every Mardi Gras season. The first suburban McKenzie's was in Gentilly, having opened in 1955. It remains in operation at this site today, featuring its iconic and instantly recognizable exterior green-paneled facade (Figure 5.26b).

At this point, the conceptual diagram first presented in Chapter 1 comes to the forefront again. Here, it drives the fundamental constructs which define the interrelationships between the built environment and public health promotion principles as they manifest in the transfusion of the catalyst site in New Orleans. The diagram's X-axis and Y-axis here each signify bipolar superordinate constructs, with the first denoting the close relationship between the URBAN/CIVIC CONTEXT and the immediate NEIGHBORHOOD, and with the second construct denoting the close relationship between the DISTRICT level spatial context and the immediate CATALYST SITE. The four specific constructs that are embedded in Figure 1.1 are reprised

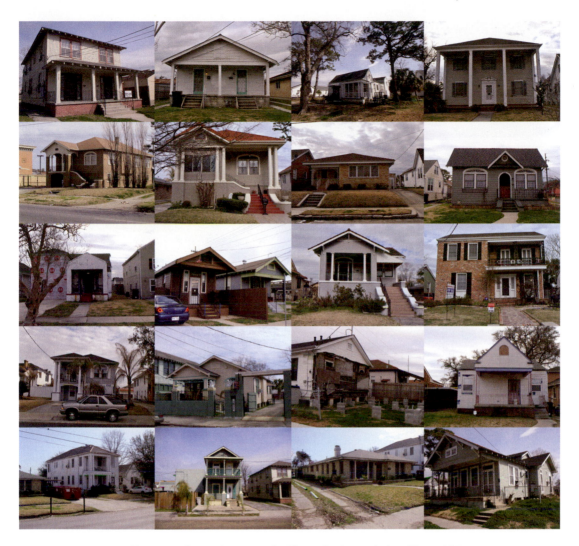

**FIGURE 5.23a–t**    Dwelling Typologies (continued). Photos by S. Verderber/Team 896

here once again relative to the Figure 1.1 X and Y governing axes and are discussed below in direct relation to the suburban transfusion initiative that is presented on the following pages. These four constructs are reprised here as follows:

## Incremental Commerce/Personal and Social Empowerment

The catalyst site and its infrastructure are redeveloped in six phases. Growth is envisioned, acknowledging the limits of the city's capacity to support and assist in its transfusion. New business ventures require substantial start up resources, so local residents will need to be skill-trained and socially re-empowered to take on the challenge, especially in the face of the city's ongoing rebuilding challenges. Expertise from both within and from outside the city will be critical. Existing small business incubators in New Orleans, i.e. the Idea Village, hold promise as resources for assisting local

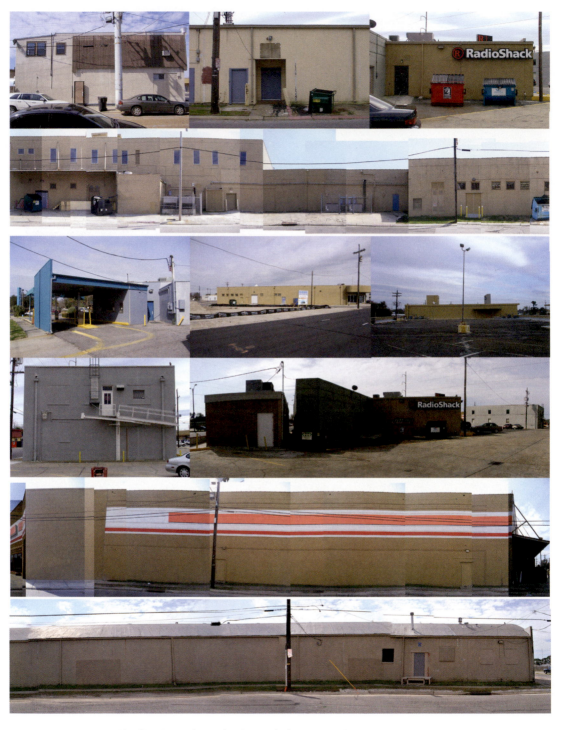

**FIGURE 5.24a–k** Residualization. Photos by S. Verderber/Team 896

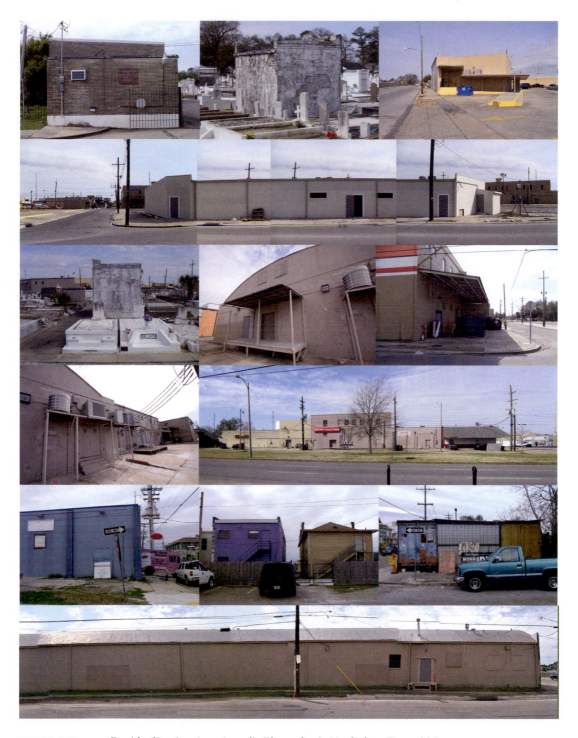

**FIGURE 5.25a–m**   Residualization (continued). Photos by S. Verderber/Team 896

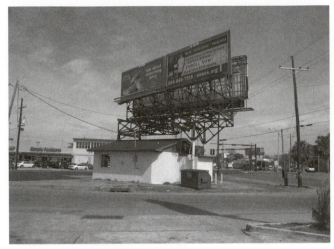

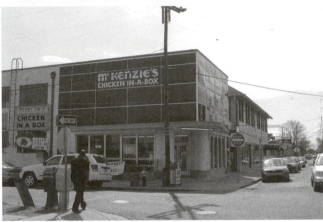

**FIGURE 5.26a–b**   Landmarks and Anomalies

entrepreneurs in Gentilly on the establishment of new businesses within the immediate area. The U.S Small Business Administration (SBA) provides low-interest loans for start-up ventures, with programs aimed at stimulating minority owned small business initiatives. However, in Katrina's aftermath, the track record of SBA loan outcomes has been mixed.[51] Local philanthropic foundations and new business incubators in New Orleans have also established grant programs for this purpose.[52] The local economy must become more diversified and self-reliant.[53] New salutogenetic-oriented business establishments will provide career opportunities. For example, a recreation/multipurpose center will provide career opportunities for staff trainers, coaches, and specialists who will offer a diverse range of health promotion and fitness classes for the immediate community.

### Place Identity and Collective Memory/Landscape Engagement

Sprawl is in most cases divorced from local cultural and vernacular building traditions because place identity and collective civic memory are often antithetical to its placeless, generic nature. The majority of sprawl machines are dismissive of historical precursors, with Las Vegas being the most well-known, wierdly notable exception in the U.S., with its borrowed, ersatz pseudo-legitimacy derived from New York City, Paris, the Great Pyramids, and so on. Sprawl's collective purpose is not to re-create any uniquely enduring memories or place-associations with, say, a specific highway strip in Toledo, Ohio, choked full with its fast food outlets, strip malls, and gas stations because it is all meant to be the same thing, everywhere. In other words, it doesn't matter where we are as long as we can find the local Wendy's outlet for lunch on that day we are traveling through Toledo.[54] Now, Gentilly's most memorable landmark will be at its epicenter. In terms of placemaking, a large public park, Gentilly Commons, is created at the center of the catalyst site, functioning as the city's first suburban example of landscape urbanism and ecological architecture. Extensive landscaping is incorporated, and an adjoining community wellness center and spa features a waterfall and hydrotherapy pool at its center, not unlike ancient Roman Bath complexes, with a multipurpose recreation center and community garden anchoring the other end of the site. The wellness center/spa, platform park, and multipurpose center will all provide vistas to the downtown skyline, surrounding neighborhoods, Lake Pontchartrain, and to its shoreline residential neighborhoods.

## Food and Nutrition/Sickness Prevention and Wellness

At present, the catalyst site is officially designated by the U.S. federal government as a food desert. There are no fresh food supermarkets where fruit and vegetables may be purchased within a short walk, bike ride, or even car trip. There is no butcher shop, nutritional health foods store, or other related businesses. The local bakery outlet remains an iconic visual landmark although its products do little to combat obesity. The area's very few convenience stores specialize in junk food. Major supermarket chains years ago abandoned this section of New Orleans. A sole market, the Economy Super Market, had operated at the main intersection of Elysian Fields and Gentilly Boulevard since the early 1950s. Flood-damaged in Katrina, it was demolished (2006) and has not been replaced.[55] In March 2011 the City of New Orleans announced a new program called the Fresh Food Retailer Initiative, which provides loans to start up fresh food grocery stores in underserved neighborhoods, including Gentilly, using $7 million in Community Development Block Grant (CDBG) funds channeled through the Hope Enterprise Corporation, a community development foundation based in Jackson, Mississippi. This is being done in conjunction with the Health Food Financing Initiative launched by the U.S. Department of Treasury, and the ASI Federal Credit Union, a local foundation created fifty years ago in support of the ship workers at the local Avondale Ship Yard. Similarly, Gentilly is equally underserved in its primary care health clinics, wellness centers, and related healthcare services.[56] For most Gentilly residents, it currently remains simply too costly and/or inconvenient to seek out fresh food stores or primary healthcare near to where they live.[57] The catalyst site will provide preventative healthcare and wellness amenities at its heart, along with the opportunity to purchase fresh food at an affordable price within close walking and biking distance.

## Walking and Cycling/Public Transport/Alternative Private Vehicles (APVs)

Gentilly, New Orleans's first 20th-century suburban area, thrived as a commercial center from the advent of the Automobile Age in the 1920s to the 1970s. Since that time, the area has suffered from "white flight" to newer suburbs outside of Orleans Parish. This disinvestment drained the area of much of its economic vitality and the volume of economic activity in its core commercial district diminished considerably. Its large parking lots were no longer needed as less and less of the local customer base could afford to own a car. Due to its excess parking capacity, all of the core commercial district's parking lots are to be demolished. One existing strip center building structure is to be retained and subsequently converted to parking for electric and allied non-fossil fuel powered vehicles. A charging station for electrically powered public transport buses is to be provided.[58] Because it is anticipated that these types of non-fossil fuel vehicles will proliferate in the coming decades, parking requirements in many sprawl communities will be radically reconfigured in the coming post-SUV age. Smaller, carbon neutralized vehicles—alternative personal vehicles (APVs)—will require less physical space compared to what conventional personal vehicles need today.[59] This will be reflected in rewritten local site planning regulations and parking requirements.[60] Multiple electro-charging stations are to be provided in the retained vestige of the 1950s strip center. In addition, utmost attention is to be devoted to walking, jogging, and cycling paths and networks linking these amenities to one another within the catalyst site and to its surrounding neighborhoods and to destination points beyond. New cycling paths are to be built that will crisscross the catalyst site neighborhood, including along the Elysian Fields neutral ground, linking the Lakefront with the Vieux Carré at the Mississippi River's edge. The long-absent Elysian Fields Avenue streetcar line is to be restored (in reference to the railroad line that once ran from the lost settlement of Milneburg at the lakefront to the CBD on this same route).[61] The Commons, located at the epicenter of the Gentilly catalyst site, is to be linked to its immediate environs via the two aforementioned pedestrian/cycling crossover bridges, one crossing over Gentilly Boulevard and a second bridge crossing over Elysian Fields Avenue.

## Implementation

Each of the four embedded constructs (a–d) are to be interpreted as a continuum from the macro scale (suburban fabric) to the micro (individual) scale. These are Incremental Commerce/Personal and Social Empowerment (a), Place Identity and Collective Memory/Landscape Engagement (b), Food and Nutrition/Sickness Prevention and Wellness (c), and Walking and Cycling/Public Transport/Alternative Private Vehicles, or APVs (d). Deployment of the various aforementioned new amenities within the catalyst site is illustrated in a series of three site/floor plans (Figures 5.27, 5.28, and 5.29). The seventy-five design considerations presented in the previous chapter are illustrated here once again in relation to the case study catalyst site as well; the individual title of each is listed here and is keyed vis-à-vis an axonometric perspective of the transfused catalyst site (see Table 5.1 and Figure 5.30).[62] This is followed by a series of six renderings illustrating selected elements of the public-health-promoting transformation of the catalyst site (Figures 5.31a–b, 5.32a–b, and 5.33a–b).

### Interval 1: Infrastructure/Health Promotion Anchors

The six phases in the transformation of the catalyst site are presented in accompanying Interval 1–6 axonometric renderings (Figures 5.34a–b, 5.35a–b, and 5.36a–b). In Interval 1, above- and below-ground infrastructural networks are constructed, and existing architectural landmarks are conserved (Figure 5.34a). The existing urban infrastructural systems within the catalyst site precinct range from inadequate to extremely poor in quality at the present time. The neighborhood is plagued year round with periodic ruptures of potable water main lines, surface water leaks, and, during the hottest summer months, periodic power grid outages. The initial redevelopment of the site necessitates the closure of two secondary streets that traverse the entire site, the reconstruction of the underground sewerage and water system, and the relocation of all above-ground electrical utilities to underground locations. Standing water is a chronic concern and this condition is rectified. The vehicular arteries to be retained

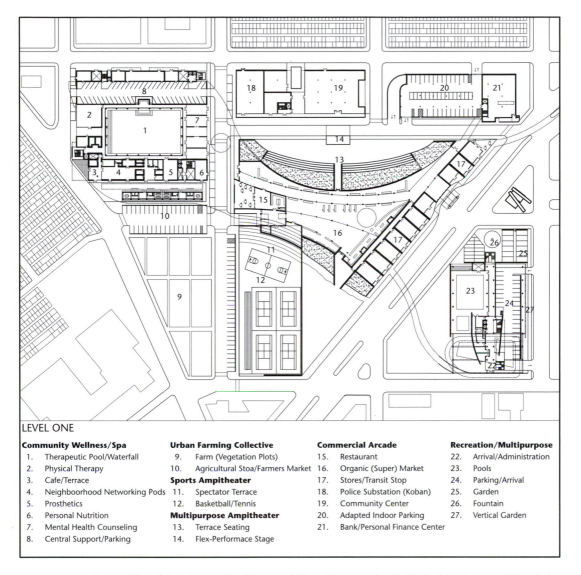

LEVEL ONE

**Community Wellness/Spa**
1. Therapeutic Pool/Waterfall
2. Physical Therapy
3. Cafe/Terrace
4. Neighboorhood Networking Pods
5. Prosthetics
6. Personal Nutrition
7. Mental Health Counseling
8. Central Support/Parking

**Urban Farming Collective**
9. Farm (Vegetation Plots)
10. Agricultural Stoa/Farmers Market
**Sports Ampitheater**
11. Spectator Terrace
12. Basketball/Tennis
**Multipurpose Ampitheater**
13. Terrace Seating
14. Flex-Performace Stage

**Commercial Arcade**
15. Restaurant
16. Organic (Super) Market
17. Stores/Transit Stop
18. Police Substation (Koban)
19. Community Center
20. Adapted Indoor Parking
21. Bank/Personal Finance Center

**Recreation/Multipurpose**
22. Arrival/Administration
23. Pools
24. Parking/Arrival
25. Garden
26. Fountain
27. Vertical Garden

**FIGURE 5.27**    Ground Level Landscape/Architectural Plan. Drawing by S. Verderber/Annette Himelick

are rebuilt, with redesigned parking, bike lanes, and pedestrian amenities. New street lighting and traffic control signals are installed. Work commences on the new Elysian Fields streetcar line. Following these steps the buildings to be retained can be stabilized and primed for reuse. Also at this time, construction is to begin on the two new health promotion anchor buildings: the Recreation/Multipurpose Center and the Community Wellness/Spa (Figures 5.31a–b, 5.32a–b, and 5.33a–b).

## Interval 2: Infrastructure/Urban Farming

The existing strip center structure at the main intersection of Elysian Fields Avenue and Gentilly Boulevard is adapted to a two-level parking deck, while the existing neighborhood bank is retained

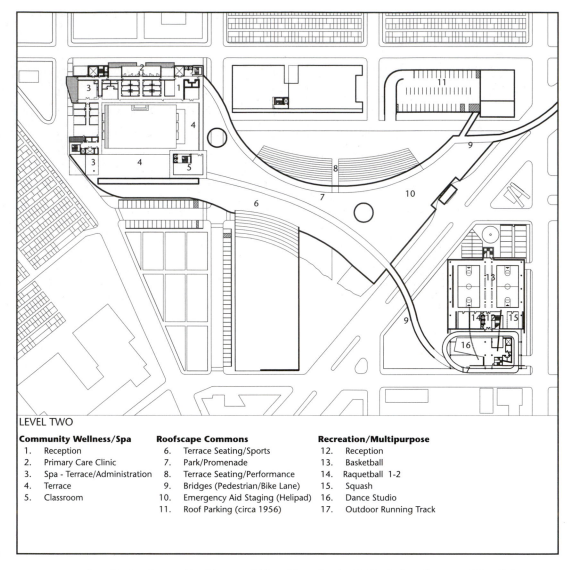

**FIGURE 5.28** Level 2 Landscape/Architectural Plan. Drawing by S. Verderber/Annette Himelick

and given further visual prominence with new signage (Figure 5.34b). The additional parking capacity in the remainder of the structure renders it feasible to demolish the existing large expanses of paving that previously dominated the front façades of the 1950s commercial strip center. The former stores on the first level become parking, and the existing roof parking deck is retained and structurally reinforced. A recharging station for electric vehicles is provided on the ground level of the parking deck within the former footprint of the reclaimed 1950s-era storefronts. A large warehouse is demolished, as are the adjoining expanses of asphalt parking lots. The 3-acre farm parcel is cleared on a triangular parcel across from the recreational/sports activity area. An irrigation system is installed and benches provided. To the north of the farm tract, construction commences for the stoa that functions as a supply storage center and a farmers' market on a seven-days-a-week basis

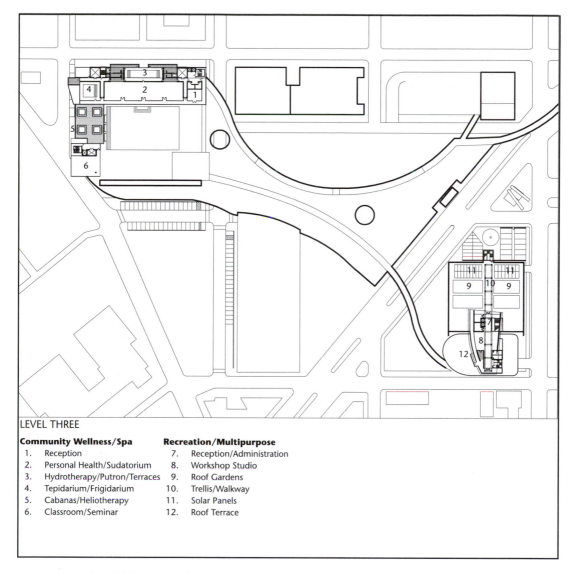

LEVEL THREE

**Community Wellness/Spa**
1. Reception
2. Personal Health/Sudatorium
3. Hydrotherapy/Putron/Terraces
4. Tepidarium/Frigidarium
5. Cabanas/Heliotherapy
6. Classroom/Seminar

**Recreation/Multipurpose**
7. Reception/Administration
8. Workshop Studio
9. Roof Gardens
10. Trellis/Walkway
11. Solar Panels
12. Roof Terrace

**FIGURE 5.29**  Level 3 Landscape/Architectural Plan. Drawing by S. Verderber/Annette Himelick

(Figure 5.31b). Landscaping is incorporated in this tract as a means to provide respite in the form of shaded pockets with benches that double as small storage bins for co-operative farming equipment and supplies.

## Interval 3: Team Sports Amphitheater

At present, the Gentilly section of New Orleans completely lacks a safe neighborhood park and related amenities for general recreational and sports activities. Residents for decades have been forced to leave Gentilly and travel to the lakefront linear park that parallels the Lake Pontchartrain levee, or to City Park, both of which are beyond easy walking distance (Figure 5.35a). The Brother Martin

**TABLE 5.1** Design Considerations 1–75

| | |
|---|---|
| Public Health in the Everyday Milieu (A1) | Heliotropic Tectonics (B12) |
| Competing Discourses (A2) | Historic Preservation (B13) |
| Sprawl and the Medically Underserved (A3) | Vertical Intervention (B14) |
| Food Deserts and Sprawl (A4) | McMansion Epidemic (B15) |
| Children, the Aged, and Sprawl (A5) | Ungate Communities (B16) |
| Reverse Infrastructural Decline (A6) | Fluid Facades (B17) |
| Landtrusting (A7) | Light Manufacturing Interwoven (B18) |
| Cyburbia (A8) | Electrocharging Stations (B19) |
| Smart Grids (A9) | Indigenous Public Health Traditions (B20) |
| Subterranean Utilities (A10) | Demise of the Megachain (C1) |
| TOADS and Sprawl (A11) | Small Box/Big Box Dialectics (C2) |
| LULUs and Sprawl (A12) | Deconstruction Strategies (C3) |
| Cell Tower Epidemic (A13) | Transparency (C4) |
| Greenfielding (A14) | Deconstruct Parking (C5) |
| Redfielding (A15) | Terracing (C6) |
| Water and Sprawl (A16) | Spacesharing (C7) |
| Water Typologies (A17) | Edge Sites as Coral Reefs (C8) |
| Transform Water Edges (A18) | Soft Surfaces (C9) |
| Recycle Stormwater (A19) | Fast Food Restaurants (C10) |
| Brownfields as Energy Farms (A20) | Sitesharing (C11) |
| Sidewalks and Sprawl (A21) | Landmarks and Anomalies (C12) |
| Pedestrians (A22) | Vertical Gardens (C13) |
| Street Furniture (A23) | Roofscaping (C14) |
| Bike Culture (A24) | Suburban Farmers' Markets (D1) |
| Social Media Parks (A25) | Microfarming (D2) |
| Light Rail/Intermodal Transit (A26) | Agrarian Stoa (D3) |
| Celebrate Public Health Achievements (A27) | Infill Agrarianism (D4) |
| Modernism and Public Health (B1) | Suburban Composting (D5) |
| Ruins and Selective Entropy (B2) | Cisterning (D6) |
| Reprise the Community Center (B3) | Horticultural Education (D7) |
| Nomadic Healthcare (B4) | Transfusion Zone Diagnostics (E1) |
| Modular Infill Buildings (B5) | LEED and Sprawl Mitigation (E2) |
| Civic Space at the Heart (B6) | Geomap Resourcing (E3) |
| Walkability (B7) | Stakeholder Engagement (E4) |
| Architectural Legibility (B8) | Gaming and Simulation (E5) |
| Bridging (B9) | Foster Innovation (E6) |
| Multigenerationality (B10) | Incremental Transfusion (E7) |
| Echo Housing (B11) | |

Catholic High School is located across the street on Elysian Fields, to the north of Gentilly Boulevard, yet access to this existing open space, including the school's baseball field, soccer field, and basketball courts, remains restricted from use by the general public. There are few basketball courts or places to have a picnic while watching children engage in a team sport, for instance. The sports amphitheater consists of a competition-level basketball court with adjacent terraced hillside seating, and four competition level tennis courts. These courts are flexibly configured to be converted to a soccer field vis-à-vis rollout artificial grass turf. A seating area parallels this space. The sports amenities are buffered by the terraced park, a retaining wall on one side and a row of trees on the side facing the urban farming collective. Lighting is installed to facilitate evening use. The 1950s-era commercial

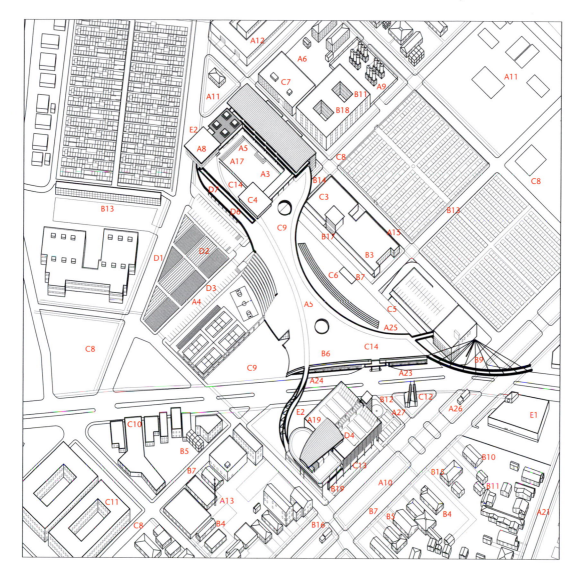

**FIGURE 5.30** Transfusion: Overview with Embedded Design Considerations 1–75. Drawing by S. Verderber/Annette Himelick

strip center structure on this site is demolished and the businesses are relocated to nearby retained buildings that currently have vacancies on adjacent parcels directly to the south of Gentilly Boulevard yet within the catalyst site.

## Interval 4: Reclaimed Residual Buildings

A second 1950s-era existing strip center structure is conserved and adapted to two new functions to serve the health promotional needs of the residents of the surrounding neighborhoods: a multi-purpose community center and a police substation (Figure 5.35b). The Community Center is available for social events, Mardi Gras functions, and activities associated with the adjacent outdoor amphitheater, including during periods of inclement weather. The large open spaces of the 1950s strip mall are ideally suited for these new functions. The police substation is modeled after the network of neighborhood-based *Koban* police substations that serve neighborhoods throughout the neighborhoods of Tokyo. Simultaneously, the catalyst site's urban infrastructural system is completed as is the urban farming collective, and the health promotion anchor buildings, and are opened for full use by the community. The farmers' market opens, directly across a driveway from the urban farm (Figure 5.31b). Also, at this time the site is cleared for the urban platform park and the park's platform base structure is constructed. This structure houses the commercial functions housed beneath the platform park, i.e. the organic fresh foods (super) market and a row of commercial storefront spaces facing Gentilly Boulevard at street grade.

### Interval 5: Landscape/Gentilly Commons

The platform base structure for the Gentilly Commons is constructed and the contoured, organically configured platform park is constructed on its roof (Figure 5.36a). This park includes the multipurpose outdoor amphitheater and stage as well as terraced seating across the grassy slope of the park, facing the stage. Entry portals connect to the street level, to the market, adjoining commercial spaces, and to restaurants below. The park's landscape features large circular light portals, allowing natural light to bathe spaces below. Winding paths transverse the green platform and its expansive lawns henceforth function as the main greenspace for the surrounding community. Landscaping is incorporated throughout, as are pockets for seating throughout the park. Its sloping contours and vistas provide topographic respite from the relentlessly flat surrounding landscape and simultaneously function as a new urban landmark for the entire city (Figure 5.31a). Direct connections are established between the platform park and surrounding new amenities as it is extended to the adjoining community health anchors—the Community Wellness/Spa and the construction of the large therapeutic pool and waterfall, all near the within its courtyard (Figure 5.32a), retained and adapted 1950s era strip center structure. At the opposing end of the park, its green space extends to the edge of Gentilly Boulevard, awaiting its connection to the Recreation/Multipurpose Center, across the street. The roof of the Multipurpose/Recreation Center features a community garden (Figure 5.33a).

### Interval 6: Path Connections

The final phase consists of completing the circulation infrastructure. This involves the construction of the two bridges that link the platform park with the surrounding neighborhoods to the east and north of the catalyst site (Figures 5.33b and 5.36b). One of the suspension bridges arcs as it crosses above the intersection of the two major vehicular arteries. This bridge connects with the far side of Elysian Fields Avenue. A second bridge arcs across Gentilly Boulevard, connecting The Commons and the Recreation/Multipurpose Center. Both bridges provide a two-way bike lane and two-way walking lane. Concurrently, ground-level biking and walking lanes are completed that now connect all surrounding blocks with the catalyst site. This system is then connected with the larger network of urban bike/walking paths in this part of the city. The newly re-established light rail streetcar line is also completed at this time and two transit stops serving the catalyst site are built in the median, i.e. neutral ground (Figure 5.32b). Lighting and related infrastructure amenities are completed. The Commons is well above the flood plain and in both pre-emergency and in post-emergency scenarios is designed to accommodate urban amphibious living in the form of temporary dwelling units, tent

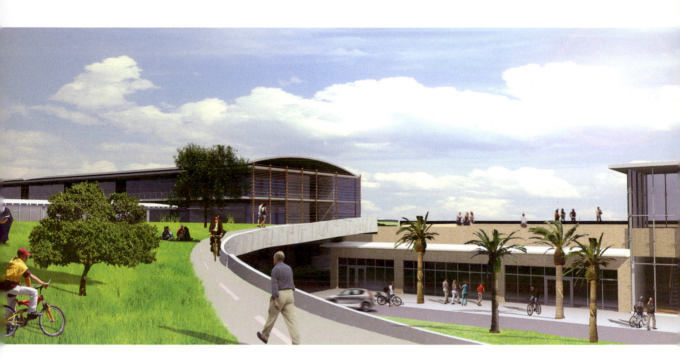

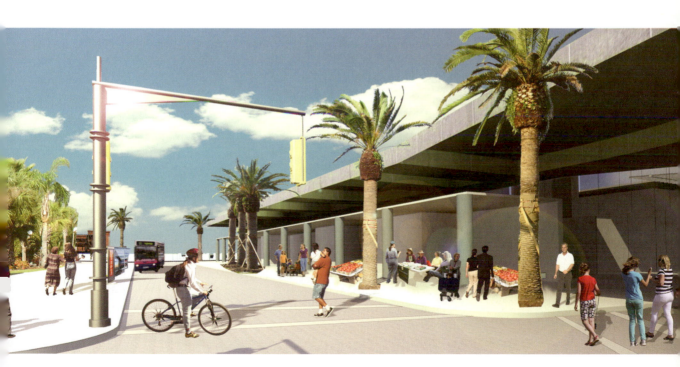

**FIGURE 5.31a–b** Gentilly Commons (Rooftop Park)—Fresh Food Market (below)/Urban Farm and Stoa. Illustrations by S. Verderber/Team 896

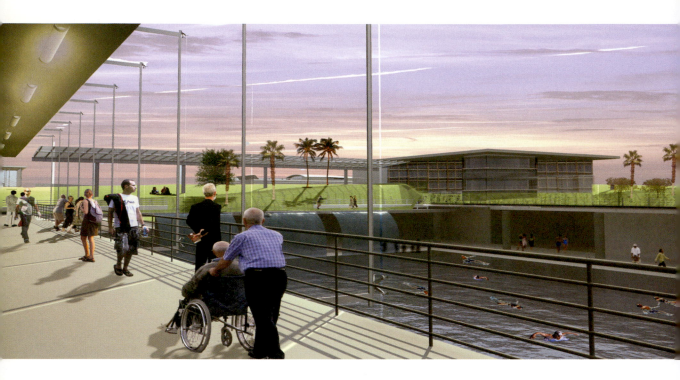

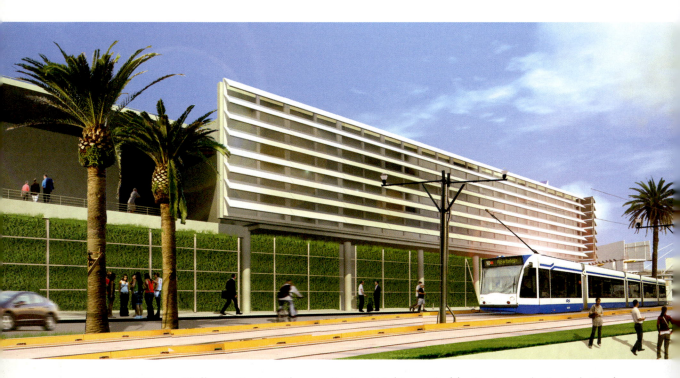

**FIGURE 5.32a–b** Wellness Center Therapeutic Spa/Multiuse Health Center and Vertical Garden. Illustrations by S. Verderber/Team 896

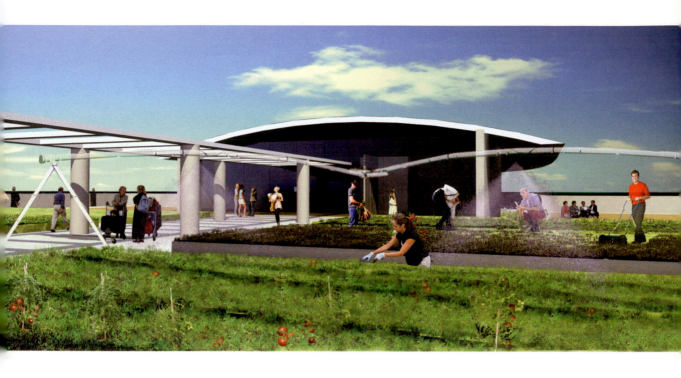

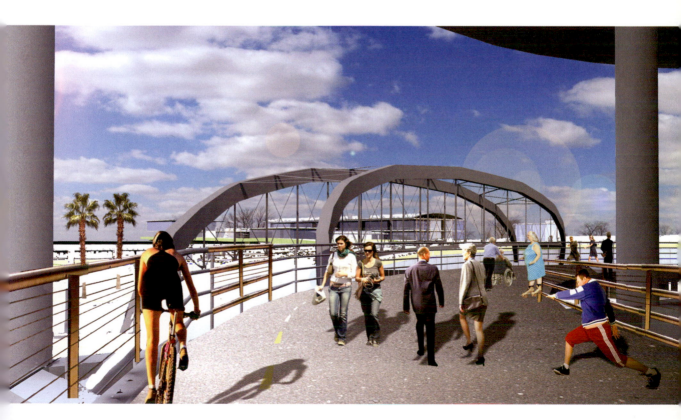

**FIGURE 5.33a–b** Rooftop Farming/Pedestrian and Cycling Paths. Illustrations by S. Verderber/Team 896

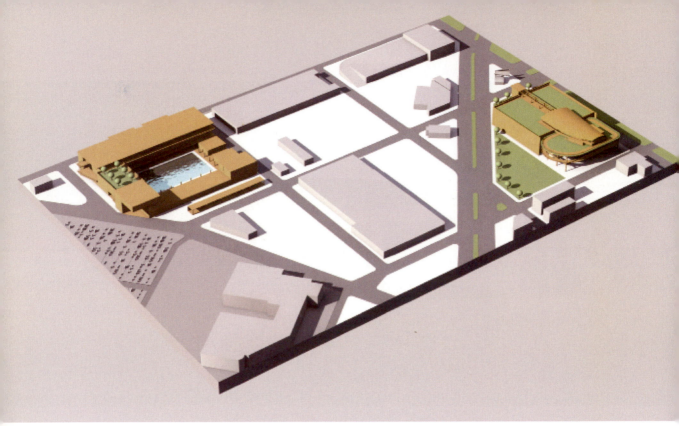

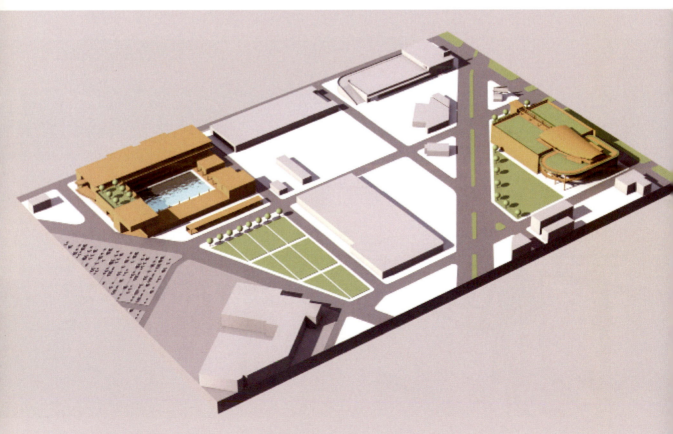

**FIGURE 5.34a–b**    Interval 1(I-1) and Interval 2 (I-2) Transfusion. Illustrations by S. Verderber/Team 896

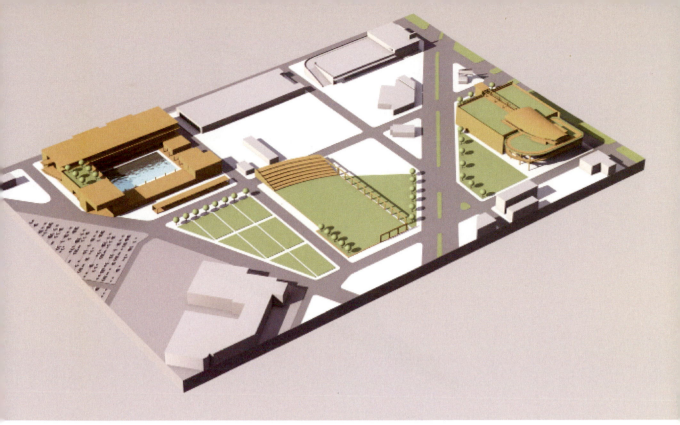

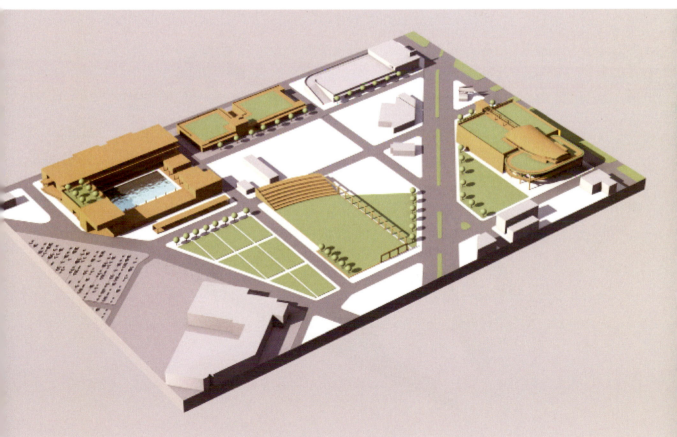

**FIGURE 5.35a–b** I–3 and I-4 Transfusion. Illustrations by S. Verderber/Team 896

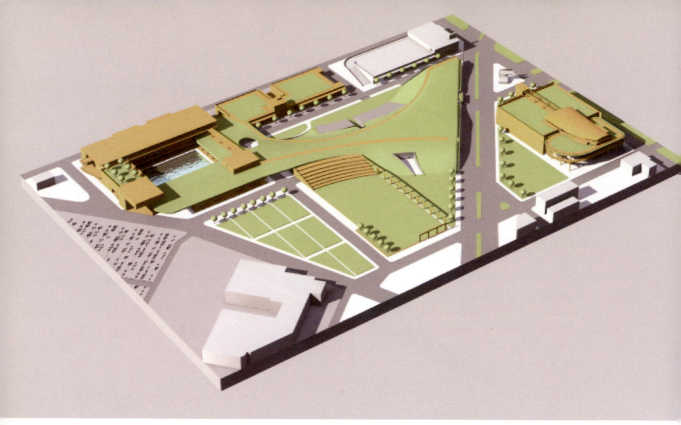

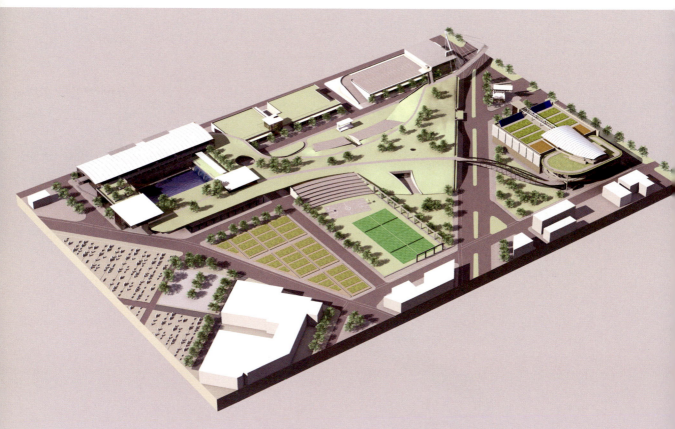

**FIGURE 5.36a–b** I–5 and I–6 Transfusion. Illustrations by S. Verderber/Team 896

clinics, and FEMA facilities as a means to provide healthcare in the aftermath of a future hurricane disaster event. Emergency backup power generator support is provided and this apparatus is housed on an elevated frame-grid directly below the landscaped park, and serves adjoining structures. The completed suburban transfusion is illustrated in Figure 5.36b.

## Transfusion, Public Health, and the Future of New Orleans

Historically, New Orleans has remained disconnected from the religiously and politically conservative American Bible Belt. It evolved its own unique live-and-let-live civic traditions since its founding in 1718. It is arguable that this unique cultural condition is the result of the city's geographic isolation as much as anything else—being surrounded by water on three sides.[63] This cultural autonomy and independence was even more pronounced during the pre-electricity, pre-interstate highway, pre-Internet eras.[64] Its citizens love to celebrate its cultural uniqueness in annual epic civic excursions such as Mardi Gras, in its culinary and musical vernacular forms that span a range of exquisite seafood dishes in the birthplace of jazz, and, more recently, through the invention of hip hop bounce music.[65] Architecturally, its most iconic styles and building typologies reflect the most prosperous periods of its long history, especially in the *sliver by the river* neighborhoods, built in the Greek Revival and Victorian styles. Much of this inventory remains intact throughout the more economically well-off neighborhoods. In stark contrast, across the less well-off neighborhoods of the city this inventory is currently under extreme risk of further disrepair and ruin, post-Katrina, including throughout the Gentilly section.[66] In a city with 64,000 vacant structures, there are simply too few preservationists or transfusionists locally to save and reinvent these historic buildings and ecological landscapes. Reinvestment is sorely needed because these buildings and landscapes are a vial part of the city's *tout ensemble*. Without substantial reinvestment, further abandonment, decay, and ruin are all but certain.[67]

Civic debates at the present time revolve around pre-hurricane citywide evacuation policies, forced relocations, resistance versus acceptance of the city's formidable geographical challenges, and political distortion of scientific facts. In the aftermath of Hurricane Katrina in 2005, when more than 1,800 persons perished and in New Orleans alone over 125,000 buildings were destroyed by floodwaters, Americans questioned the city's continued viability as a place to live. Katrina stands as the costliest disaster in United States history, having surpassed $5.5 billion in damage payouts and reconstruction (as of December 2010).[68] The lowest-lying neighborhoods below sea level—Lakeview, Gentilly, and the Lower Ninth Ward—experienced the most severe devastation from a one–two knockout punch of the combination of extreme flood and wind damage.[69] Gentilly has only had mixed success in its reconstruction to date. The Upper and Lower Ninth Ward was the poorest of these three neighborhoods and as a result has experienced the sparsest rebirth of any section of the city.[70] It is, in a way, an artificial existence, made possible solely by civil engineering feats.[71] Richard Campanella summarizes this chronic dilemma:

> Should we remain in eroding marshes and continue centuries of tradition, or end our way of life and move inland so that aggressive coastal restoration may commence? Should we maintain all low-lying, far-flung neighborhoods and trust that levees will protect us? Or should we concede these areas to nature and build only on higher ground? Should we try to save everyone, at the risk of losing everyone? Or should we ask some to sacrifice everything so that others may maintain something? Shall we strive toward the probable survival of half the society, or the possible survival of the entire society?[72]

Campanella cites the arguments of three competing camps—the abandonists, the concessionists, and the maintainers—over the future of the city, post-Katrina. The call for open resettlement basically everywhere within the flood footprint quickly became the clarion slogan of then-mayor C. Ray Nagin (Mayor for two terms, 2002–2010).[73] Nagin had previously speedily assembled the aforementioned Bring New Orleans Back (BNOB) initiative.[74] The ad hoc policy from City Hall was a call for all people to return as they wished to whatever neighborhoods they wished. The city has since been forced to react to the ad hoc patterns of resettlement as have occurred haphazardly ever since. This very loose resettlement "policy" has resulted in a highly uneven reconstruction of the city across its most severely damaged neighborhoods, including Gentilly, in a city whose population has contracted by more than 125,000 persons since 2005.[75] At the end of the day, it will be up to private citizens, and not the government, to shape a healthier, more active, prosperous future for their city.

## Notes

1  The most notable of these former paths is the Atchafalaya Basin, about 85 miles west of the current path of the Mississippi.
2  Campanella, Richard (2009) *Bienville's Dilemma: A Historical Geography of New Orleans*. Lafayette: Center for Louisiana Studies. Its port was the major reason for the city's expansion, as it was a nexus for the cotton, sugar cane, and myriad commodities imported and exported across the globe.
3  Duffy, John (1974) 'Nineteenth century public health in New York and New Orleans: A comparison,' *Louisiana History: The Journal of the Louisiana Historical Association*, 15(4): 325–337.
4  Ibid., p. 332.
5  McNabb, Donald and Madère, Jr., Louis E. "Lee", *A History of New Orleans*. Online. Available at http://www.madre.com/history.html (accessed 1 February 2011). Today, the city's Sewerage and Water Board maintains a set of six pumping stations, all of which were built nearly 100 years ago. Improvements have been made to these pumping stations but a single major rainstorm can easily overwhelm their collective capacity to pump rainwater out from the below sea level bowl into Lake Pontchartrain.
6  United State Army Corps of Engineers (1996) *A History of New Orleans Drainage*. Online. Available at http://www.usace.army.mil/pdf/history/abt_nodrainagechap3.pdf (accessed 30 January 2011). Also see Baudier, Roger (1954) *A Historical Sketch of the St. Louis Cathedral of New Orleans, Metropolitan Church Built in 1794: The First Ursuline Convent and the Mortuary Chapel*. New Orleans: A.A. Laborbe & Sons, pp. 14–18.
7  Ibid., pp. 12–14.
8  The first suburb was Faubourg Marigny, named for Bernard de Marigny, a wealthy Creole landowner aristocrat. This was following by Bywater, and later the Upper and Lower Ninth Wards. See Donze, Frank (2011) 'Streetcar service along Rampart, St. Claude is getting a green light,' *The Times-Picayune*, 25 January. Online. Available at http//:www.nola.com/business/index.ssf/2011/01/streetcar_service_along.html (accessed 29 January 2011).
9  Hardee, Thomas Sydenham (1878) *Topological and Drainage Map of New Orleans and Surroundings from Recent Surveys and Investigations*. Lithograph with Watercolor. Accession Number 00.34a. The Historic New Orleans Collection, 2000 (reprinted).
10  McNabb and Madère, Jr., *A History of New Orleans*, pp. 12–14.
11  Ibid., p. 15.
12  Ibid., pp. 16–17. Most slaves were not used for manual labor, but were instead mainly household servants. Ten years earlier (1850) slaves represented 16 percent of the total population but their numbers declined due to their high value as plantation workers outside the city. In 1860, in the New Orleans slave market, the center of the Mid-South slave trade, slaves sold for $2,000 apiece, skilled slaves for $2,500, and women sold for approximately $1,800 apiece (all in 1860 dollars).
13  Ibid., p. 18. The streets fanned out from the river in a pie-shaped circular configuration, with the various street grids "colliding" at their upper ends, or apexes. These large boundaries had drainage canals and later streets with wide neutral grounds (grassy medians) would be lined with stately residences by the families of prosperous merchants and professionals. Street patterns influenced racial geographies. Whites resided along

the major streets and boulevards that formed super blocks. African-American neighborhoods, until the 20th century, were small and geographically distinct from one another.

14  Lewis, Pierce (2003) *New Orleans: The Making of an Urban Landscape.* Charlottesville: University Press of Virginia, p. 15. Also see Colten, Craig (2004) *An Unnatural Metropolis: Wrestling New Orleans From Nature.* Baton Rouge: Louisiana State University Press.

15  LaWare, Margaret (1998) 'Encountering visions of Aztlan: Arguments for ethnic pride, community activism, and cultural revitalization in Chicano murals,' *Argumentation and Advocacy*, 34(3): 33–43.

16  In 1943 this establishment was then the Walter Patrolia Beer Parlor. The cost of signs such as this was often split 50/50 between the brewery and the proprietor. Its visibility at night was minimal compared to the enormous roof-mounted billboards in the CBD during this period. This mural had been covered for sixty-five years. A long tradition exists of mural painting in New Orleans. Commercial murals were commissioned in far more socially acceptable contexts, such as the large murals in the Sazrac Lounge at the Roosevelt Hotel (1937), in the CBD, the Pontchartrain Hotel on St. Charles Avenue (1938), and, more recently, the street scenes (1994) painted at the Mid-City Rock n' Bowl Lanes on Carrollton Avenue. Prominent publicly sponsored murals include the Lakefront Airport's main terminal (1939), the Amtrak Station (1954), and in the original 1952 terminal at Moissant Field (now Louis Armstrong International Airport), created in 1995. The city's commercial strips were once lined with wonderful drive-ins and various commercial establishments that featured aesthetically elaborate, and at times provocative, neon signs. These included the Half Moon bar's neon sign on Magazine Street (1934), the original Rock n' Bowl exterior neon sign (1946), the Kopper Kettle diner's neon sign (1952), and the Meal-a-Minit Diner (1949), both on Tulane Avenue near downtown. A large neon sign was perched on top of Lambert's Bakery (1947) on Elysian Fields Avenue in Gentilly. The Pat Gilliam Bowling Lanes on Airline Highway in Metairie featured a large boomerang neon sign (1954). This one had a serialized neon bowling ball "rolling" down the lane. The eponymously named "Flowers" shop on Claiborne Avenue uptown had an iconic neon sign in front (1951), as did the neon "sugar bowl" on the roof of the Sugar Bowl Motel (1946), on Airline Highway in Metairie. Every one of these neon signs is gone except for the Half Moon's iconic neon sign.

17  First there were Bayou St. John and the new Basin Canal, and the Industrial Canal was created prior to World War II. Additional drainage arteries included those at the London Avenue Canal and the 17th Street Canal. The portions of the canals that originated in the old city were eventually covered. This network included drainage canals beneath major thoroughfares, including Claiborne Avenue, Nashville Avenue, and Louisiana Avenue.

18  Pre-1940 railroad lines within the city included the lines along the river, serving the Port of New Orleans. The City of New Orleans train linked the downtown to points west and north, terminating in Chicago.

19  The interrelationship between open green spaces with tree planting yielded tree-shaded neutral grounds along the city's major arteries. This canopy is most mature in the older sections, with far less planting having occurred after 1945.

20  *New Century New Orleans Master Plan.*

21  Alexander Milne, a Scottish man who arrived in 1775, held much of the remaining land. Although he believed New Orleans would grow towards the north, to the lakefront, this would remain impossible until the Pontchartrain railroad was built in 1831. This railroad connected Lake Pontchartrain with Vieux Carré and ran along the present-day Elysian Fields Avenue. Milneburg closed in 1930 after a new seawall built there displaced the existing structures.

22  Its developers sought to create a "gentile" community—or community of gentiles—that upheld the so-called virtues of "pride of ownership, personal and family dignity, and civic purpose."

23  Gentilly Terrace Company (1909) *Gentilly Terrace—Where Homes Are Built on Hills.* Brochure produced by the Gentilly Terrace Company. New Orleans Special Collections, Howard-Tilton Memorial Library, Tulane University. Excerpts reproduced with permission.

24  Preservation Resource Center of New Orleans (2002) *Living with History in New Orleans' Neighborhoods: Gentilly Terrace.* New Orleans: Preservation Resource Center.

25  DPZ and the Congress for the New Urbanism. Community Planning Charrette for District Six (2006), Final Reprt, May 2006, p 4.

26  Ibid., pp. 26–27, 66.

27  I videotaped the proceedings, as I sensed it would be of historic value. Duany et al. proffered images of bucolic streetscapes rendered in pastels while most in the audience remained homeless and/or displaced from the city.

28  DPZ Gentilly Final Report, May 2006, p. 27. A green building and conservation plan was outlined, including bioswales, greenspace retention and recharge areas, and evaporative transpiration

techniques. Finally, the team called for special areas to be treated separately, with phased redevelopment, focusing on affordable housing, reconditioning of salvageable existing housing, with new infill development.

29  Jones, Anthony (2006) 'HUD approves $4.2B for Louisiana's "Road Home" program,' *USA Today*, 11 July. Online. Available at www.usatoday.com/news/nation/2006-07-11-hud_x.htm (accessed 14 January 2011). Also see Duany, Andres (2007) 'Restoring the real New Orleans,' *Metropolis* 18(2): 132.

30  Gentilly Terrace Company, *Gentilly Terrace*, p. 14.

31  Bazile, Karen Turni (2006) 'St. Bernard moves to adopt guidelines,' *The Times-Picayune*, 18 March, p. B-8.

32  Griswold, Kent (2008) 'Katrina cottages,' *Tiny House Blog*. Online. Available at http://tinyhouseblog.com/stick-built/katrina-cottages/html (accessed 12 January 2011).

33  Lukez, Paul (2007) *Suburban Transformations*. New York: Princeton Architectural Press.

34  Kunstler, James Howard (1996). *The Geography of Nowhere*. New York: Simon & Schuster.

35  Kelbaugh, Douglas (1997). *Common Place: Toward Neighborhood and Regional Design*. Seattle: University of Washington Press.

36  Rossi, Aldo (1982) *The Architecture of the City*. Cambridge, MA: MIT Press.

37  Lukez, *Suburban Transformations*, p. 12.

38  Ibid., p. 13.

39  Ibid., pp. 13–14.

40  Ibid., p. 15.

41  Lukez proceeds in subsequent chapters of his book to delineate a series of operative steps expressed within an iterative process. The elements of this equation consist, in part, of eradication (complete), eradication (partial), etching, excision, entropy, and excavation. These operations are used in his procedural model to gather, compile, map, and analyze information and to express its myriad formal and spatial permutations, where, in the broadest terms, Identity = Site + Time.

42  Mayor's Office, City of New Orleans (2006) *Bring New Orleans Back Commission, Final Report*, January. Also see Curtis, Wayne (2007) 'The savior of New Orleans?' *Architect Magazine*, 6 August. Online. Available at www.architectmagazine.com/educational-projects/the-savior-of-new-orleans.aspx.html (accessed 15 January 2011).

43  Venturi, Robert, Scott Brown, Denise, and Izenour, Steven (1972) *Learning from Las Vegas*. 1st Edition. Cambridge, MA: MIT Press.

44  Gandelsonas, Mario (1991) *The Urban Text*. Cambridge, MA: MIT Press.

45  Ibid., pp. 3–8.

46  Jervis, Rick (2010) 'Pipes, pumps trouble Big Easy,' *USA Today*, 16 December. Online. Available at www.usatoday.com/news/nation/2010-12-16-nosewer_N.htm (accessed 16 January 2011).

47  Verderber, Stephen (2010) 'Five years after: Three New Orleans neighborhoods,' *Journal of Architectural Education*, 64(2): 107–121.

48  Verderber, Stephen (2010) 'The *un*building of historic neighborhoods in post-Katrina New Orleans,' *Journal of Urban Design*, 14(3): 257–277.

49  DPZ Gentilly Report, May 2006, p. 49.

50  Roach, Joseph (1996) *Cities of the Dead*. New York: Columbia University Press.

51  Weiss, Mitch (2010) 'SBA's Katrina loans criticized for mismanagement, bias,' *Huffington Post*, 24 August. Online. Available at www.huffingtonpost.com/2010/08/24/sbas-katrina-loans-critic_n_692940.html (accessed 11 March 2011).

52  Quillen, Kimberly (2010) 'Idea Village launches business accelerator program', *The Times-Picayune*, 16 August. Online. Available at www.nola.com/business/index.ssf/2010/08/idea_village_launches_business.html (accessed 11 March 2011).

53  Liu, Amy (2010) *The State of New Orleans Five Years after Hurricane Katrina*. Washington, D.C.: The Brookings Institution. Also see Anglin, Roland, Liu, Amy, Mizelle Jr., Richard M., and Plyer, Allison (2011) *Resilience and Opportunity: Lessons from the U.S. Gulf Coast after Katrina and Rita*. Washington, D.C.: The Brookings Institution.

54  Verderber, Stephen (2009) *Delirious New Orleans: Manifesto for an Extraordinary American City*. Austin: University of Texas Press, ch 6.

55  Ibid., pp. 203–233.

56  Mowbray, Rebecca (2011) 'Food deserts targeted by $7 million federal grant,' *The Times Picayune*, 9 October. Online. Available at www.nola.com/business/index.ssf/2011/10/asi_federal_credit_union_to_st.html (accessed 10 October 2011). Also Barrow, Bill (2010) 'Governor Bobby Jindal, Mayor Mitch Landrieu announce continuance of New Orleans community clinic network,' *The Times-Picayune*,

22 September. Online. Available at www.nola.com/health/index.ssf/2010/09/gov_bobby_jindal_mayor_mitch_I.html (accessed 12 February 2011).

57  Verderber, Stephen (2005) *Compassion in Architecture: Evidence-Based Design for Health in Louisiana*. Lafayette: Center for Louisiana Studies.

58  Jones, Mark (2010) 'Proterra selects Greenville, SC. as location for R&D, assembly of hybrid vehicles', *Reliable Plant*, 26 August. Online. Available at www.reliableplant.com/read/22684/Proterra-Greenville-assembly-hybrid-vehicles.html (accessed 11 March 2011).

59  Hincha-Ownby, Melissa (2010) 'Predicting sales of alternative fuel vehicles', *Mother Nature Network*, 8 March. Online. Available at www.mnn.com/green-tech/transportation/stories/predicting-sales-of-alternative-fuel-vehicles.html (accessed 9 March 2011).

60  Vairani, Franco (2011) 'Bit Car: Concept of a stackable car', *MIT Media Lab*. Online. Available at www.web.mit.edu/francov/www/citycar/html (accessed 9 March 2011).

61  McNabb and Madère, *A History of New Orleans*, p. 56.

62  Verderber, *Compassion in Architecture*.

63  Lewis, *New Orleans*, pp. 44–47.

64  Baumbach, Jr., Richard O. and Borah, William E. (1980) *The Second Battle of New Orleans: A History of the Riverfront Expressway Controversy*. Tuscaloosa: University of Alabama Press.

65  Verderber, *Delirious New Orleans*, pp. 101–136.

66  Verderber, 'The *un*building of historic neighborhoods in post Katrina New Orleans', p. 273.

67  Verderber,, *Delirious New Orleans*, pp. 203–234.

68  Liu, *Five Years After*, p. 22.

69  Verderber, Stephen, 'Five years after: Three New Orleans neighborhoods', p. 112.

70  Other neighborhoods, particularly Broadmoor, also experienced significant flooding damage. It is situated at the bottom of the bowl that constitutes New Orleans's urban topography.

71  Campanella, Richard (2008). *Bienville's Dilemma: A Historical Geography of New Orleans*. Lafayette: Center for Louisiana Studies.

72  Ibid., p. 44.

73  In January 2006, Nagin had turned against the advice of national experts, most notably the prestigious Urban Land Institute (ULI). Acting as first responders, the ULI had conducted a study in the fall of 2005 led by a nationally prominent planning firm, Wallace Todd Harrison, which recommended shrinking the total urban footprint. This sparked an intense controversy.

74  This effort consisted of a series of blue-ribbon panels each charged with a facet of recovery: schools, businesses, neighborhoods, infrastructure, and so on.

75  Robertson, Campbell (2011) 'Smaller New Orleans after Katrina, census shows', *The New York Times*, 3 February. Online. Available at www.nytimes.com/2011/02/04census.html?_r=1&ref=hurricanekatrina (accessed 5 February 2011). Also see Gill, James (2011) 'Hurricane Katrina changes becoming permanent', *The Times-Picayune*, 9 February. Online. Available at www.nola.com/opinions/index.ssf/2011/02/hurricane_katrina_changes_beco.html (accessed 12 February 2011).

# 6

# THE FUTURE

A General Electric television commercial in the U.S. in 2011 began by showing hundreds of people walking across a picturesque rural landscape holding a giant Claus Oldenburg pop-art-like power cord high above their heads. They plugged this cord into a giant, mock-up wall socket sited in the middle of the rural landscape. Magically, the lights of a distant metropolis came to life. Interestingly, no intervening sprawl was included in the scene. Would including the sprawl machine between the country and the city center have had a contaminating effect on GE's marketing message? Of course. Where were all the fast food franchises, Wal-Marts, roadside motels, and assorted accruements? Corporations such as Wal-Mart are given carte blanche to erect their oppressive superstores on cheap land on open greenfield sites virtually everywhere. They then promptly run nearly every local merchant out of business and the local economy is severely dislocated in the process, all because an unsuspecting public craves ultra cheap products (including GE products) without realizing the devastating collateral costs. In James Howard Kunstler's words:

> The local merchants who were put out of business had been the (town's) caretakers. They often owned at least two buildings in town—their home and the building in which they did business—and they generally took good care of both. The physical decrepitude that is now the most visible characteristic of American towns is the direct result of extirpating that class of local people. . .they sat on the library boards, the school and hospital boards, the planning board. They ran the local charities. They were invested in the history of the place. . .and the prospects of the generations to come after. Every virtue that grew out of these local relations between person and place was traduced by the big-box national retail corporations, and the American public was absolutely complicit.[1]

More than 80 percent of everything ever manufactured in America was made in the years after World War II. The American manufacturing economy became far-flung and increasingly non-local. It is axiomatic that within diffuse, non-local economies, locally based economic activity suffers. The local employees of multinational corporations are too often treated less equitably and less compassionately than had they remained employed by a locally owned business. We live in a time of prosperity without theoretical limits. But we are fast becoming painfully aware that sprawl is utterly dependent on decreasing reserves of fossil fuel, natural gas, coal, and uranium. Because of this, stagnant, non-growth economies may become a permanent fixture of everyday life and this goes hand in hand with steeply rising oil prices, the exhaustion of fresh water reserves, and the slow death of the world's oceans.[2] The net effect? Society is held in check.[3] Prior to all this, few had bothered to quantitatively measure the deleterious effects of a community's *sprawlness* to any serious extent. But it is not too late. For example, the systematic empirical study of pedestrian flow and typologies, *pedestrianism*, is rapidly evolving and applies metrics in the study of the efficacy of public rights of ways, how they are regulated, and associated user attributes and preferences.[4]

As for land use, a new wave of *urban sharecropping* has arisen in the past decade. In Brooklyn, BK Farmyards secured its first farm acreage in 2009 after Stacey Murphy, a former architect, stood on a street corner shouting aloud that she wanted to farm someone's/anyone's yard in the neighborhood. Adrienne Fisher, a foundation grant manager and mother of three with a three-story Victorian house and a large backyard, heard her plea and took her up on her offer to share the initial costs of planting a large vegetable garden. The first harvest was divided among six neighbors, with each having invested in partial ownership. Urban sharecroppers are now selling their produce and poultry to local restaurants, and with notable success.[5] Urban sharecropping has garnered attention recently in the media, in academia, and in community activism circles. It is a strategy to help protect open land in economically distressed neighborhoods against excessive gentrification.

A *land trust* is another neighborhood grassroots vehicle/tool that has proven to be effective in the long-term preservation of open space (see Chapter 4). A land trust removes land from contradictory market-driven pressures and archaic local zoning laws, and can function as a buffer against profit-driven real estate pressures.[6] The California Infill Builders Association is a professional group that endeavors to promote smart growth.[7] In Detroit, the Community Development Advocates of Detroit (CDAD) have defined eleven new neighborhood types to guide the city's future redevelopment. These include urban homestead shelters, naturescapes, green venture zones, spacious residential transition zones, village hubs, city hubs, and green thoroughfares.[8]

Collective change begins with each individual taking responsibility for his or her actions at the local level. Similarly, an individual takes responsibility—ownership—for maintaining and improving one's own personal health at that point in time when the private automobile becomes a high luxury and when more people will have to walk and bike out of necessity (and not choice). It may no longer be a matter of walking and biking only for recreational exercise, or as some casual, elective activity to ensure that we remain physically fit.[9] It is noteworthy that global bicycle production, averaging 94 million units per year from 1990 to 2002, climbed upwards to 130 million units produced by 2007, far outstripping automobile production in that same year (70 million units). In 2009, the Italian national government incentivized individual citizens' purchase of bicycles and electric bikes as a means to improve urban air quality and to lessen the volume of auto traffic on the country's congested streets and highways. These direct payments now cover up to 30 percent of the purchase cost of a bicycle.[10] Against this backdrop of community-based change, here are some suggestions for coping with sprawl mitigation from a public health perspective:

## Be Engaged

It is useless to stand passively on the sidelines. Work with others to save places of cultural meaning and importance in your local community. Hold onto historic buildings and landscapes in suburbia. Mix caution with optimism in the forging of new networks of collaborators at the grassroots level. Further the aims of suburban transfusion with others who are willing to fight the fight. Align with public health activists, i.e. epidemiologists, physicians, and community health advocates, social scientists, and demographers, and other advocates for the improvement of public health. It is they who are currently on the front lines but they often have no skills in coping with experienced, entrenched, recalcitrant developers and other pro-sprawl special interests. These pro-sprawl special interests often do not seek out nor want change. Sprawl serves their aims quite nicely—and keeps everyone driving everywhere for everything. Do not silently surrender, as was the case in the 1950s with regards to well-heeled automobile manufacturers and their lobbyists, who bullied their way into ridding American cities of virtually all light rail public transport infrastructure.

### Do Not Trust Those in Charge to Do the Right Thing

It is naïve to expect self-interested politicians and corporations to think and act in the public's best interest when it comes to sprawl. Do not look to your elected officials to lead the way. The record shows that, in general, they will act to mitigate the deleterious consequences of sprawl when there is absolutely no other option. They are controlled by local power brokers—special interests—those in control of the local "economic development" apparatus. The status quo often prevails. Auto dependency prevails. Megachains such as Wal-Mart, shopping mall owners, fast food empires, and the mega-oil companies are the major winners. Wall Street, for its part, loves sprawl. Sprawl machines are the products of Wall Street's shareholder-first ideology—expand, expand, expand. Growth for it own sake mantras, place, too often, suburban commercial vernacular and housing typologies at great risk because they become subject to demolition at precisely that point in time they are on the threshold of having acquired historic landmark stature. Often, these buildings and places are lost just when they are needed most.

### Be Wary of the Parachuting Outside Expert

As shown in the previous chapter, it can be naïve to rely on outside experts who travel from afar to assist because they risk dismissal by the locals who live and work there. These outside expert teams, for their part, remain cool and do not get flustered when the locals start to question their parachuting-in credentials. Their smug approach is typically "Now things will be done right." The "outside expert syndrome" was in full throttle in the aftermath of Hurricane Katrina (see Chapter 5). It is far more prudent to construct a team with a blend of local and outside "expert" professionals, together with representatives of local grassroots neighborhood organizations. Try to not get caught in the middle of intractible, ideological turf wars either, such as that currently waging between the New Urbanism and landscape urbanism camps (see Chapter 2).

### Overcome Barriers of Race, Class, and Unhealthy Lifestyles

Progressive communities naturally take pride in their racial and ethnic diversity. They take pride in their openness to a broad spectrum of ideological viewpoints and opinions. These values are often deeply embedded and manifest in their constructed built environment. The recent controversy against the construction of a mosque near Ground Zero in New York City personified the opposite end of this spectrum. Intolerance prevails only where allowed to do so. Divergent opinions in time become suppressed to the extent of being literally banned by the majority viewpoint. This occurred repeatedly throughout the 20th century and continues to be worrisome in light of global population growth and racial diversity, environmental degradation, and rapidly disappearing natural resources. In the United States, the 2010 census painted a portrait of a nation significantly more diverse than only ten years prior although

55 percent of Americans continue to not possess a "reasonable understanding" of Islam.[11] Misinformation campaigns waged by unscrupulous special interests seek to obfuscate, skew, and otherwise distort the truth every step of the way.

## Avoid Paralysis through Over-analysis

There comes a point where analysis and over-analysis ad infinitum become an excuse to not do anything at all. The process itself becomes paralyzed when this happens. Obfuscation and over-analysis can be used either to achieve a positive outcome or as a means to promote a surreptitious agenda. People looking for the "perfect" solution probably should not become involved in endeavors requiring a decisive action, be it in sports, the arts, business, urban redevelopment, construction, or even politics: "perfect" solutions are elusive, few and far between. Indecision and gridlock serve no one in the end—where nothing happens at all except the continued decline of the suburban built environment, further exacerbating unhealthful, sedentary lifestyles in suburbia such as increased chronic disease and high obesity rates. In addition, infighting within organizations and with opposing factions can be debilitating. Indecision gridlock is most unfortunate and ironic when it occurs within professional teams attempting to "do the right thing." The result is long delays and missed opportunities to transform, for instance, a dead mall into an entropic nature preserve. The more controversial the initiative, the more susceptible it will be to unfortunate, counterproductive delays including NIMBY-ism on the part of pro-sprawl special interests.

## Treat Sprawl Mitigation like a Marathon

Reinventing suburbia is not unlike a military campaign. Both require strategic planning, tactical skill in outmaneuvering the opponents, conscientious planning, and the determination, resources, and capacity to follow through with precise plans of action. Both require overcoming difficult, well-funded political headwinds, pockets of pro-sprawl local opposition, and misinformation campaigns. The most costly aspect is the phased reconstruction of physical infrastructural systems, a process that can take years: creating smart grids, building public transit networks, constructing electrocharging stations, pedestrian and cycling networks, landmarks preservation and adaptive use, and new infill construction. Generic "how to" and "sprawl repair" directives run the real risk of being too narrow and prescriptive.[12] For the foreseeable future, banking institutions will remain conservative in their lending practices. Before, the money flowed. Lending institutions, private philanthropists, foundations, local private citizens, and local elected officials need to be much better educated on how to define and start transfusion projects although there is more than one way to achieve the desired outcome of healthier communities.[13] A full court press is on in many suburban locales to singularly adopt CNU form-based *Smart Codes* but there are other means of achieving the desired end result that may be equally or more effective.[14]

## Sprawl Transfusion—Going Forward

Architecture as a profession should not be looking in its rear-view mirror. There is not time for that. Disciplinary boundaries are blurring with landscape design/planning firms increasingly functioning as the project coordinator and with architects serving as team members in a somewhat less dominant role. As discussed in previous chapters, landscape architecture is experiencing a renaissance with its recent fusion of infrastructural design with ecological imperatives. One outcome of this is the architect of the future may no longer always be the universal go-to orchestrator, or, in Gwen Webber's words, the "king of the mountain."[15] As discussed in Chapter 2, the era of architecture-as-monument-building is coming to a close. Regardless, no building can lobby to save itself from destruction. It requires humans motivated to speak up. It takes people working together to save significant places and buildings—the shopping malls, supermarkets, gas stations, and fast food outlets located out on the post-World War II suburban highway strip. Strong examples of these everyday building typologies of the mid-to-late 20th century will increasingly be threatened because they are viewed as either too ugly or as not old enough to quality for historic landmark protections. The classic Tastee Freeze drive-in out on the old pre-Interstate two-lane road into town lives on in a nebulous in-between vortex. This maddening dilemma often results in the premature destruction of iconic modernist churches, libraries, schools, housing, and industrial-age architecture that could have been meaningfully reborn as part of a transfused suburbia. Leadership is urgently needed from within the professional design community. The preservation of mid-20th-century historic buildings and places in the everyday suburban milieu is the central focus of the International Committee for the Documentation and Conservation of Buildings, Sites, and Neighborhoods of the Modern Movement (DOCOMOMO).[16]

It is one thing to fight to save a historic mid-20th century building, but can a parking lot be considered historic? Beloved cities and neighborhoods share one thing in common the world over: the distinct absence of massive parking lots. Perhaps it is time that minimum parking requirements in suburbia died their long-overdue death. According to Tom Vanderbilt, writing in *Cities*:

> What makes the whole thing so weird is that there is no obvious powerful lobby to agitate for the perpetuation of these requirements. Developers would love to be able to determine for themselves how much parking was optimal, and it's not like Big Parking Lot has a massive [lobbying] presence in Washington; even the automakers don't really have much of a dog in this fight. So why *are* these regulations so very persistent?[17]

The main problem with endless free parking in suburbia is that it comes with a high environmental and public health price tag in the form of environmental degradation and the high healthcare costs tied to the obesity epidemic and related non-communicable diseases.[18] Meanwhile, the hallowed search for happiness in suburbia has become a frenzied and hectic regimen, having de-evolved into a zombie-like mania to have the latest Apple product, eat of the newest restaurant in the mall's food court, or have the latest pair of jeans from Gap. Mania is defined as a "dysphonic state of activity and mood." Sprawl spawns consumer zombies who mindlessly crave more and more without knowing why they really want it in the first place. In this relentless pursuit, the utopian promise of life in suburbia deteriorates into a dystrophic grind. It is a living fiction. In recent decades, economic output per person in the United States has risen sharply, but there has been no corresponding increase in overall levels of life satisfaction; peoples' distrust and depression have increased substantially during this same period as America became a suburban nation, in an era of endless free parking.[19]

A community is a collection of people who share a common purpose. If so, then people become isolated from one another in suburbia's horizontalism undermining any possible genuine sense of community.[20] Meanwhile, social scientists' and market researchers' measurements of personal happiness are often equated with economic productivity in what might be termed the more-is-always-better syndrome. The standard measurement of economic output in the U.S., the Gross Domestic Product (GDP), has been under attack recently as being badly flawed as a metric to portray the nation's collective economic well being. There are many shortcomings in the metrics currently used to compute GDP in the U.S. Alternative metrics, such as the Human Development Index, take a more inclusive approach to measuring economic well being.[21] Unfortunately, the GDP brand of economic wealth produced by sprawl machines has not as of yet translated into improved public health.

Capitalism feeds on zombie-like mass consumerism. This syndrome persists and it is associated with both environmental decline and the decline of personal health. Private consumption expenditures in the U.S. represent about 70 percent of the country's total GDP, with most of it in consumer spending.[22] It is the business of big business to keep households believing in carrying on as good consumers by creating zombie-like desires for an endless stream of material possessions. Since 1970, the size of a new American home has increased by more than 70 percent, municipal solid wastes generated per capita have increased by 33 percent, and 80 percent of all new homes built have been built in suburbia. But even all these ever-larger homes could not warehouse all of our material possessions, and in America the self-storage industry has boomed as a result.[23]

What about better education on the merits of green consumerism as this contributes to healthier personal lifestyles? How can we reduce our carbon footprint? Being *green* denotes a predilection to recycle. As for the built environment, buildings currently consume more than 40 percent of all non-renewable energy on the planet. A single building consumes a tremendous amount of energy. Yet it remains interesting that in the U.S., of 20,000 LEED-registered projects as of mid-2011, no study has yet empirically proven that a single LEED-certified building has actually resulted in encouraging its inhabitants to engage in significantly more walking and biking, for instance (see Chapter 4). Further, no study has yet definitively proven that LEED-certified buildings actually significantly reduce energy consumption.[24]

As for the role of consumer product manufacturers, up to very recently they have had no real incentive to engage in more sustainable business practices than before.[25] There is some evidence, however, that zombie consumers who live within sprawl machines might be willing to switch to a hybrid or an all-electric car, and consume less water, gas, and drive less. But sadly, a large percentage of U.S. consumers still do not regularly purchase green products and they do not yet wish to trade off the status quo of comfort, convenience, or their low everyday Wal-Mart prices.[26] And this remains beautiful music to the ears of those who control sprawl machines. The "rebound" effect also comes into play here, whereby the consumer conserves in one area yet increases consumption in another. Another concern is the growing number of opportunistic companies who deceptively seek to exploit the trendiness of being green in order to make money although their products are not "greener" in any real sense.[27]

Sprawl machines are only about the perpetuation of mass consumer consumption (see Appendix). The homebuilding industry created America's aforementioned zombie-like craving for McMansions. The local Best Buy outlet wants us to buy a larger and more expensive TV. Our possessions, whether a house or any other consumer object, becomes one cog in an illusive craving for more and more. This constant craving for more and more was at the root of the U.S. housing bubble that burst in 2008.[28] Mass consumer culture's insatiable need for more and more has been termed *Affluenza*: it is like an embedded chip in the memory of every sprawl machine, not all that unlike the uranium embedded in the core of a nuclear reactor. It is what makes the machine work. *Affluenza* is like an insatiable thirst.[29] Zombie mass consumerism within sprawl machines channels our:

> [d]esires, our insecurities, our need to demonstrate our worth and our success, our wanting to fit in and to stand out increasingly through material things—into bigger homes, fancier cars, grander appliances, exotic vacations. But in the background. . .we know we're slighting the precious things. . .that truly make life worthwhile. . .if we don't wake up we will soon lose the chance to return to reclaim ourselves, our neglected society, our battered world, because if we are not more careful [there will be] nothing left to return to. . .many people are now trying to fight

back. . .marketers tell us [to] create social [and built] environments where over-commercialization is viewed as silly, wasteful, ostentatious. Create commercial-free zones. Buy local. . .simplify your life. Shed possessions. Downshift. Build consumer-owned cooperatives.[30]

Of the 100 largest economies in the world, fifty-three are actually corporations. Exxon Corporation alone is bigger than 180 nations on the planet.[31] Much recent criticism has been leveled at these large multinationals and at the globalization movement they represent. Its countermovement—*antiglobalization*—seeks to combat what more and more people see as destructive global economic policies and dangerous geopolitical trends. To its critics, is appears unlikely that globalism will ever be more than always seeking cheaper ways to make more money, and new ways to exploit low wage workers in the process.[32] Are its forces willing to throw the world into an environmental upheaval, threatening its very survival? If so, the result would be a hapless world of rampant inequality, the erosion of trust and caring, diminished personal and societal public health, and failed planetary life support systems. It would be a world of centrally planned corporate-controlled economies, having replaced individualism, cultural diversity, and the virtues of placemaking. In its place, vacuous strategic self-interests, global greed unleashed, and hyper-materialism.[33]

The implications for public health and personal well being would be profound.

Uncontrolled sprawl is a lot like an offshore oil and gas–drilling zone. Both are constructed painstakingly (and carelessly, witness the BP Deepwater Disaster in 2010) over time, usually over many years. Both are then exhaustively used and consumed by vested corporate interests in the name of maximizing profit. These interests methodically use up all the available resources and then abandon them. In both examples, what once were pristine resources held in the public domain—ocean, wetland, and land—become no more than used-up remnants of abuse, and exploitation. Do we wish to allow ourselves to be tricked by manipulative corporations who seek to maximize profit at any environmental, architectural or public health cost? The challenges of global climate change alone are vexing enough.[34] In light of this, the deconstruction of sprawl machines will become necessary in many places as a means to redirect increasingly scarce natural and human resources in critically vital new directions. Many experts on the subject of the future of capitalist societies see globalism headed for disaster anyway due to four prevailing intersecting crises: the crisis of overproduction combined with excess capacity, the crisis of global social polarization and mistrust, the crisis of the unraveling of centralized political authority, and the crisis of environmentally unsustainable policies and practices. Underlying structural breakdowns will be compounded by the basic inability of any given government to maintain global law and order.[35] This is precisely why the future of the euro is in such peril at this time: no given government in the EU is in charge of this central currency's future. In the face of such developments it will be necessary to reaffirm the legitimacy and supremacy of eco-humanist values.

There is no quick fix to solving these unsettling trends, and certainly not in the form of a state-controlled capitalism such as how China is attempting to grow its economy within the parameters of a "softer" Communism. The simultaneous strengthening of global human capital, global public health, and global environmental well being will require, as Kunstler argues, a recovery of the time-tested attributes of successful pre-modern societies. Such societies valued equally the unity of work and life, society and community, the individual and the collective enterprise, culture and politics, and economy and morality.[36] And, as discussed in previous chapters, this will likely require new forms of land ownership and regulatory control. Municipal, state, and national public land trusts, as discussed in Chapter 4, will be needed to operate for the highest common good. Peter Barnes has explored this line of reasoning in depth in his book *Capitalism 3.0*.[37] Individuals and communities whose health is at increasing risk will demand new solutions. They will demand suburban transfusion. The political and economic system that spawned sprawl for over half a century will be deconstructed and rebuilt. But it may be impossible to achieve one or the other alone without rebuilding both.

The main reason why this degree of radical change may be inevitable is because hypercapitalism no longer enhances everyday life for the people who live and work amid sprawl. People are increasingly dissatisfied and looking for more meaningful alternatives. This will only grow in intensity and therefore force massive change. Antiglobalism will likely become more pronounced and therefore also play a role in this coming transformative period. Weakened democracies and their failed environmental and capitalist economic polices will be transformed out of sheer necessity. The prevailing winds are shifting. Innovation, it is hoped, will guide this process along an upward trajectory.[38] In affluent societies a breaking point has already been reached where prosperity, as defined by materialism, has reached its logical limits. In the most affluent societies, people and communities unsatisfied with their endangered health status will no longer be interested in or able to trade off—in effect sell—their health for material gain per se. Against this backdrop, in a field such as urban planning, so obsessed with generating quantifiable data, why has there been so little leadership forthcoming? And what about all the sprawl makers who have taken the money and run? This list is getting longer by the day and includes Michael Mastro, a prominent developer who fled the U.S. in 2011 after having been forced into bankruptcy in New York City.[39]

New paradigms are needed. Otherwise, future generations will be shocked and dumbfounded by our having remained so brazenly indifferent to the gravity of our multidimensional dilemma. Where the right to plunder nature was once unquestioned, societies in the future will be forced to revere and respect planet earth. The consequences of inaction will be untenable. The path towards an ecologically sustainable and salutogenetic planet will be interwoven into our everyday life. Can we continue to have developing nations such as China, India, and Indonesia pollute at exceedingly high rates and for this to be justified simply because they should be allowed to do so because the developed nations exercised their own sovereign right to plunder the earth in decades past?[40] It is equally indefensible to deny the facts associated with global climate change.[41] Meanwhile, for coastal communities such as New Orleans and Venice as much as for remote island-nations in the South Pacific, time is running out.[42]

Eco-humanism calls for a transformational worldview to facilitate the transition from today to tomorrow. In James G. Speth's words this will require:

> Changing from seeing humanity as something apart from nature, transcending and dominating it, to seeing ourselves as part of nature. . .and wholly dependent on its vitality. . .from seeing nature in strictly utilitarian terms. . .[and as] humanity's resource to exploit as it sees fit. . .to seeing the natural world as having value independent of people and rights. . .[thereby] creating the duty of ecological stewardship. . .from discounting the future, focusing severely on the near term, to empowering future generations economically, politically, and environmentally and recognizing duties to yet unborn human and natural communities well into the future. . .from hyperindividualism, narcissism, and social isolation to powerful community bonds reaching from the local to the cosmopolitan and to profound appreciation of interdependence both within and among countries. . .from parochialism, sexism, prejudice, and ethnocentrism to tolerance, cultural diversity, and human rights. . .from materialism, consumerism, getting, the primacy of possessions. . .from gross economic, social, and political inequality to equity, social justice, and human solidarity.[43]

Genuine grassroots civic activism equates with genuine social capital.[44] Global change starts at the local level. In the case of sprawl mitigation and its relationship to global public health, neither true democracy nor environmental stewardship is possible when citizens anywhere are forced to compete with one another with no allegiances beyond their own narrow self-interests. *Salutogenetic* models of public health need further development in this regard to devote far more emphasis and fiscal resources to health promotion versus conventional hospital-based disease-treatment policies and practices. Unfortunately, the surest path at present to paradigmatic change is through having to react suddenly to cataclysmic events that shake and rattle us, reshaping how we see things and in so doing, delegitimizing the status quo. Many have made this point. In recent years, 9/11, Hurricane Katrina, the earthquakes in Haiti and Japan, and the recent global economic meltdown all possessed this transformative power. Each event can spark profound positive change. And when such change does finally happen it usually occurs in spite of—not because of—inspired leadership demonstrated on the part of elected politicians.

There is mounting evidence that people are ready for something better than the status quo. A growing number of political scientists believe that otherwise, an irrevocable rise of political inequality will occur. It will so greatly impair our existing democratic institutions as to render the ideals of democracy and social equality to be largely irrelevant.[45] By extension, a diminished standard of daily living, the endangerment of public health, and an overall decline in the quality of everyday life are unacceptable alternatives. Disenchantment with the status quo must overcome our collective insecurities, fears, attitudes, and routine patterns of behavior. Will we have the courage to create healthful, health-promoting architecture, public places, and communities for persons of all ages, income levels, and backgrounds? Will we have the courage to realize the promise of sprawl mitigation and improved public health through suburban transfusion?

## Notes

1  Kunstler, James Howard (2005) *The Long Emergency*. New York: Grove Press, p. 189.
2  Ibid., p. 192.
3  Ibid., p. 260.
4  Blomley, Nicholas (2010) *Rights of Passage: Sidewalks and the Regulation of Public Flow*. London: Routledge.
5  McLaughlin, Katy (2010) 'The rise of the lazy locavore,' *The Wall Street Journal*, 13–14 November, p. C1.
6  Kotkin, Joel (2010) 'The rise of the efficient city,' *The Wall Street Journal*, 26 November, p. A10.
7  Stephen, John (2011) 'New professional group promotes infill development,' *California Planning and Development Report*, 16 February.
8  Berg, Nate (2010) 'The 11 types of Detroit neighborhoods,' *The New Urban Network*. Online. Available at www.newurbannetwork.com/article/11-types-detroit-neighborhoods-13422.html (accessed 12 December 2010).
9  Kunstler, *The Long Emergency*, p. 265.
10  Brown, Lester R. (2010) 'The return of the bicycle,' *IPS News*. Online. Available at www.ipsnews.net/interna.asp?idnews=52066.html (accessed 7 July 2010).
11  Ghosh, Bobby (2010) 'Islamophobia: Does America have a Muslim problem?' *Time*. 19 August. Online. Available at www.time.com/time/nation/article/0,8599,2011798-2,00.html (accessed 11 May 2011).
12  Tachieva, Galina (2010) *Sprawl Repair Manual*. Washington, D.C.: Island Press, p. 87. For example, in the section on community-level repairs, four key procedural steps are outlined: comprehensive thoroughfare standards for roadway realignments attuned to "context-sensitive design," a single-point main street business management vehicle, marketing protocols that show various options and their cause-effects, and the adoption of LEED-Neighborhood Development criteria. Under "Step Four, Secure Incentives for Implementation," specific recommendations consist of the following: permitting by right, state and federal funding for design and construction of parking structures and transit infrastructure, the transfer of development rights (TDR), Tax Increment Financing (TIF) districts, the establishment of a Business Improvement

District (BID) or a Business Improvement Area (BIA), state and federal grants such as Community Development Block Grants (CDBG), and Energy Efficiency and Conservation Block Grants (EECBG). Additional steps outlined for the implementation of sprawl repairs at the community level consist of sprawl repair tax credits, special purpose sales taxes, state tax credits for workforce housing, bonuses to developers for the creation of civic/pubic spaces, and federal grants earmarked for regional planning.

13 Laetz, Emily (2010) 'A return to physical planning,' *Planetizen.com*. 25 October. Online. Available at www. planetizen.com.html (accessed 10 November 2010).

14 Tachieva, Galina (2010) 'Sprawl repair: What it is and why we need it,' *Planetizen.com*. 18 October. Online. Available at www.planetizen.com.html (accessed 10 November 2010).

15 Webber, Gwen (2011) 'Contested ground,' *The Architect's Newsletter*, August, p. 42.

16 The web site of this not-for-profit organization based in Barcelona, Spain, is www.docomomo.com/html. Also see Verderber, Stephen (2009) *Delirious New Orleans: Manifesto for an Extraordinary American City*. Austin: University of Texas Press.

17 Vanderbilt, Thomas (2010) 'Why do minimum parking requirements still exist?' *Cities*. 24 June. Online. Available at www.blogs.reuters.com/felix-salmon/2010/06/24/why-do-minimum-parking-requirements-still-exist/html (accessed 8 August 2010). Also see Owen, David (2010) *Green Metropolis: Why Living Smaller, Living Closer, and Driving Less are the Keys to Sustainability*. New York: Riverhead Books.

18 Motavalli, James (2010) 'The high cost of free parking,' *emagazine.com*. Online. Available at www. emagazine.com/view/?2418.html (accessed 10 August 2010).

19 McKibben, Bill (2007) 'Reversal of fortune,' *Mother Jones*, March–April, pp. 39–40.

20 Myers, David G. (2004) 'What is the good life?' *Yes! A Journal of Positive Futures*, p. 15. Also see Myers, David G. (2000) *The American Paradox: Spiritual Hunger in an Age of Plenty*. New Haven and London: Yale University Press.

21 United Nations Development Program (1998) *Human Development Report*. New York: Oxford University Press.

22 Speth, James G. (2008) *The Bridge at the End of the World*. New Haven and London: Yale University Press, p. 144.

23 Ibid., p. 148.

24 Liu, Michael (2011) 'The shadow government,' *Architecture Boston*, Summer. Online, Available at www. architects.org/architectureboston/articles/shadow-government.html (accessed 7 June 2011).

25 Bahamón, Alejandro and Sanjinés, Camila (2010) *Rematerial: From Waste to Architecture*. New York: Wiley.

26 Speth, *The Bridge at the End of the World*, p. 151.

27 Ibid., p. 154.

28 Anon. (2011) 'The housing illusion,' *The Wall Street Journal*, 2 June, p. A18.

29 de Graff, John et al. (2005) *Affluenza: The All-Consuming Epidemic*. San Francisco: Berrett-Koehler.

30 Speth, *The Bridge at the End of the World*, p. 162.

31 Ibid. p. 170.

32 Cavanagh, John and Mander, Jerry (2004) *Alternatives to Economic Globalization: A Better World is Possible*. 2nd Edition. San Francisco: Berrett-Koehler Publishers, p. 17.

33 Ibid., p. 4.

34 Heilbroner, Robert L. (1985) *The Nature and Logic of Capitalism*. New York: W.W. Norton, pp. 143–144.

35 Robinson, William (2004) *A Theory of Global Capitalism: Production, Class, and State in a Transnational World*. Baltimore: Johns Hopkins University Press, p. 147.

36 Hamilton, Clive (2004) *Growth Fetish*. New York: Pluto Press, p. 212. Also see Hamilton, Clive (2006) *Affluenza: When Too Much is Never Enough*. New York: Allen & Unwin.

37 Barnes, Peter (2006) *Capitalism 3.0: A Guide to Reclaiming the Commons*. San Francisco: Berrett-Koehler.

38 Davis, Stephen et al. (2006) *The New Capitalists: How Citizen Investors Are Reshaping the Corporate Agenda*. Boston: Harvard Business School Press. Also see Wolf, Martin (2007) 'The new capitalism,' *Financial Times*, 19 June, p. 11.

39 Laplante, Martin (2010) 'Evidence-based urban planning,' *Planetizen.com*. 1 November. Online. Available at www.planetizen.com.html (accessed 10 November 2010). Also see Brown, Eliot (2011) 'Creditors seek missing developer,' *The Wall Street Journal*, 21 September, p. C8.

40 Dahl, Robert A. (2007) *On Political Equality*. New Haven and London: Yale University Press, pp. 114–116. Also see Reich, Charles A. (1970) *The Greening of America*. New York: Random House.

41 Shaw, Rajib and Sharma, Anshu, eds. (2011) *Climate and Disaster Resilience in Cities*. London: Emerald Group Publishing. Also see Klein, Naomi (2008) *The Shock Doctrine: The Rise of Disaster Capitalism*. London and New York: Picador/Macmillan.

42 Schleifstein, Mark (2010) 'State urged to buy up flood-prone property,' *The Times-Picayune*, 17 March, p. A-5.

43 Speth, *The Bridge at the End of the World*, p. 207. Also see Kellert, Stephen R. and Farnham, Timothy J., eds. (2002) *The Good in Nature and Humanity: Connecting Science, Religion, and Spirituality with the Natural World*. Washington, D.C.: Island Press; Merchant, Carolyn (1992) *Radical Ecology: The Search for a Livable World*. London: Routledge; and Ferkiss, Victor (1993) *Nature, Technology, and Society: Cultural Roots of the Current Environmental Crisis*. New York: New York University Press.

44 Alperovitz, Gar (2005) *America Beyond Capitalism: Reclaiming Our Wealth, Our Liberty, and Our Democracy*. Hoboken, NJ: John Wiley & Sons.

45 Dahl, *On Political Equality*, p. 139.

# APPENDIX: MALL TYPOLOGIES

Early on in the research phase Team 896 documented the formal compositional properties and sprawl machine contexts of twenty shopping malls. These were located in North and South Carolina and in Georgia. In each case, ten variables were documented: walking/biking amenities, pedestrian amenities, parking-pavement, figure-ground relationships, landscape, vehicular traffic arteries, volume levels, signage, proximity to residential neighborhoods, and degree of economic vitality. The data obtained were instrumental in subsequent phases of the research. Eight of these case studies are summarized below and on the following pages. All photos by S. Verderber/Team896.

1. Clemson Place
Location: Clemson, South Carolina
Date of Construction: 1963
Type: Boomerang
Status: Dying

2. Dutch Square Mall
Location: Columbia, South Carolina
Date of Construction: 1971
Type: Revolver
Status: Dying

3. Eastland Mall
Location: Charlotte, North Carolina
Date of Construction: 1974
Type: Battleship
Status: Dead

4. St. Andrews Shopping Center
Location: Charleston, South Carolina
Date of Construction: 1985
Type: Dogleg
Status: Alive

5. Tunnel Road and River Hills Mall
Location: Asheville, North Carolina
Date of Construction: 1978
Type: Bumpercar
Status: Dying

6. Village Square
Location: Charleston, South Carolina
Date of Construction: 1981
Type: Boxcar
Status: Alive

7. West Broad Mall
Location: Athens, Georgia
Date of Construction: 1961
Type: Shoebox
Status: Dead

8. South Windermere Center
Location: Charleston, South Carolina
Date of Construction: 1956
Type: Camshaft
Status: Alive

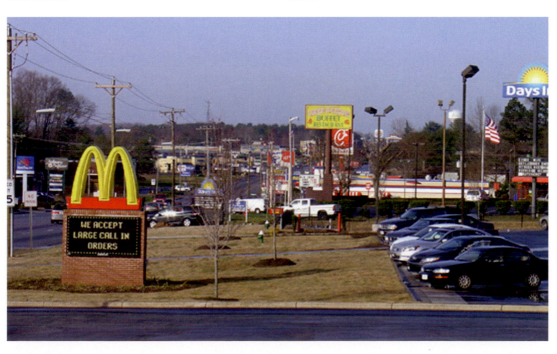

## 1. Clemson Place

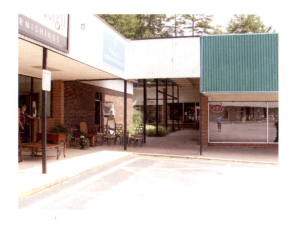

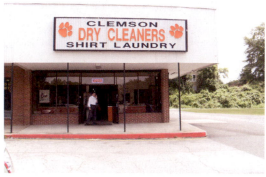

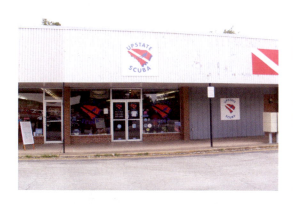

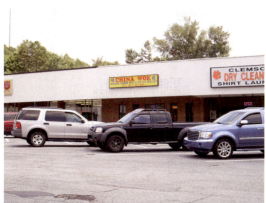

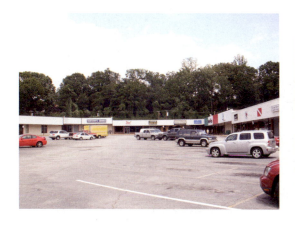

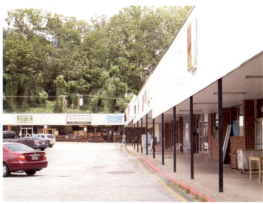

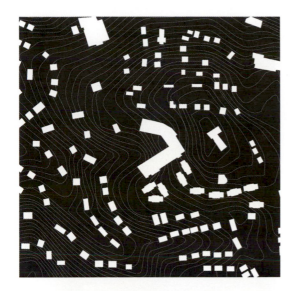

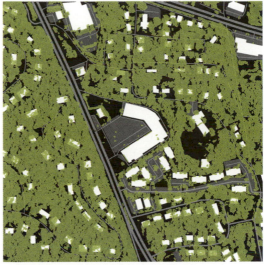

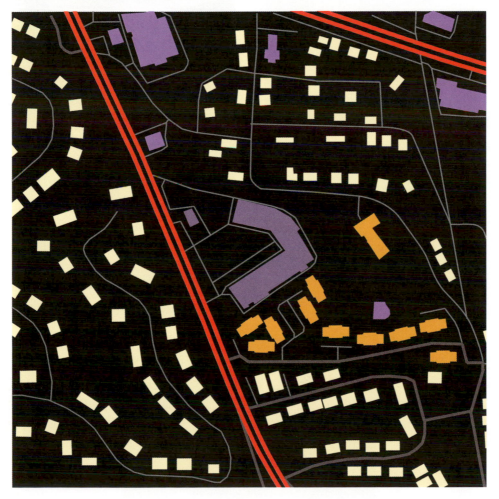

## 2. Dutch Square Mall

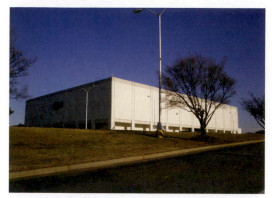

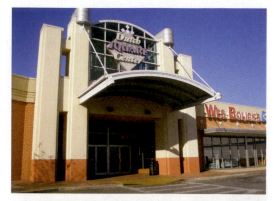

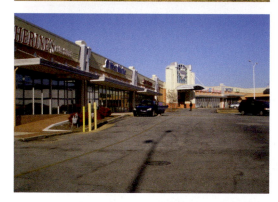

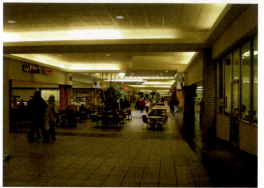

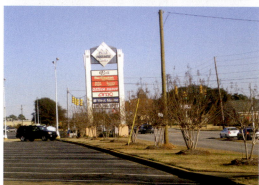

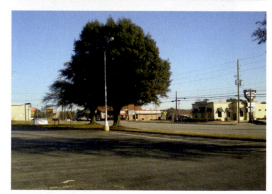

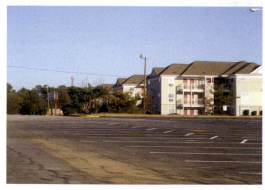

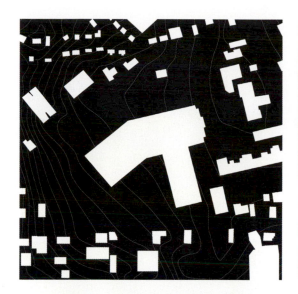
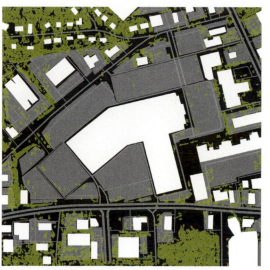
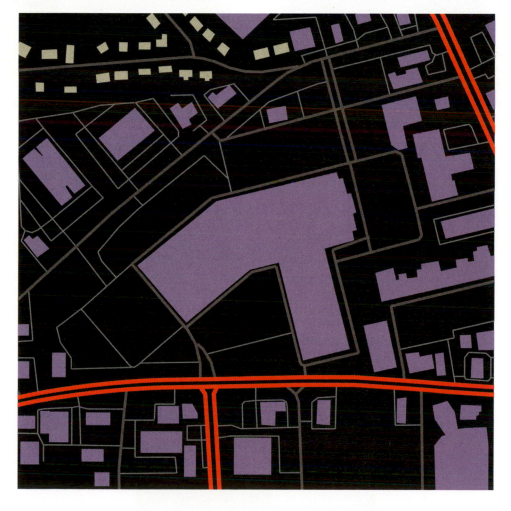

## 3. Eastland Mall

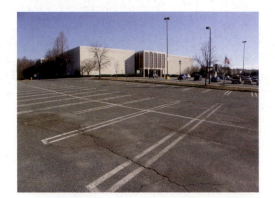
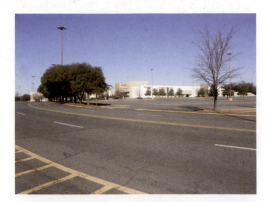
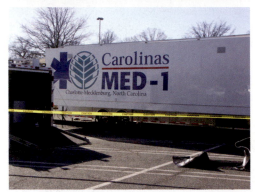
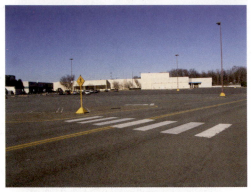
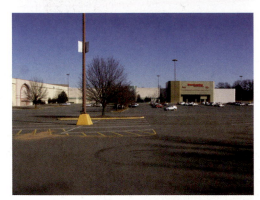
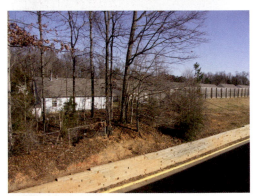
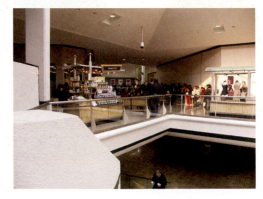

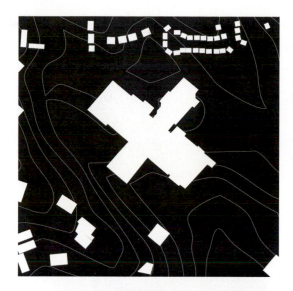

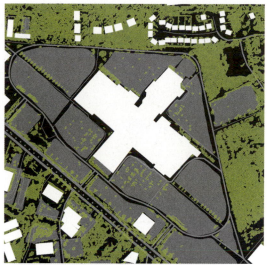

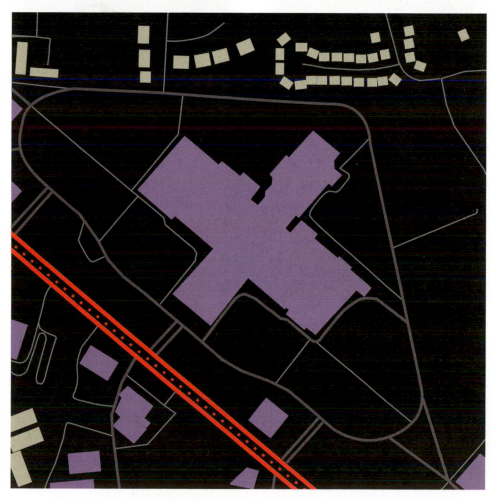

## 4. St. Andrews Shopping Center

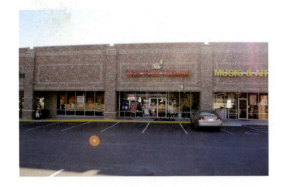

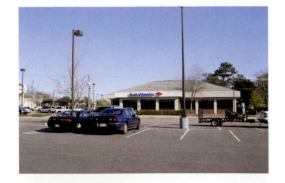

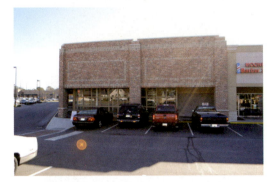

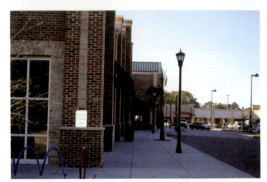

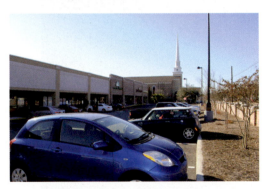

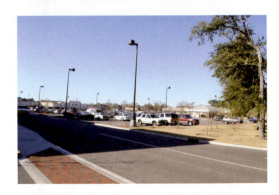

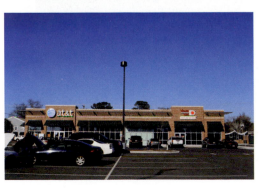

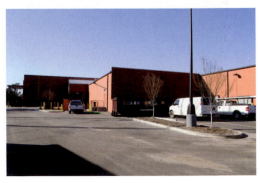

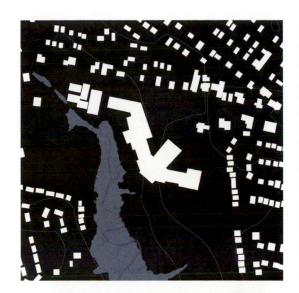
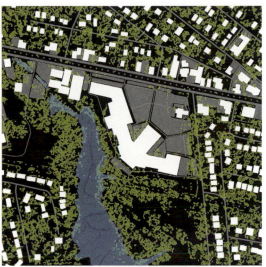
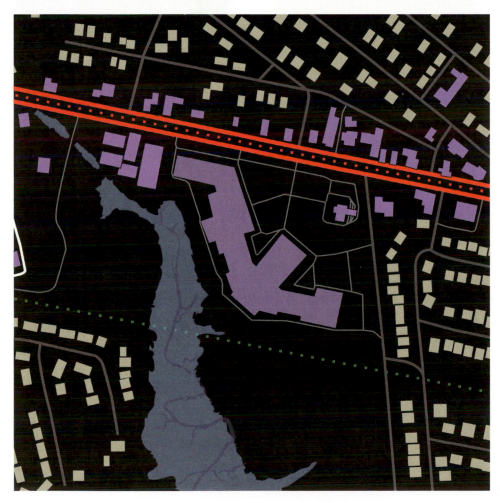

## 5. Tunnel Road and River Hills Mall

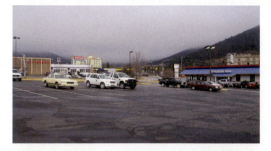
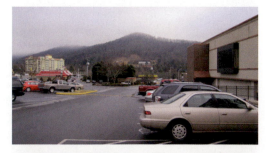

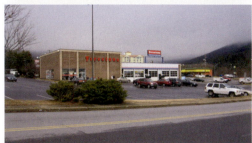
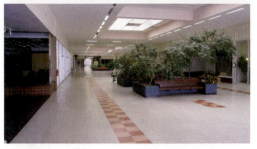

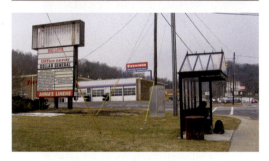
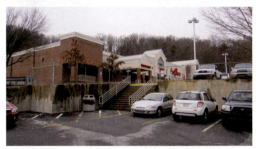

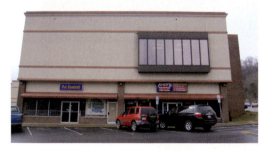
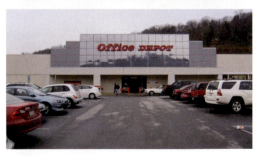

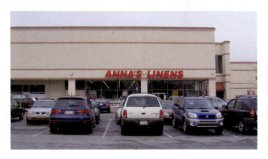

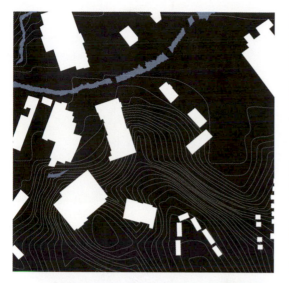
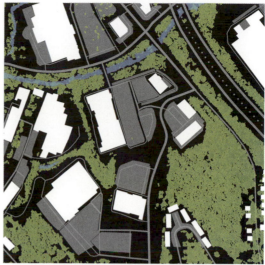

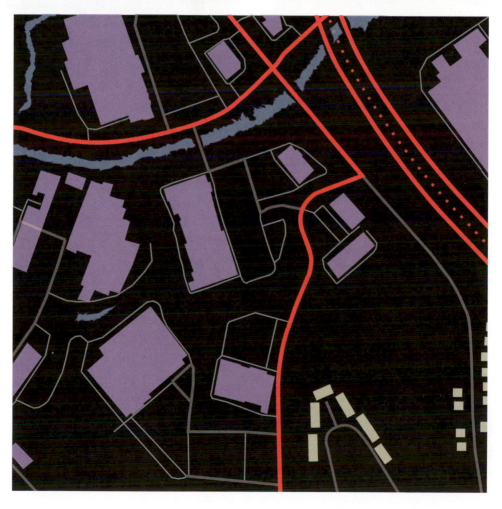

## 6. Village Square

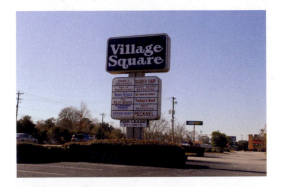

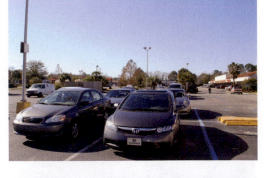

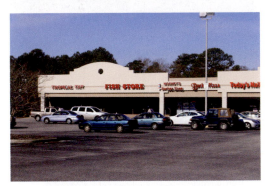

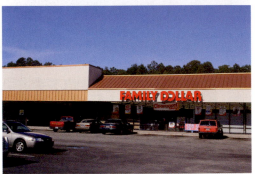

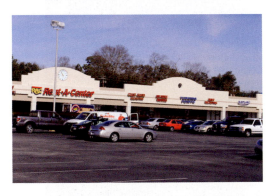

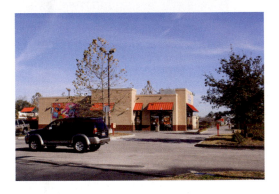

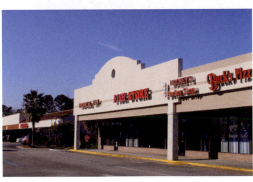

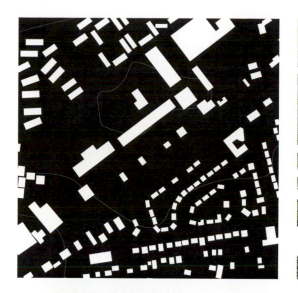

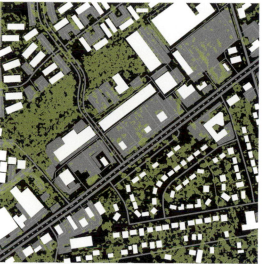

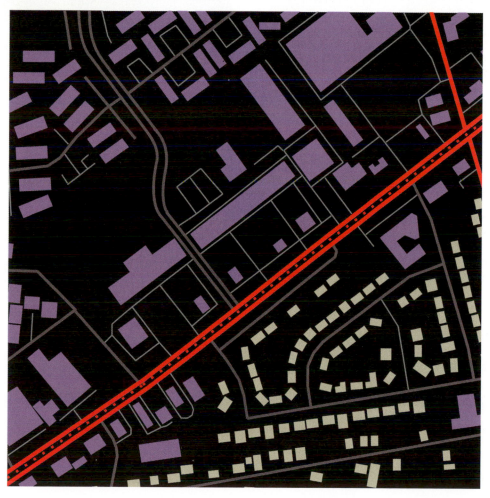

## 7. West Broad Mall

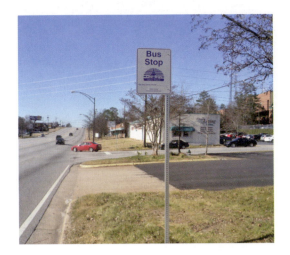

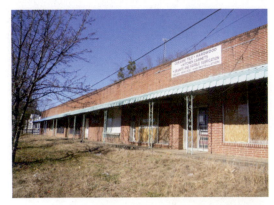

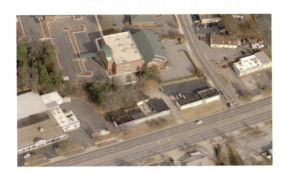

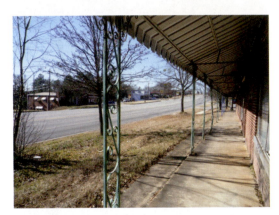

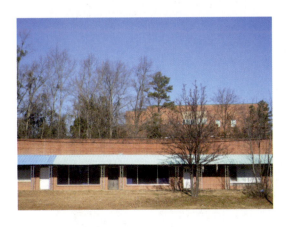

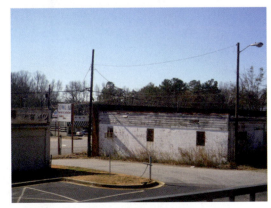

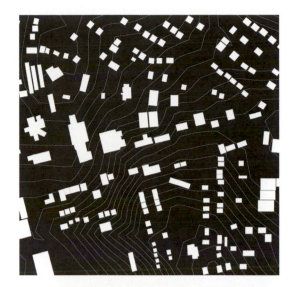

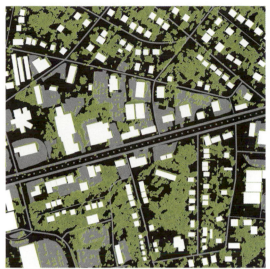

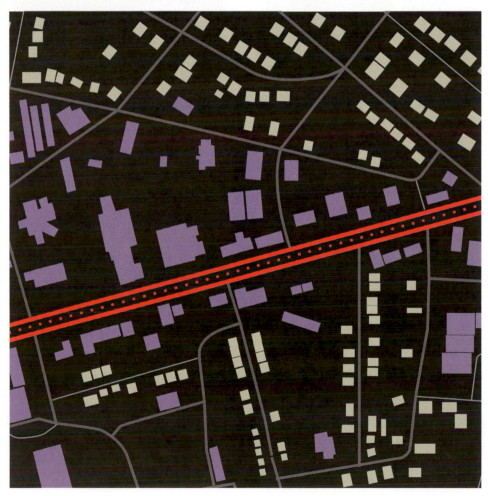

## 8. South Windermere Center

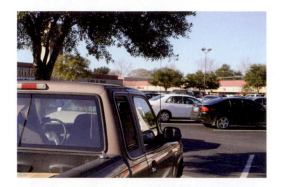
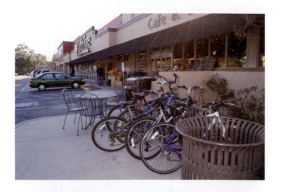

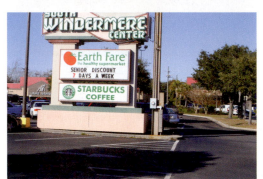
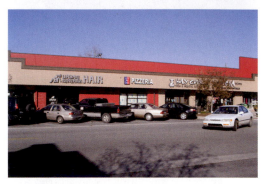

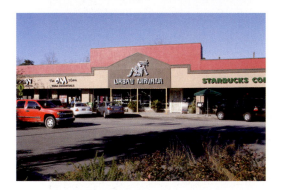
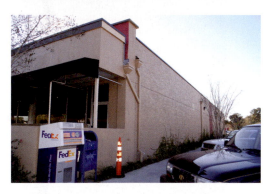

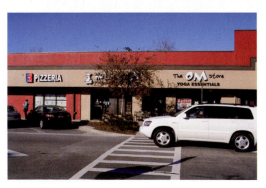
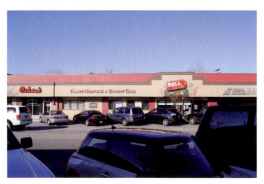

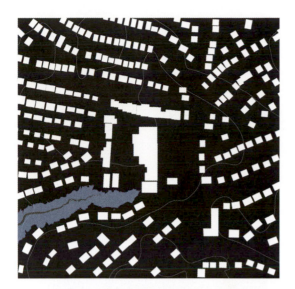

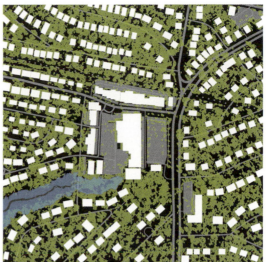

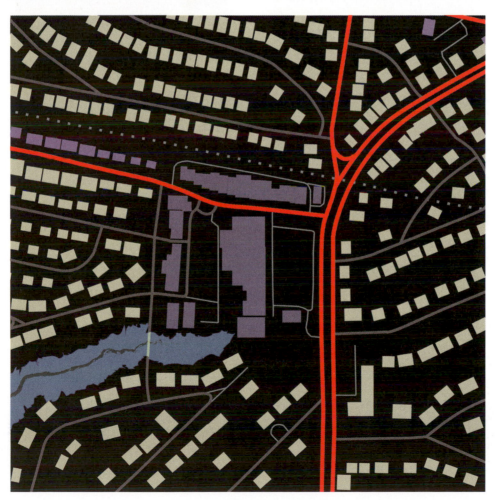

# INDEX

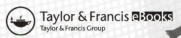

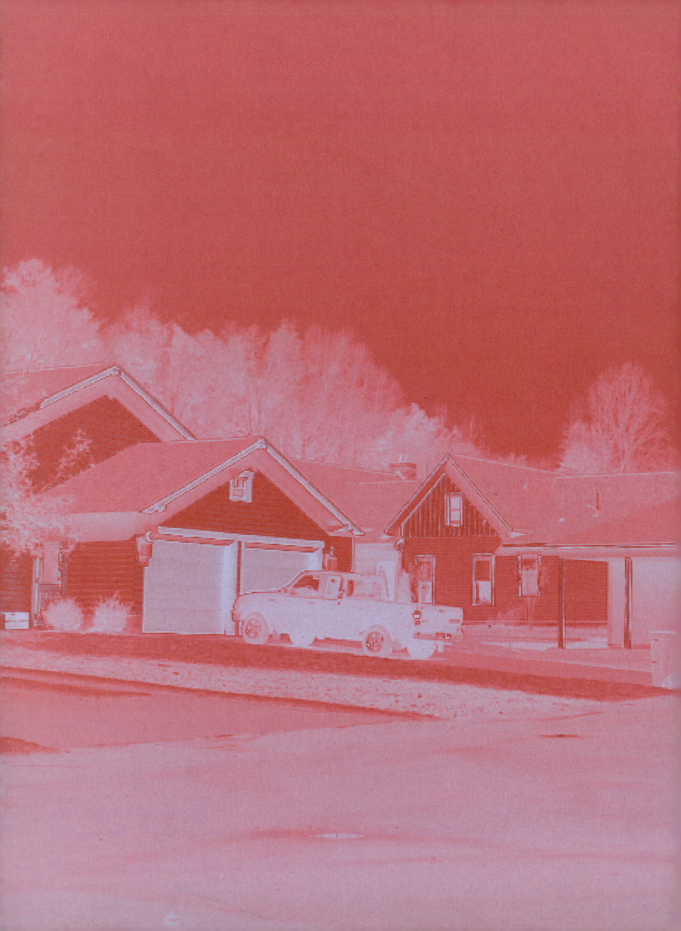

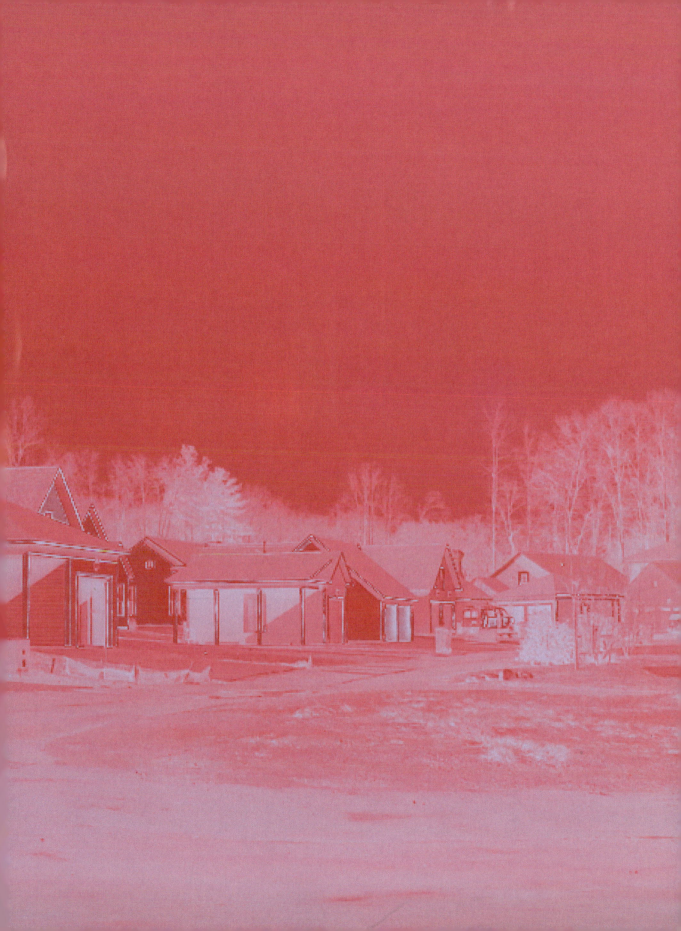